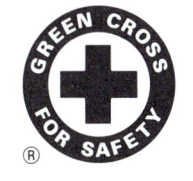

National Safety Council

First Aid Essentials

Consulting Editor
Alton L. Thygerson
Brigham Young University

JONES AND BARTLETT PUBLISHERS
BOSTON   PORTOLA VALLEY

Library of Congress Cataloging-in-Publication Data

Thygerson, Alton L.
  First aid essentials.

  At head of title: National Safety Council.
  1. First aid in illness and injury. I. National
Safety Council. II. Title.
RC86.7.T475 1989   616.02'52   88-8340
ISBN 0-86720-116-9

Copyright © 1989 by Jones and Bartlett Publishers, Inc.

All rights reserved. No part of the material protected by this copyright notice may be reproduced or utilized in any form, electronic or mechanical, including photocopying, recording, or by any information storage and retrieval system, without permission from the copyright owner.

Editorial, sales, and customer service offices:
  Jones and Bartlett Publishers, Inc.
  20 Park Plaza
  Boston, MA 02116

ISBN: 0-86720-116-9

Typing and Word Processing: Sherry I. Littler
Illustrator: Chris Young
Illustrator of Flow Charts: Greg Kyle
Text and Cover Design: Rafael Millán
Typesetting: Publication Services, Inc.

Printed in the United States of America

10 9 8 7 6 5 4 3 2

The first aid and emergency care procedures in this book are based on the most current recommendations of responsible medical sources. The author, the publisher, and the National Safety Council, however, make no guaranty as to, and assume no responsibility for, the correctness, sufficiency or completeness of such information or recommendations. Other or additional safety measures may be required under particular circumstances.

Preface

Several circumstances justify this book:

- With more than 140,000 Americans annually dying from injuries and one person in three suffering a nonfatal injury, everyone at some point in life will encounter a situation demanding first aid.
- With significant medical advances impacting first aid knowledge and procedures, the public deserves accurate and understandable information.

First Aid Essentials meets these demands. The National Safety Council endorsement brings sanctioning from an organization recognized as one of the most reliable sources of accidental injury information. Every effort was made to present currently accepted medical facts.

Moreover, the book's design gives clear, complete, and systematic directions for proper first aid.

Special features include:

- Comprehensive and accurate information and procedures
- Superior drawings
- Unexcelled flowcharts
- Attractive information tables
- Multi-color printing
- Full color injury photographs
- Self-checks for each chapter

Those successfully completing a first aid course using this book can acquire a National Safety Council certification card.

TO INSTRUCTORS

First Aid Essentials allows a "customized" course to fit:

- Available time (i.e., 4, 8, 16, 20, etc., hours)
- Available resources (i.e., videos, films, etc.)
- Various instructional formats (i.e., small groups, individualized study, lecture, etc.)
- Sponsoring organization's needs
- Instructor's preferences
- Student's needs

This flexibility greatly differs from the rigid "multi-media" courses.

Each chapter contains self-check questions using different formats to avoid boredom. These self-checks provide immediate, periodic feedback and ensure an active learning process rather than a passive one. Perforated pages allow their submission to the instructor and permit the student to keep the book as a reference after the course completion.

A comprehensive first aid teaching package is available to all instructors from the publisher. This four-part package is designed to aid the instructor and to challenge, motivate and reinforce first aid procedures and concepts for the students. This package includes:

- *Teaching First Aid Resource Book* — an indispensable 400 page book containing everything an instructor needs to know to effectively teach a first aid course.
- *Trauma Slide Set* — consists of 120 35mm color slides of various injuries a first aider might encounter.
- *Overhead Transparencies* — consists of 54 color acetate transparencies of flow charts that depict common injuries and recommended responses.
- *First Aid Test Bank* — consists of over 700 multiple choice test questions and answers covering all topics in first aid.

Further information on this excellent teaching package and the certification cards is available by contacting **Jones and Bartlett Publishers, Inc.**

ALTON THYGERSON

Table of Contents

1. **Introduction** 1
   Activity 1: Statistics 4
   Activity 2: How to Get Quick Emergency Help 5

2. **Victim Assessment** 7
   Activity: Victim Assessment 15

3. **Respiratory and Cardiac Resuscitation** 17
   Activity 1: Adult Resuscitation 28
   Activity 2: Adult Choking 29
   Activity 3: Child and Infant Resuscitation 30
   Activity 4: Child and Infant Choking 31

4. **Shock** 43
   Activity 1: Hypovolemic Shock 50
   Activity 2: Anaphylactic Shock 51
   Activity 3: Fainting 52

5. **Bleeding** 53
   Activity 1: External Bleeding and Wounds 68
   Activity 2: Infection and Tetanus 69
   Activity 3: Amputation 69
   Activity 4: Animal Bites 70

6. **Specific Body Area Injuries** 71
   Activity 1: Head Injury 98
   Activity 2: Eye Injury 98
   Activity 3: Nosebleeds 100
   Activity 4: Dental Injuries 100
   Activity 5: Chest Injuries 100
   Activity 6: Abdominal Injuries 102
   Activity 7: Foreign Objects 102
   Activity 8: Hand and Finger Injuries 103
   Activity 9: Blisters 103

7. **Poisoning** 105
   Activity 1: Ingested Poison 127
   Activity 2: Insect Stings 128
   Activity 3: Snakebites 128
   Activity 4: Spider Bites and Scorpion Stings 129
   Activity 5: Tick Removal 129
   Activity 6: Poison Ivy, Oak, and Sumac 130
   Activity 7: Carbon Monoxide Poisoning 130

8. **Burns** 131
   Activity 1: Thermal Burns 140
   Activity 2: Chemical Burns 141
   Activity 3: Electrical Burns 141

9. **Exposure to Cold and Heat** 143
   Activity 1: Frostbite 155
   Activity 2: Hypothermia 155
   Activity 3: Heat-Related Injuries 156

10. **Bone, Joint, and Muscle Injuries** 157
    Activity 1: Fractures 175
    Activity 2: Spinal Injuries 175
    Activity 3: Joint Injuries 176
    Activity 4: Muscle Injuries 176

11. **Medical Emergencies** 177
    Activity 1: Heart Attack 191
    Activity 2: Stroke 191
    Activity 3: Diabetic Emergencies 192
    Activity 4: Epilepsy 193
    Activity 5: Asthma 193

12. **First Aid Skills** 195

13. **Moving and Rescuing Victims** 209

Answers to Self-Check Questions 219

Quick Emergency Index 220

1 Introduction

- Injury: Magnitude of the Problem
- Need for First Aid Training
- Legal Aspects of First Aid

INJURY: MAGNITUDE OF THE PROBLEM*

Injuries are the most serious public health problem. Injuries are the leading cause of death and disability in children and young adults. They destroy the health, lives, and livelihoods of millions of people, yet they receive scant attention, compared with diseases and other hazards.

- Each year, more than 140,000 Americans die from injuries, and one person in three suffers a nonfatal injury.
- Injuries kill more Americans aged 1–34 than all diseases combined, and they are the leading cause of death up to the age of 44.
- Preceded by heart disease, cancer, and stroke, injury is the fourth leading cause of death among all Americans.
- Injuries cause the loss of more working years of life than all forms of cancer and heart disease combined. See Figure 1-1.
- One of every eight hospital beds is occupied by an injured patient.
- Every year, more than 80,000 Americans join the ranks of those with unnecessary, but permanently disabling, injury of the brain or spinal cord.
- Injuries constitute one of our most expensive health problems, costing $75–$100 billion a year directly and indirectly.

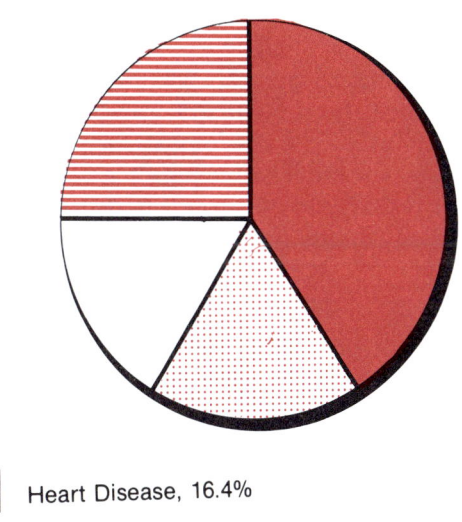

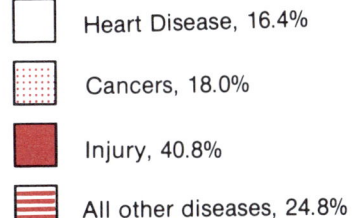

☐ Heart Disease, 16.4%
▦ Cancers, 18.0%
▦ Injury, 40.8%
▦ All other diseases, 24.8%

---

*Committee on Trauma Research of the National Research Council and the Institute of Medicine, *Injury in America: A Continuing Public Health Problem* (Washington, D.C.: National Academy Press, 1985).

1-1. Percentages of years of potential life lost to injury, cancer, heart disease, and other diseases before age 65. Modified from Centers for Disease Control.

- Injury is the leading cause of physician contacts. And more than 25% of hospital emergency room visits are for the treatment of injuries.

NEED FOR FIRST AID TRAINING

With the size and magnitude of the injury problem, everyone must expect sooner or later to be on hand when an injury or sudden illness strikes. The outcome of such misfortune frequently depends not only on the severity of the injury or illness, but on the first aid rendered. Therefore, first aid knowledge and skills are essential in our society. Every person should be trained in first aid.

First aid is the immediate care given to an injured or suddenly ill person. First aid does not take the place of proper medical treatment. It consists only of furnishing temporary assistance until competent medical care, if needed, is obtained, or until the prognosis for recovery without medical care is assured. Remember that most injuries and illness are corrected with only first aid care.

A knowledge of first aid, when properly applied, may mean the difference between life and death, rapid recovery and long hospitalization, or temporary disability and permanent injury.

LEGAL ASPECTS OF FIRST AID

Duty to Act

No one is required to render aid when no legal duty to do so exists. For example, even a physician could ignore a stranger suffering a heart attack or a fractured bone. There may be moral obligations, but this is not always the same as a legal obligation to render aid.

Duty to act may occur in the following situations:

1. When under a contractual duty. In other words, if a preexisting relationship exists between two people (e.g., teacher-student, physician-patient, parent-child, lifeguard-swimmer, driver-passenger), there is a duty to render first aid.

2. When beginning first aid. Once you start first aid, you cannot stop. Duty to give first aid is usually questioned only when a person fails to act.

Standards of Care

Standards of care ensure quality care and protection for injured or suddenly ill victims. The elements making up a standard of care include:

- *The type of provider*. For example, a first aider should provide the level and type of care expected in a reasonable person with the same amount of training and in similar circumstances.
- *Published recommendations*. Emergency care-related organizations and societies publish recommended first aid procedures. For example, the American Heart Association publishes procedures for administering CPR.

Obtain Consent

First aiders should obtain the victim's consent to receive first aid or they may risk incurring charges of technical assault and battery.

- Consent should be an informed consent. Oral consent is valid. The victim must understand that you are a first aider.
- Consent should be obtained from every conscious, mentally competent adult.
- Consent is implied for emergency lifesaving first aid to the unconscious victim.
- Consent should be obtained from the parent or guardian of a victim who is a child, or of one who is an adult but is mentally incompetent. If a parent or guardian is not available, emergency first aid to maintain life may be given without consent.
- Psychiatric emergencies present difficult problems of consent. Under most conditions, a police officer is the only person with the authority to restrain and transport a person against that individual's will. However, if the victim is not violent, the situation is similar to that for minors.

Abandonment

First aiders must remain with the victim until the victim is under the supervision of others of equal or greater competence, or until the victim refuses treatment and transportation. This may seem like an obvious requirement, but there have been cases where critically ill or injured victims were left.

The Right to Refuse Care

A perplexing problem is that of the conscious, rational, adult victim who is suffering from an actual or potential life-threatening injury or illness, but who refuses treatment or transportation. In such a situation, you should make every reasonable effort to convince the victim, or anyone who can influence the victim, to accept first aid and/or transportation. When a victim refuses to consent, you may not give first aid or transport the victim.

Should consent be refused, you should document this refusal on paper. Attempt to obtain the victim's signature and that of an impartial witness. It is hazardous to attempt to force the victim to submit to first aid; those who do may be subject to suits for assault.

Parent Refusing Permission to Help a Child
Very rarely will a first aider encounter a parent who refuses permission—usually on moral, ethical, or religious grounds—to care for a seriously injured or ill child. When a parent refuses permission to treat a child, every effort must be made to convince the parent of the seriousness of the problem and the necessity of the first aid. If you do not succeed, you should summon the police.

The Intoxicated or Belligerent Victim
As a first aider, you may encounter people who are in some stage of drug or alcohol intoxication and are injured. If an intoxicated victim refuses treatment, make every effort to persuade the individual to consent to first aid care. If refused, make sure to document the situation and attempt to have it signed by the victim and by an impartial witness.

If the intoxicated person consents to first aid, take the greatest possible care. Alcohol and drugs may mask vital symptoms, so that the seriously injured may also have a higher-than-average risk of death or disability.

Many first aiders may be repulsed by the intoxicated victim's appearance or attitude. If such is the case, you may overlook important symptoms that could be vital.

Good Samaritan Laws

Starting in the early 1960s, a number of states enacted statutes that were designed to provide freedom from liability to individuals who stopped and helped at the scene of an emergency. There are notable differences in the range of these laws among different states. First aiders are covered by a Good Samaritan law in some states, but this is not the situation in most cases. Some state laws cover only physicians and nurses, or only automobile accidents. It is recommended that you look carefully at your state law. Volunteer first aid personnel are usually given protection because there is no profit or expectation of payment involved.

The Good Samaritan legislation only protects those acting in good faith and without gross negligence or willful misconduct.

SELF-CHECK QUESTIONS

Activity 1: Statistics

Directions: In the left column list your estimate of the appropriate information. Your estimate should be for the entire United States for a period of one year. After you have completed your estimate, fill in the right column with information from your instructor or the National Safety Council's annual publication, *Accident Facts*.

		Estimate	The Facts
1.	Annual number of deaths from all causes	_____	_____
2.	Annual number of accidental deaths	_____	_____
3.	Annual number of disabling injuries	_____	_____
4.	The 4 leading causes of death	a _____ b _____ c _____ d _____	a _____ b _____ c _____ d _____
5.	The 6 leading causes of accidental death	a _____ b _____ c _____ d _____ e _____ f _____	a _____ b _____ c _____ d _____ e _____ f _____
6.	The two most dangerous regions for accidents in the United States	1 _____ 2 _____	1 _____ 2 _____
7.	Sex of most accident victims	_____	_____
8.	Age group of most accident victims	_____	_____
9.	Most accidental deaths occur in motor vehicles. Where do most injuries occur?	_____	_____
10.	Day of the week on which accidental deaths and injuries occur most frequently	_____	_____
11.	Months of the year in which accidental deaths and injuries occur most frequently	_____ _____ _____	_____ _____ _____

Activity 2: How to Get Quick Emergency Help*

To receive the best emergency medical help fast, you should keep a list of the following phone numbers near your telephone. If you have no such list, clip this section from the book and write in the appropriate phone numbers.

In many communities, to receive emergency assistance of every kind you just dial 911. Check to see if this is true in your community.

  1. The Rescue Squad _____
Often part of the local fire department, these specially trained paramedics are likely to respond swiftly and competently.

  2. The Police _____
They may or may not be able to respond with medically trained personnel; however, they can get someone to the hospital quickly.

  3. Ambulance Service _____
Some services have trained paramedics; others do not.

  4. Your Doctor _____
Your own doctor may not be available, but he or she should be alerted if an emergency has occurred.

  5. Poison Control Center _____
In some communities, this service will give information to doctors only. Call before an emergency occurs to find out.

_____
*Adapted from Consumer's Union, *Consumer's Reports*.

Give the following information over the phone:

  1. *The victim's location.* Give city or town, street name, and street number. If calling at night, describe the building. This is probably the single most important piece of information.

  2. *What has happened?* Tell the nature of the emergency—woman is bleeding badly, child has fallen and is unconscious, man has a heart attack, and so on.

  3. *Identify yourself.* Give your name. If it is different from the name of the homeowner or the apartment dweller, give that person's name as well.

  4. *Give your phone number.* This information is required not only to help prevent false calls but, more important, to allow the center to call back for additional information.

  5. *Tell them if they will need extra help.* Tell them if the victim is overweight, if there are several flights of stairs and no elevator, number of people involved, and so on.

  6. *Ask for questions and advice.* Let the person on the other end of the line ask you questions and tell you what to do until help arrives.

  7. *Always be the last to hang up the phone.* The police, ambulance, or fire department may need to ask more questions about how to find you. They may also tell you what to do until help arrives.

  8. *Speak slowly and clearly.* Shouting is difficult to understand.

Emergency Telephone Numbers

Your Home Address   _____

    Home Telephone   _____

Nearest Intersection   _____

Doctor's Name and Telephone   _____

Doctor's Name and Telephone   _____

Doctor's Name and Telephone   _____

Dentist's Name and Telephone   _____

Fire   _____

Police   _____

Poison Control Center   _____

Ambulance Service   _____

Hospital Emergency Room   _____

Life Support Unit   _____

Drugstore Name and Telephone   _____

Drugstore Name and Telephone   _____

Relative's Name and Telephone   _____

Neighbor's Name and Telephone   _____

Children's Names and Birthdays   _____

Additional Numbers   _____

THE NATIONWIDE EMERGENCY TELEPHONE NUMBER IS: 9–1–1

Does your community have a 9–1–1 number?   Yes   No

2
Victim Assessment

- Physical Examination • History-Taking • Vital Signs
- Head-to-Toe Examination

Examining a victim is essential to determine the extent of a victim's injury and/or illness in order to provide adequate first aid. Such exams are, however, subject to error; and treatment, whether by a first aider or a physician, should not be founded upon the results of a single examination. Any examination that could affect someone must be repeated at least twice before it can be considered valid. Exception to this "two-time test rule" naturally occurs when a life threatening situation exists and time is crucial.

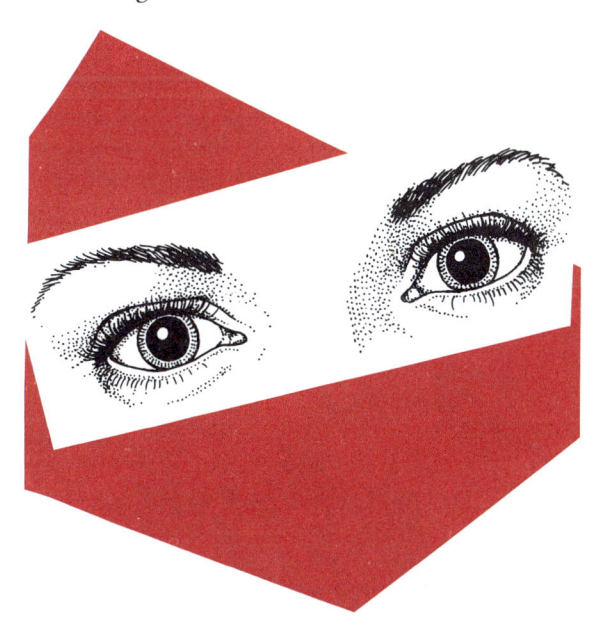

Injury victims, conscious or unconscious, should always be surveyed. Injury victims may have obvious as well as not-so-obvious injuries. Every unconscious person should also be examined, regardless of whether coma has been produced by injury or illness.

To find out the needs of an injured or suddenly ill person, first you must ask important questions and then examine the person carefully. You should look for signs and symptoms that help you tell how the person is and what kind of problem he or she may have.

There are certain basic things to ask and to look for in anyone who is sick or injured. Certainly, those with extensive experience in the field of emergency care may have their preferences as to what to ask and what to look for. However, the intent is to focus on the basics which are pertinent to the first aider level. The things the victim feels or reports (symptoms), as well as things you notice on examining him (signs), are the basics of a victim examination. Signs can be especially important in victims unable to talk.

A victim assessment has the following purposes:

• Gain the victim's confidence and thereby relieve some of the victim's anxiety due to discomfort and pain.

• Identify the victim's problem(s) and establish which problem(s) require immediate first aid.

- Obtain information about the victim that may not be readily available later in the hospital but could be useful to the attending medical personnel.

The information a first aider gains through a victim assessment depends largely on the way in which these procedures are performed. Victim assessment must be unhurried and systematic; a hasty approach always leads to omissions.

Urgent first aid may be required before you can stop to ask questions or perform a thorough examination, as in the case of a victim with an obstructed airway.

Having completed the primary survey and attended to any problems it uncovers, take a closer look at the victim and make a systematic examination from head to toe. This examination is called the secondary survey.

The secondary survey is done to discover problems that do not pose an immediate threat to life but may do so if they remain uncorrected. The secondary survey has three parts:

- History-taking
- Vital signs
- Head-to-toe examination

PHYSICAL EXAMINATION

The physical examination of either an injured victim or a medically ill victim is divided into two steps:

- Primary survey
- Secondary survey

Physical assessment begins with the primary survey, which covers the following areas:

A — Airway
B — Breathing
C — Circulation
H — Hemorrhage

The primary survey is the first step in the first aider's assessment of the victim and always takes precedence over all other aspects of the physical examination. Its purpose is to find and correct life-threatening conditions. Many times the primary survey will be completed in short order: when, for example, you encounter the alert victim with medical problems. Other times, however, close examination will be required to accomplish the primary survey: when the victim, for example, is unconscious or suffering from a major injury. If the primary survey uncovers any findings, such as an obstructed airway or massive bleeding, you must attend immediately to those injuries before proceeding with the victim assessment.

HISTORY-TAKING

History-taking begins as soon as you see the victim; before asking a single question, evaluate the victim's environment. History-taking may involve the victim, the victim's family, and bystanders. In general, if the victim is able to communicate, it is best to question him or her rather than the others. The victim is thus reassured that he or she is the center of interest. If you need to question others, do so one at a time.

When taking a history, obtain the victim's chief complaint — the problem that prompted the need for help. Often, it will be obvious; for example, the man who lies bleeding in the street after being struck by an automobile. However, there may be unexpected findings. The victim may have an obvious fracture of the left leg, and yet his chief complaint may be, "I can't breathe." Most chief complaints are characterized by pain, abnormal function, some change from a normal state, or an observation made by the victim.

After finding out about the chief complaint, obtain any pertinent information about the victim's past medical history that relates to the current problem. It is, for example, not especially relevant to learn whether the victim underwent a hernia operation five years earlier or had measles as a child, when the problem is a second-degree burn over the back of the victim's body. In general, you will want to determine the following:

• Does the victim have any major underlying medical problems (for example, diabetes or a serious condition that has required a doctor's care)?

• Does the victim take any medication regularly? If so, what are they? Medications may give important clues to a victim's underlying condition.

• Does the victim have known allergies?

Two mnemonic devices might help you identify the victim's problem: taking a S-A-M-P-L-E history and P-A-I-N.

*S*ymptoms (chief complaint)
*A*llergies
*M*edications
*P*revious illnesses (relating to the problem)
*L*ast meal (in case of surgery)
*E*vents prior to emergency

*P*eriod of pain (How long? What started it?)
*A*rea (Where?)
*I*ntensity
*N*ullify (What stops it? Rest, a certain position, medication?)

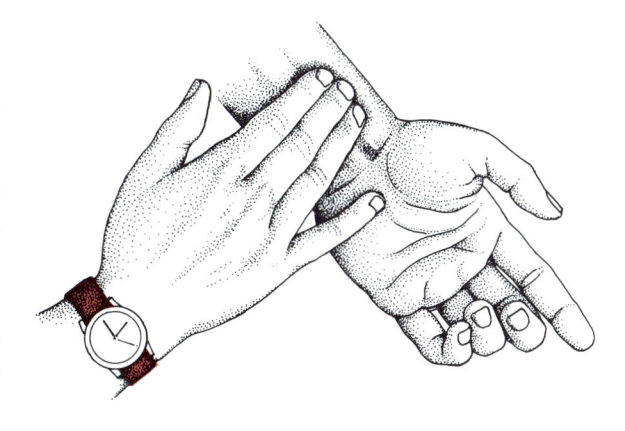

2-1. Palpating the radial pulse

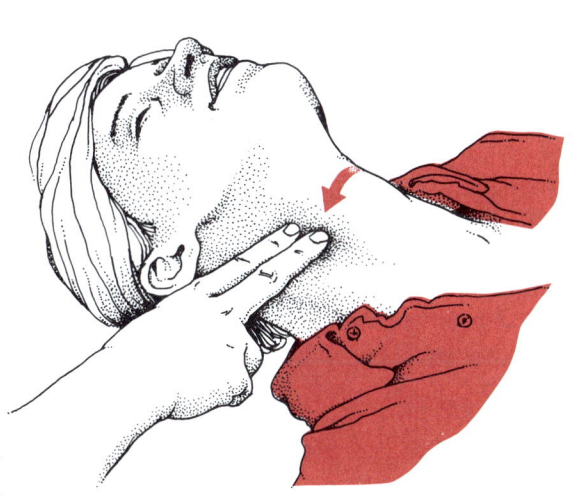

2-2. Palpating the carotid pulse

VITAL SIGNS

Pulse

A fingertip held over an artery where it either crosses a bone or lies close to the skin surface can easily feel characteristic pulsations as the pressure wave of blood causes the vessel wall to expand; hence the term pulse. Do not use your thumb to feel for the pulse—it has its own pulse.

The pulse rate can be determined at a number of points throughout the body, but the usual method is to palpate the radial point at the wrist (*see* Figure 2-1) or use the carotid point (*see* Figure 2-2) at the neck if you cannot feel the radial pulse. Do not palpate both carotid arteries at the same time. Pulsations are usually visible at the carotid artery in a victim lying down; pulsations disappear as the victim is elevated to a sitting position (usually a 45° angle). Never put too much pressure or massage the carotid, especially in victims who have had a heart attack—the heart's electrical conduction system may be disturbed.

Normal pulse at rest for adults is from 60 to 80 beats per minutes. (Refer to Table 2-1.) For children, it is 80 to 100; and for babies, it is 100 to 140 beats per minute. As a general rule, the pulse increases 20 beats per minute for each degree rise in fever.

TABLE 2-1. Normal Pulse Rates

60–70	Men
70–80	Women
80–90	Children over seven years
80–120	Children from one to seven years
110–130	Infants

Pulse Classified in Adults

60 and below	Slow or subnormal
60–80	Normal (men, women)
80–100	Moderate increase
100–120	Quick
120–140	Rapid
140 and above	Running (hard to count)

Source: U.S. Public Health Service, *The Ship's Medicine Chest and Medical Aid at Sea.*

Respiration

The only concern for respiration during a primary survey is that the victim is breathing through an unobstructed airway. In the secondary survey, you should be concerned with the rate of respirations.

Count the number of breaths per minute. Between 12 and 20 breaths per minute is normal for adults and older children. Up to 30 breaths per minute is normal for children, and 40 is normal for babies.

As you determine the rate of respirations, also listen for sounds, for example,

- A whistle or wheeze and difficulty breathing out can mean asthma.
- A gurgling or snoring noise and difficult breathing in an unconscious person may mean the tongue, mucus, or something else is stuck in the throat and does not let enough air get through.

Temperature

Body temperature measurement is important, as in cases of heat stroke or high fever. It is often wise to take a victim's temperature, even if he or she does not seem to have a fever.

Body temperature is often recorded when a person cannot receive medical care for some time, as in a rural area when snow or high water prevents the immediate transfer of a sick or injured person to a medical facility. If the victim is very sick, take the temperature at least four times each day and write it down.

Body temperature is measured with a thermometer that is held for a short time under the tongue, within the rectum, or in an armpit. The techniques are referred to as oral, rectal, and axillary (armpit), respectively. A standard glass thermometer should not be used when there is any chance that the victim will bite through it. Temperature at the axilla is usually a degree lower than that measured under the tongue, and rectal temperature is generally a degree higher.

Although 98.6°F is considered to be normal, the body temperature of healthy individuals may vary from 97°F to 99°F. (Refer to Table 2-2.)

If there is no thermometer, you can get an idea of the temperature by putting the back of one hand on the victim's forehead and the other on your own or that of another healthy person. If the victim has a fever, you should feel the difference. Fingertips may be somewhat insensitive because of calluses.

TABLE 2-2. What Body Temperatures Mean

Fahrenheit (F)		Centigrade (C)
108°	Usually Fatal	42.2°
107	Critical Condition	41.7
106		41.1
105		40.6
104	High Fever	40.0
103		39.4
102		38.9
101	Moderate Fever	38.3
100		37.8
99		37.2
98.6	Healthy (Normal) Temperature in Mouth	37.0
98	Subnormal Temperature	36.7
97		36.1
96		35.6
95		35.0

Source: U.S. Public Health Service. *The Ship's Medicine Chest and Medical Aid at Sea.*

Skin Color

The color of the skin, especially in Caucasian victims, reflects the circulation immediately underlying the skin as well as the oxygen saturation of the blood. In darkly pigmented individuals, these changes may not be apparent in the skin, but may be assessed by examining the mucous membranes (mouth, inner eyelids, and nailbeds). If the skin vessels constrict or heart output drops, the skin becomes pale, mottled, or cyanotic (a bluish discoloration). If the blood vessels of the skin dilate or blood flow increases, the skin becomes warm and pink.

Table 2-3 identifies possible medical conditions related to pulse, respirations, temperature, skin color, and pupil signs.

HEAD-TO-TOE EXAMINATION

Once as much pertinent information as possible has been obtained, the first aider should move to a head-to-toe examination of the victim, looking for other signs of injury or disease. Be careful not to aggravate injuries or contaminate wounds. Take great care not to move the victim because there could be undetected neck and spinal injuries.

Removal of clothing from the victim during the head-to-toe examination is not usually necessary.

Head and Neck

Check the scalp for lacerations and contusion. Is there blood in the hair? Where is it coming from? Do not move the head during this procedure. Pay particular attention to the area over the mastoid bone, just behind the ear. Bluish discoloration of this area is called Battle's sign and indicates a probable basal skull fracture.

Check the ears and nose for discharge of clear fluid or blood. Blood draining from the ears may be a sign of skull fracture; clear fluid draining from the nose or ears may be cerebrospinal fluid (CSF), again indicating a skull fracture. Do not attempt to stop the flow.

Inspect the mouth for blood or foreign materials such as broken dentures. The lips should be observed for cyanosis in victims with trauma or suspected cardiorespiratory problems.

Eyes

Pay attention to the size of the pupils (*see* Figure 2-3). Very large pupils can mean a state of shock; very small pupils can mean poison or the effect of certain drugs.

A difference in the size of the two pupils is almost always a medical emergency. Unequal pupils may be due to a stroke or a head injury. However, this unequal condition occurs normally in 2% to 4% of the population.

Use a small bright light source (beam of a flashlight) to determine if the pupils are reactive. If there is no flashlight, cover the eye with your hand and notice the pupil reaction when the eye is uncovered. No pupil reaction to light could mean death, coma, cataracts in older persons, or an artificial eye.

While inspecting the pupils of the eye, look at the inner surface of the eyelids. They are pink in all normal, healthy people regardless of skin color. If the eyelids are pale in color, it may indicate anemia or blood loss. Remember that eyelids should be pink in color.

Chest

Check the chest for cuts, bruises, penetrations, and impaled objects. Warn the victim that you are going to apply pressure to the sides of the chest. Pain from squeezing or compressing the ribs may indicate possible rib fracture(s). Check to see if both sides of the chest expand normally when the victim breathes.

Abdomen

If something is protruding from the abdomen, it will be obvious. Less obvious and perhaps even difficult to see will be a wound produced by a small caliber bullet or a long thin weapon such as an ice pick.

If a person has pain in the abdomen, try to find out exactly where it hurts. When you examine the abdomen, first look at it for any unusual swelling or lumps.

The location of the pain often gives a clue to the cause (for example, pain in the upper right quadrant may be from a gallbladder). First, ask the person to point with one finger where it

TABLE 2-3. Diagnostic Signs

Observation	Examples
1. Pulse	
a. **Rapid, strong:**	fright, apprehension, heat stroke
b. **Rapid, weak:**	shock, bleeding, diabetic coma, heat exhaustion
c. **Slow, strong:**	stroke, skull fracture
d. **None:**	cardiac arrest, death
2. Respirations	
a. **Shallow:**	shock, bleeding, heat exhaustion, insulin shock
b. **Deep, gasping, labored:**	airway obstruction, chest injury, diabetic coma, heart disease
c. **None:**	respiratory arrest due to any number of illnesses/injuries
d. **Bright, frothy blood coughed up:**	lung damage possibly due to fractured ribs or penetrating objects
3. Skin temperature	
a. **Cool, moist:**	shock, bleeding, heat exhaustion
b. **Cool, dry:**	exposure to cold
c. **Hot, dry:**	heat stroke, high fever
4. Face color	
a. **Red:**	high blood pressure, heat stroke, diabetic coma
b. **Pale/white/ashen:**	shock, bleeding, heat exhaustion, insulin shock
c. **Blue:**	heart failure, airway obstruction, some poisonings

Note: Blue results from poor oxygenation or circulating blood. For people with dark skin pigmentation, blue may be noted around the finger nails, palms of hands and mouth.

5. Pupils of the eyes	
a. **Dilated:**	shock, bleeding, heat stroke, cardiac arrest
b. **Constricted:**	opiate addiction
c. **Unequal:**	head injury, stroke
6. State of consciousness	
a. **Confusion:**	most any illness/injury, fright, apprehension, alcohol, drugs
b. **Coma:**	stroke, head injury, severe poisoning, diabetic coma
7. Inability to move upon command — an indicator of paralysis.	
a. **One side of the body:**	stroke, head injury
b. **Arms and legs:**	damage to spinal cord in neck
c. **Legs:**	damage to spinal cord below neck
8. Reaction to physical stimulation — an indicator of paralysis.	
a. **No sensation in arms and/or legs:**	damage to spinal cord as indicated above
b. **Numbness in arms and/or legs:**	damage to spinal cord as indicated above

Note: No sensation or indication of pain when there is an obvious injury can also be due to hysteria, violent shock, or excessive alcohol or drug use.

Source: National Highway Traffic Safety Administration, *Emergency Medical Services: First Responder Training Course* (Washington, D.C.: U.S. Superintendent of Documents).

hurts. Then, beginning on the opposite side from the spot the victim has pointed to, press gently on different parts of the abdomen to see where it hurts the most. Feel for any abnormal lumps and and hardened areas in the abdomen, but be extremely careful about pushing too deeply—lightly palpate the victim's abdomen. The victim who has tenderness may guard the painful area by tightening the abdominal muscles. Palpate the four abdominal quadrants.

If a person has a constant pain in the abdomen, with nausea and has not been able to move his bowels, put an ear on the abdomen and listen for gurgles in the intestines. If you hear nothing after about two minutes, this is a danger sign of an abdominal emergency.

Other procedures could be performed, but the ones discussed here form a basis to help first aiders determine what a particular victim's problem is.

Extremity Assessment

In the trauma victim, the first aider should inspect the extremities for bruises and deformities, always checking for the presence of a pulse, sensation, and motion. Circulation to the extremities may also be gauged by the warmth of the limb and the degree of capillary refill in the nailbed. To assess capillary refill, you should exert gentle pressure on the nailbed sufficient to whiten the underlying tissue. Then, release the pressure and observe the rate at which the nailbed become pink again. If there is good circulation of the extremity, the capillaries should refill almost instantly, with prompt return of a pink coloring beneath the nail. Refill time greater than two seconds is definitely abnormal.

The first aider should check the victim's pulses. A normal pulse is full, easily felt, and equal to the corresponding pulse on the opposite side. The first aider should use the radial and pedal pulses to check circulation of the extremities. The sudden disappearance of a pulse in one extremity, together with sharp, sudden, severe pain in the limb may indicate occlusion of an artery in that extremity.

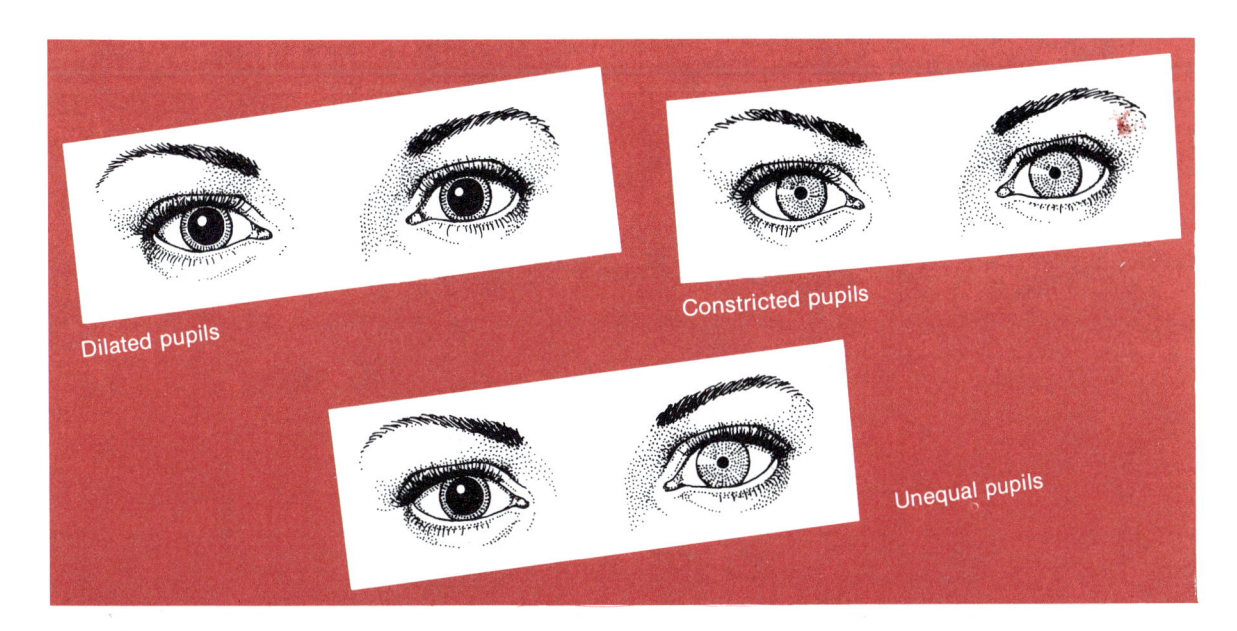

2-3. Changes in pupil size can have medical significance.

14 FIRST AID ESSENTIALS

In injured victims, the first aider should look for abnormal positioning of the legs. For example, a leg that is externally rotated suggests a hip fracture.

Assessment of the Back

When examining the back, remember to avoid excessive movement of the victim. In all victims with possible spinal injury as well as those with suspected stroke, the first aider should check strength and sensation in all extremities. The victim with a spinal injury may show paraplegia (paralysis of both legs) or quadriplegia (paralysis of all four extremities); the stroke victim is more likely to have hemiplegia (paralysis of an arm or leg on the same side of the body). The loss of movement in the extremities is usually accompanied by a loss of sensation in those extremities. It is very important that the first aider recognize this finding and appropriately immobilize the victim.

Putting It All Together

The physical exam will be influenced by whether the victim is suffering from a medical problem or is injured, whether the victim is conscious or unconscious, and whether life-threatening conditions are present. Table 2-4 shows the suggested sequence for conducting a victim assessment. Remember to first conduct the primary survey and correct any problems it uncovers before continuing on to the secondary survey.

TABLE 2-4. Victim Assessment

Primary Survey

- A—Airway?
- B—Breathing?
- C—Circulation: pulse?
- H—Hemorrhage?

Secondary Survey
History-Taking

- S— Symptoms (chief complaint)
- A— Allergies
- M— Medications
- P— Previous illnesses (relating to the problem)
- L— Last meal (in case of surgery)
- E— Events prior to emergency

- P— Period of pain (how long? what started it?)
- A— Area (where?)
- I— Intensity
- N— Nullify (what stops it? rest, a certain position, medication?)

Vital Signs

- Pulse rate
- Respiration rate
- Temperature
- Skin color

Head-to-Toe Examination

- Head and neck—Bleeding? Deformity? CSF? Cyanosis?
- Eyes—Pupils equal? Pupils react? Eyelid color?
- Chest—Pain? Wounds?
- Abdomen—Pain? Wounds?
- Extremities—Deformity? Pulses? Sensation?
- Back—Extremities checked for sensation and movement
- Medical Alert Symbols—check for tags, bracelets, etc.

SELF-CHECK QUESTIONS

Activity: Victim Assessment

A. Mark the following true (T) or false (F).
 1. ☐ If you find severe bleeding during a victim evaluation, continue your examination and come back to the bleeding later.
 2. ☐ Use your thumb to feel for a victim's pulse.
 3. ☐ A pulse can be felt at either the wrist's radial point or the neck's carotid point.
 4. ☐ Feel for both carotid points at the same time.
 5. ☐ Normal adult pulse rate is 60–80 beats per minute.
 6. ☐ Normal adult respiration rate is between 12 and 20 breaths per minute.
 7. ☐ Clear fluid draining from the nose or ears may be cerebrospinal fluid (CSF).
 8. ☐ Very small (pinpointed) eye pupils can mean a state of shock.
 9. ☐ Unequal eye pupils may result from a head injury.
 10. ☐ All normal, healthy people (regardless of skin color) have a pink inner eyelid surface.
 11. ☐ The capillary refill technique can indicate the quality of blood circulation in an arm or leg.

B. Designate which of the following are signs (with an A) and which are symptoms (with a B).
 1. _____ Sherry states that she feels dizzy.
 2. _____ Matt says he feels like throwing up.
 3. _____ Steve's skin is red and blistered.
 4. _____ Jim says that he has no feeling in his right arm.
 5. _____ Scott's pulse rate is 88 beats per minute.
 6. _____ Joni's oral temperature is 104°F.
 7. _____ Justin's pupils are unequal.
 8. _____ Mike begins to vomit.
 9. _____ Blood is spurting from Tom's leg.
 10. _____ Carla has a fruity odor on her breath.
 11. _____ Glen has an impaled object in his eye.
 12. _____ Cerebrospinal fluid is coming from Joann's ear.
 13. _____ Wes has a deformity in his wrist after falling on it.
 14. _____ Liz is wheezing while breathing.
 15. _____ After falling, Whitney's ankle becomes swollen.

3

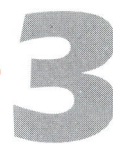

Respiratory and Cardiac Resuscitation

- Adult Resuscitation • Child and Infant Resuscitation

Sudden death from heart disease accounts for the most prominent medical emergency today. Prompt action providing early entry into the emergency medical services (EMS) system, cardiopulmonary resuscitation (CPR), or both can prevent a large number of deaths.

Successful resuscitation offers the only survival chance for a substantial number of persons experiencing cardiac arrest. Early bystander CPR remains the critical element in the prevention of sudden death. When coupled with an efficient emergency medical service (EMS) system and advanced cardiac life support capability, the chances increase to over 40% for survival. Larger numbers of trained lay people and a rapid response system of well-trained paramedical personnel could save an estimated 100,000 to 200,000 lives each year in the United States. In addition, prompt and proper application of CPR could save a number of victims who die of drowning, electrocution, suffocation, and drug intoxication.

The first two hours after the onset of symptoms represent the greatest risk of death from heart attack. Lay people, both those recognized to be at high risk and their immediate family and friends, must first be educated to recognize the unusual manifestations of heart attack. They then must know how to gain access to the EMS system. The use of a universal emergency telephone number, such as 911, represents the fastest way for an emergency medical team to respond.

Young adults who are not often exposed to high-risk individuals compose the majority of lay people taking CPR courses. An emphasis, however, must be placed on the need to train families, neighbors, and coworkers of high-risk individuals.

Most CPR training emphasizes one-rescuer CPR by the lay individual. Two-rescuer CPR is seldom, if ever, used by lay rescuers, because when help is summoned it most often comes in the form of EMS personnel who then relieve the lay rescuer. Learning the skills of two-rescuer CPR adds complexity, likely leading to decreased retention of the main techniques of one-rescuer CPR.

First aiders should initiate CPR to the best of their knowledge and capability in cases they recognize as cardiac arrest. First aiders should continue resuscitation efforts until one of the following occurs:

1. Effective circulation and ventilation have been restored.
2. Resuscitation efforts have been transferred to another responsible person who continues efforts to resuscitate.
3. A physician or a physician-directed person or team assumes responsibility.
4. The victim is transferred to properly trained personnel charged with responsibilities for emergency medical services.

18 FIRST AID ESSENTIALS

5. The rescuer is exhausted and unable to continue resuscitation.

No instance is known in which a lay person who has performed CPR reasonably has been successfully sued.

The following procedures are based upon the Standards and Guidelines for Cardiopulmonary Resuscitation (CPR) and Emergency Cardiac Care (ECC). (*JAMA*, June 6, 1986, American Heart Association.)

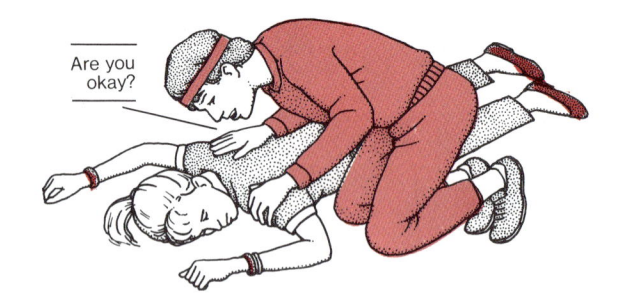

ADULT RESUSCITATION

Airway

1. *Check for Unresponsiveness.* Quickly check the person by tapping or gently shaking the person and shouting, "Are you okay?" (*See* Figure 3-1.) Move a head or neck injured person only if absolutely necessary because paralysis may result.

2. *Shout for Help.* If the person does not move or answer, call out for help. If someone responds, send him or her to phone the emergency medical services (EMS) system for help.

3. *Position the Victim.* Place the person onto his or her back on a firm, flat surface. Inadequate blood flow to the brain happens if the head is higher than the chest.

4. *Open Airway.* Immediately open the victim's airway. Use the head-tilt/chin-lift technique (*see* Figure 3-2).

    a. Place your hand closest to the victim's head on his or her forehead and apply firm, backward pressure to tilt the head back.

    b. Place the fingers of the other hand under the bony part of the lower jaw near the chin to lift the chin forward until the teeth are nearly together. Do not close the mouth.

If a neck injury sign appears, moving the lower jaw forward without tilting the head represents the safest way to open the airway. Rest your elbow on the surface which the victim is laying. Move the lower jaw forward with both hands, one on each side. Do not tilt the head in any direction.

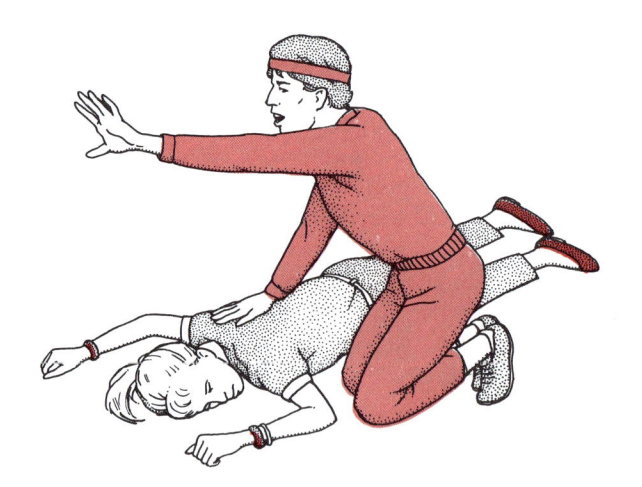

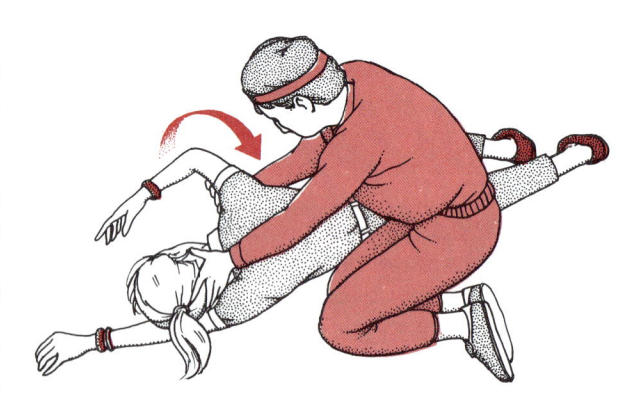

3-1. Initial steps of cardiopulmonary resuscitation. Top, Determining unresponsiveness; center, calling for help; bottom, positioning the victim.

Breathing

5. *Check for Breathlessness.* While maintaining an open airway, place your ear near the victim's mouth. (*See* Figure 3-3.) Then,

   a. *look* for the chest to rise and fall;

   b. *listen* for breathing; and

   c. *feel* for air coming out of the victim's nose and mouth.

Check for only 3 to 5 seconds.

6. *Give Two Full Breaths.* Keep the airway open by the head-tilt/chin-lift method. Gently pinch the victim's nose shut by using the thumb and index finger of the hand on the forehead. Seal your lips tightly around the outside of the victim's mouth. Give two full breaths with pauses long enough between breaths for you to take another breath. Each breath should make the victim's chest rise. Listen and feel for air escaping as the victim's chest falls. (*See* Figure 3-4.)

If unsuccessful, reposition the victim's head and try giving the two full breaths again. If still unsuccessful, use proper foreign body obstruction maneuvers. Refer to later sections on choking.

Circulation

7. *Check for a Pulse.* Keeping the head tilted, place two or three fingers on the Adam's apple. Then slide these fingertips into the groove at the side of the neck nearest you. Do not use your thumb because you may feel your own pulse. This carotid pulse check should take 5 to 10 seconds. (*See* Figure 3-5.)

If you locate a pulse but no breathing exits, give one breath every 5 seconds (after the initial two full breaths).

If you feel no pulse, begin chest compressions after the initial two full breaths.

8. *Phone the EMS System.* If someone responded to your call for help, send him or her to activate the EMS system. If still alone, perform breathing or CPR for about 1 minute and then you should telephone for help. If unable to alert the EMS system, your only choice is to continue resuscitating the victim.

9. *Compress Chest.*

   a. *Hand Position.* Locate the lower edge of the rib cage on top of the "notch" (xiphoid process) where the ribs meet the breastbone (sternum) in the center of the lower part of the chest. Place the middle finger on the notch, then the index finger next to it.

Place the heel of your other hand on the breastbone next to the index finger you used to find the "notch."

Remove the hand from the "notch" and place this hand directly on top of the hand already on the victim's breastbone.

Keep fingers up off the chest.

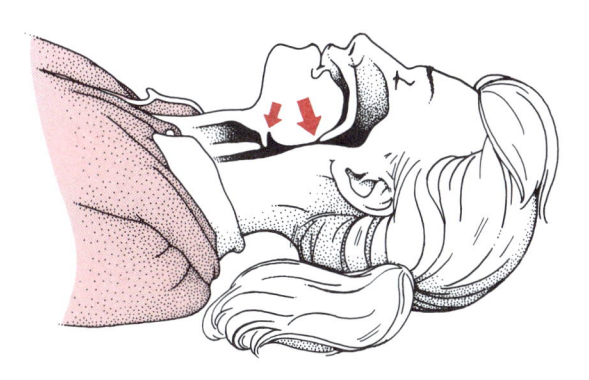

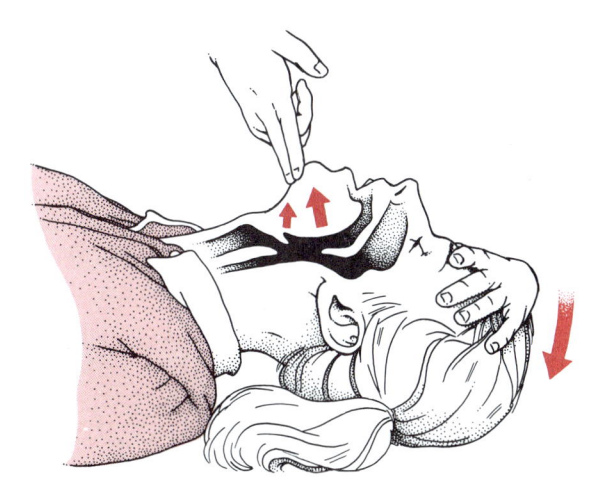

3-2. Opening the airway. Above, Airway obstruction produced by tongue and epiglottis; right, relief by head-tilt/chin-lift.

20 FIRST AID ESSENTIALS

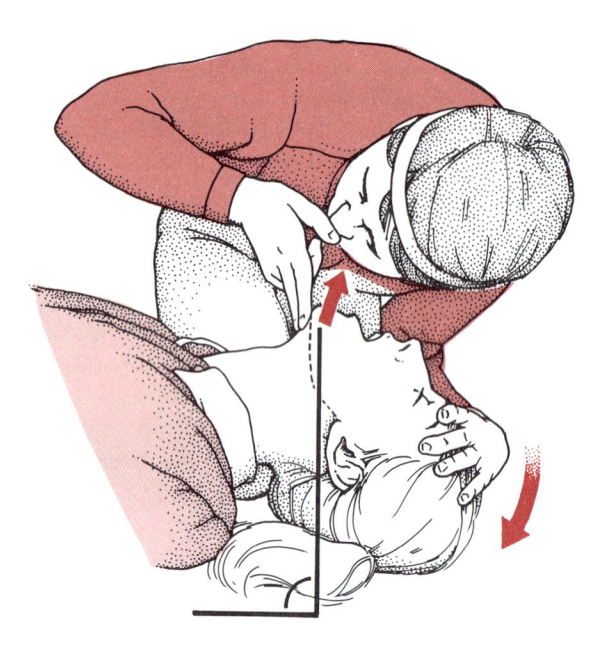

3-3. Determining breathlessness.

Rescuers with arthritic conditions may find grasping the wrist of the hand on the breastbone more acceptable.

    b. *Compression Technique.* Place shoulders and weight directly over hands, keeping elbows straight. Pushing straight down with smooth and even compressions, press downward 1½ to 2 inches at a rate of 80 to 100 compressions per minute. Avoid lifting the hands from the chest. Follow 15 compressions with two breaths, then repeat cycle again. (*See* Figure 3-6.)

Stop and check pulse and breathing every few minutes. Do not interrupt CPR for more than 7 seconds except in special circumstances.

Check carotid pulse for 5 seconds. If absent, continue CPR. If present, check breathing for 3 to 5 seconds. If present, give breathing once every 5 seconds.

3-4. Rescue breathing. Top, Mouth-to-mouth; center, mouth-to-nose; bottom, mouth-to-stoma.

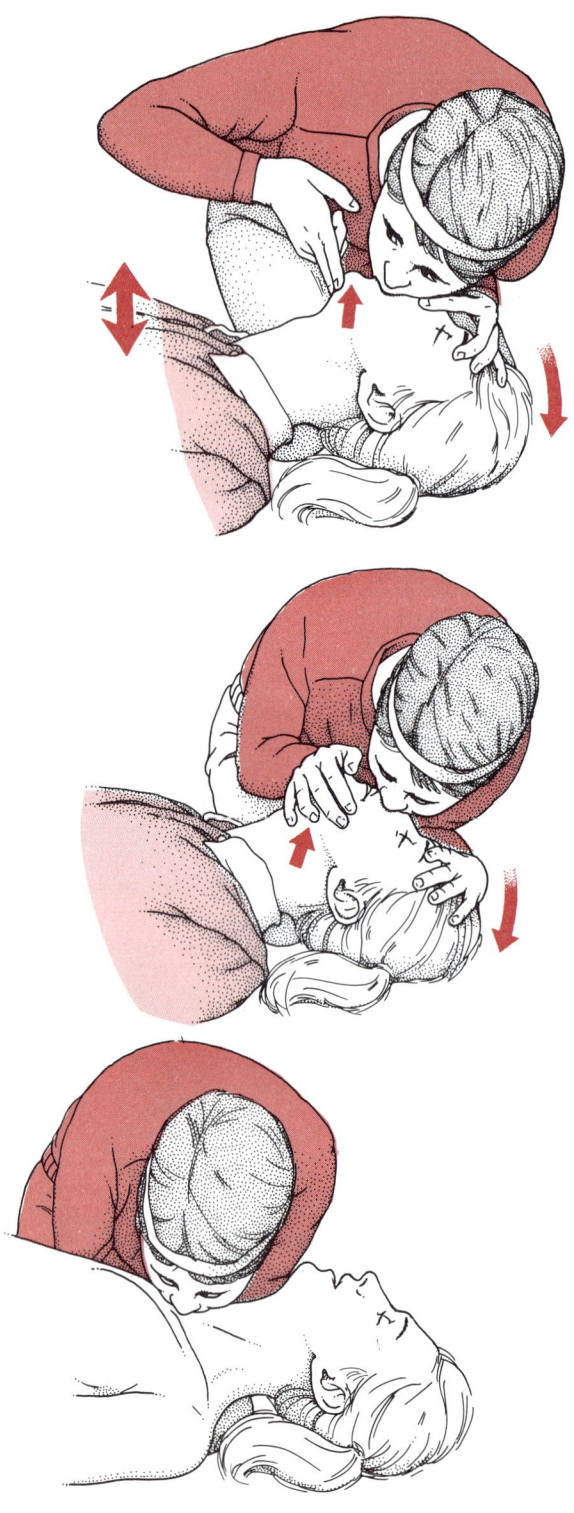

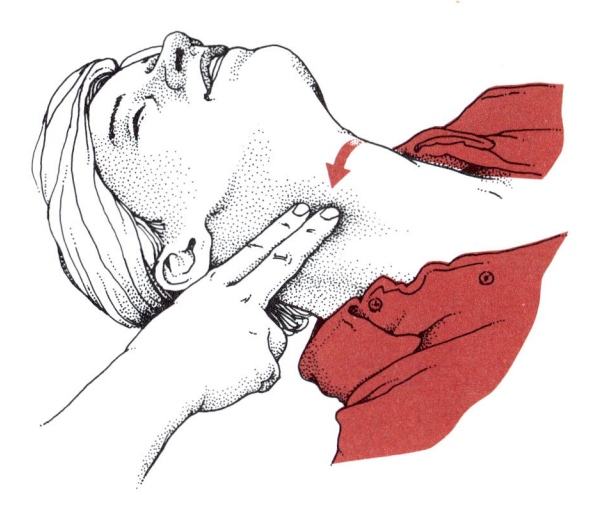

3 / RESPIRATORY AND CARDIAC RESUSCITATION 21

son clutching the neck with one or both hands represents the universal distress signal for choking. (*See* Figure 3-7.)

First Aid for Choking

Attempt the Heimlich maneuver to relieve choking. This maneuver forces air from the lungs through an artificial cough capable of moving an

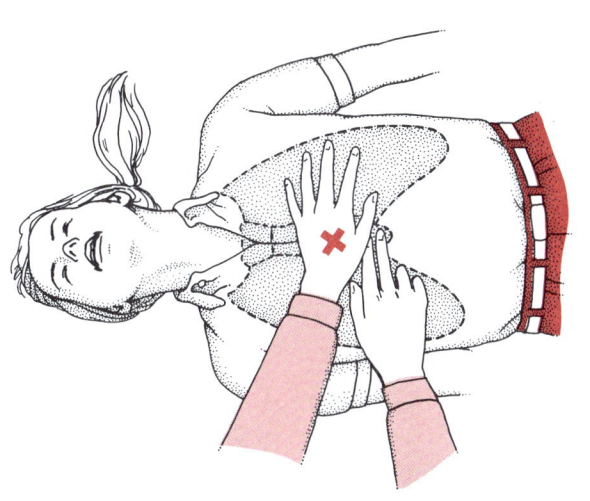

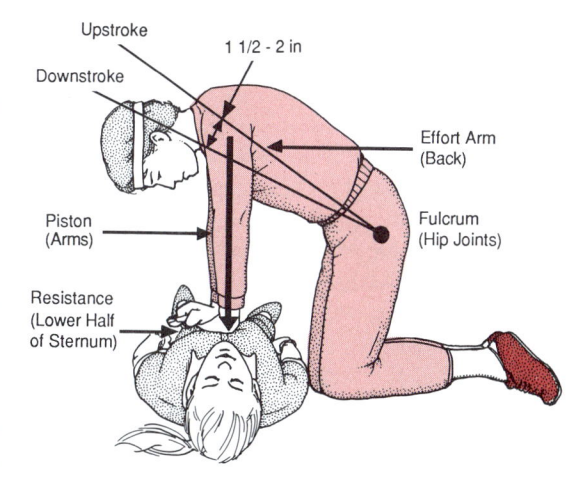

3-5. Determining pulselessness.

ADULT CHOKING

Causes

The National Safety Council reports about 3,000 deaths yearly due to choking. Choking results from:

- Swallowing large, poorly chewed pieces of food.
- Elevated blood alcohol affecting eating and swallowing of food.
- Wearing dentures (false teeth), making chewing food difficult.
- Laughing and talking while chewing and swallowing food.
- Walking, running, or playing with food or other objects in the mouth.

Recognizing Choking

Allow victims with partial airway obstruction involving "good air exchange" to cough. Wheezing between coughs may occur. Do not interfere with the victim's attempt to breathe and cough.

A weak, ineffective cough plus a high-pitched noise while breathing identifies a person with "poor air exchange." Treat these victims as though they have a complete airway obstruction.

A person unable to speak, breathe, or cough identifies a complete airway obstruction. A per-

3-6. External chest compression. Top, Locating the correct hand position on the lower half of the body; bottom, Proper position of the rescuer, with shoulders directly over the victim's sternum and elbows locked.

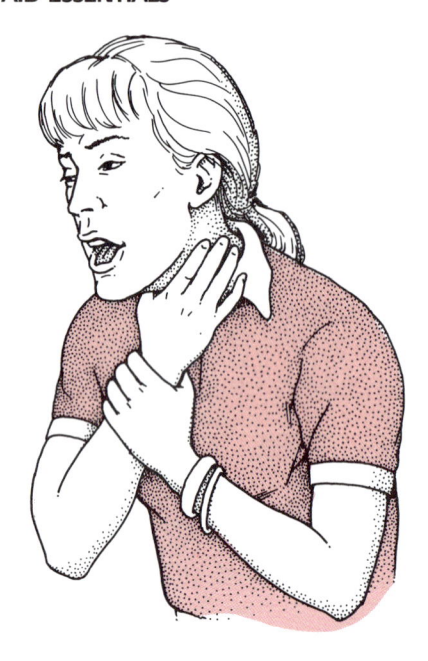

3-7. Universal distress signal for foreign-body airway obstructions.

obstructing foreign object. Repeating the maneuver 6 to 10 times may be necessary. Never place the hands on the tip of the breastbone nor on the lower edges of the ribs. The hands should be slightly above the navel.

Victim Standing or Sitting
Stand behind the victim and wrap your arms around the victim's waist. Make a fist with one hand. Place the fist thumb side against the victim's abdomen, slightly above the navel and well below the tip of the breastbone. Grasp your fist with the other hand. Press the fist into the victim's abdomen with a quick upward thrust. (See Figure 3-8.)

Victim Lying
Place the victim on his or her back with the face up. Straddle the victim's thighs. Place the heel of one hand against the victim's abdomen, slightly above the navel and well below the tip of the breastbone. Place the other hand directly on top of the first hand. Press into the abdomen with a quick, upward thrust. (See Figure 3-9.)

Finger Sweep
Use this maneuver only on unconscious victims. With the face up, open the victim's mouth and grasp both the tongue and lower jaw between the thumb and fingers. Lift the jaw. This procedure draws the tongue from the throat and may by itself relieve the obstruction. Slide the index finger of the other hand into the mouth down along the inside of the cheek to the base of the tongue. Use a hooking action to dislodge and maneuver the object so it can be removed. Do not force the object deeper into the airway.

Chest Thrusts with Standing or Sitting Victims
Use only on those in the late stages of pregnancy or a greatly overweight victim. Stand behind and wrap your arms around the chest. Place the thumb side of your fist on the middle of the breastbone. Be sure your fist is not near the lower tip of the breastbone. Then grab your fist with the other hand and give backward thrusts until the foreign body is cleared.

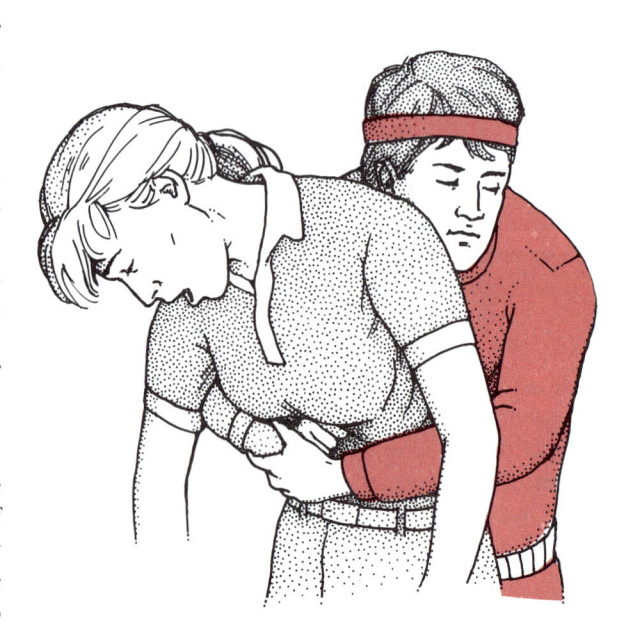

3-8. Heimlich maneuver administered to conscious victim of foreign-body airway obstruction.

Chest Thrusts with Victim Lying
Use only on those in the late stages of pregnancy or a greatly overweight victim. Place the victim on his or her back with the face up. Kneel next to the victim with your hands placed as though giving CPR.

CHILD AND INFANT RESUSCITATION

Events necessitating resuscitation in children include: (1) injuries, (2) suffocation caused by foreign objects, (3) smoke inhalation, (4) sudden infant death syndrome, (5) infections of the respiratory tract, and (6) drownings.

1. *Check for Unresponsiveness.* Check a child's or an infant's unconsciousness by gently shaking him or her and shouting.

2. *Shout for Help.* If the first aider is alone and the child is not breathing, perform CPR for one minute before calling for help.

3. *Position the Victim.* Carefully position the child on his or her back on a firm, flat surface. If a head or neck injury is suspected, carefully place the child on his back. Turn the entire body as one unit, with the head and neck firmly supported. Don't let the head roll, twist, or tilt backward or forward, especially if you think the head or neck is injured.

4. *Open the Airway.* Open the child's airway so air can get to his or her lungs. How you do this depends on whether you think the child's neck may be injured:

• *If there is any sign of neck injury*, the safest way to open the airway is to move the lower jaw forward without tilting the head. Rest your elbows on the surface the child is lying on. Place two or three fingers under each side of the child's jaw, just beneath the ears, and lift the jaw upward. (*See* Figure 3-10.)

• *If you are sure the neck is not injured*, place one hand on the child's forehead and hook the fingers, not the thumb, of the other hand under the bony tip of the child's chin. Lift the chin gently while pressing down on the forehead. Tilt the head gently back, taking care not to close the mouth. (*See* Figure 3-11.)

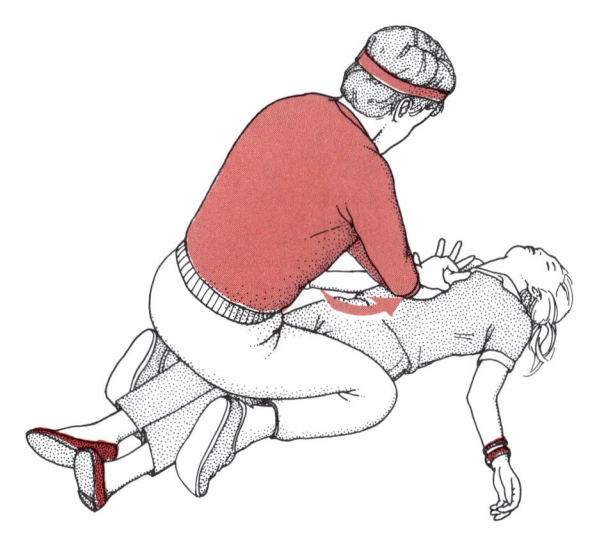

3-9. Heimlich maneuver administered to unconscious victim of foreign-body airway obstruction.

5. *Check for Breathlessness.* If you are unsure whether the child is breathing, place your ear close to his mouth and nose. Listen and feel for exhaled air. At the same time, look at the chest and stomach for movement.

6. *Give Two Breaths.* If the child is breathing, keep the airway open. If he is not breathing, you must breathe for him.

• *For an infant*, cover the mouth and nose with your mouth. Be sure your lips make a tight seal. Also be sure to support the tip of the baby's chin with your finger. (*See* Figure 3-12.) Without this support, you won't be able to get air into the baby's lungs. Gently blow a little air into the

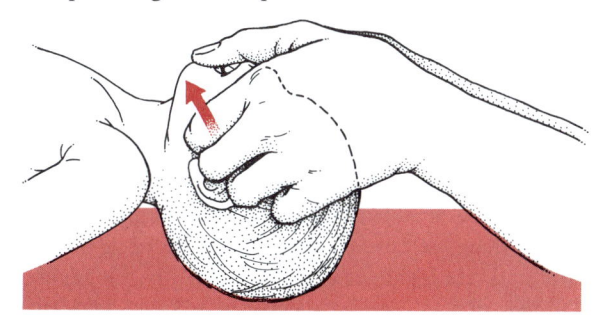

3-10. Jaw-thrust.

24 FIRST AID ESSENTIALS

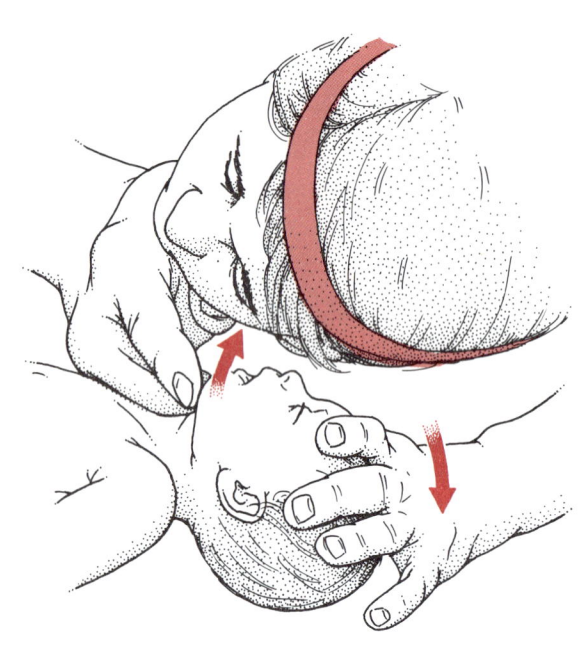

3-11. Head-tilt/chin-lift.

infant's mouth and nose—just enough to make the baby's chest rise. If you breathe too hard, you may hurt the infant's lungs. Breathe slowly to give enough air at the lowest possible pressure. Give two slow breaths to the child, between 1 and 1½ seconds per breath—then pause to give yourself time to take another breath. Repeat.

• *For an older child,* pinch the nose tightly with the fingers of the hand resting on the forehead. Take a breath and seal the child's mouth with yours. (*See* Figure 3-13.) Give two slow breaths to the child—between 1 and 1½ seconds per breath—and pause to give yourself time to take another breath. Repeat.

  7. *Check for a Pulse.*

• *For an infant:* Infants younger than one year of age have short, chubby necks making the carotid pulse difficult to locate. Therefore, use the pulse in the upper arm (brachial pulse) instead. Its location can be found on the inside of the upper arm between the elbow and the shoulder. (*See* Figure 3-14.) Place your thumb on the outside of the arm and press gently with your index and middle fingers on the inside of the arm to feel the pulse. Do this for 5 to 10 seconds.

• *For an older child:* Check the carotid pulse the way you would for an adult. Locate the Adam's apple with the index and middle fingers of one hand while keeping the head tilted back with a hand on the forehead. Then slide your fingers toward you into the groove next to the windpipe at the side of the neck. Gently press to feel for a pulse. Do this for 5 to 10 seconds. (*See* Figure 3-15.)

  8. *Phone the EMS System.* If a person arrives to help, have him call the local emergency telephone number. If this person is trained, he or she could relieve you while you call for help. If unable to telephone for help, the only option is to continue CPR.

  9. *Compress the Chest.*

• *For the infant.* If there is no pulse, place two fingers on his or her breastbone, one fingerwidth below the nipple line, and give five chest compressions for every breath. (*See* Figure 3-16.) Compressions should be a half to one inch deep. All five should be given in the three-second interval between each breath (100 times per

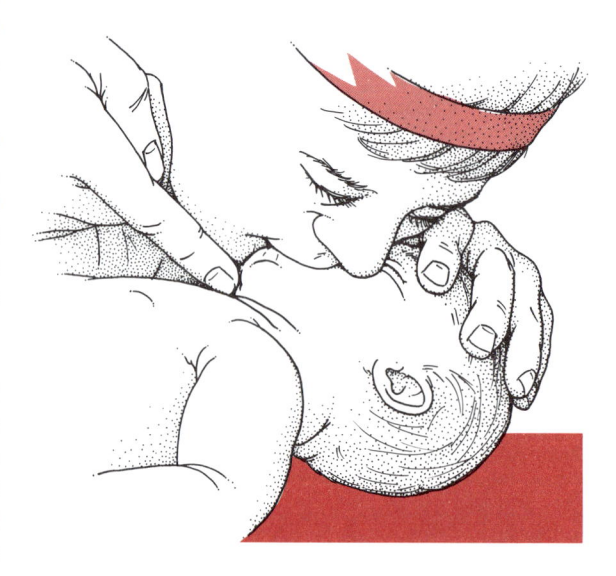

3-12. Mouth-to-mouth and nose seal.

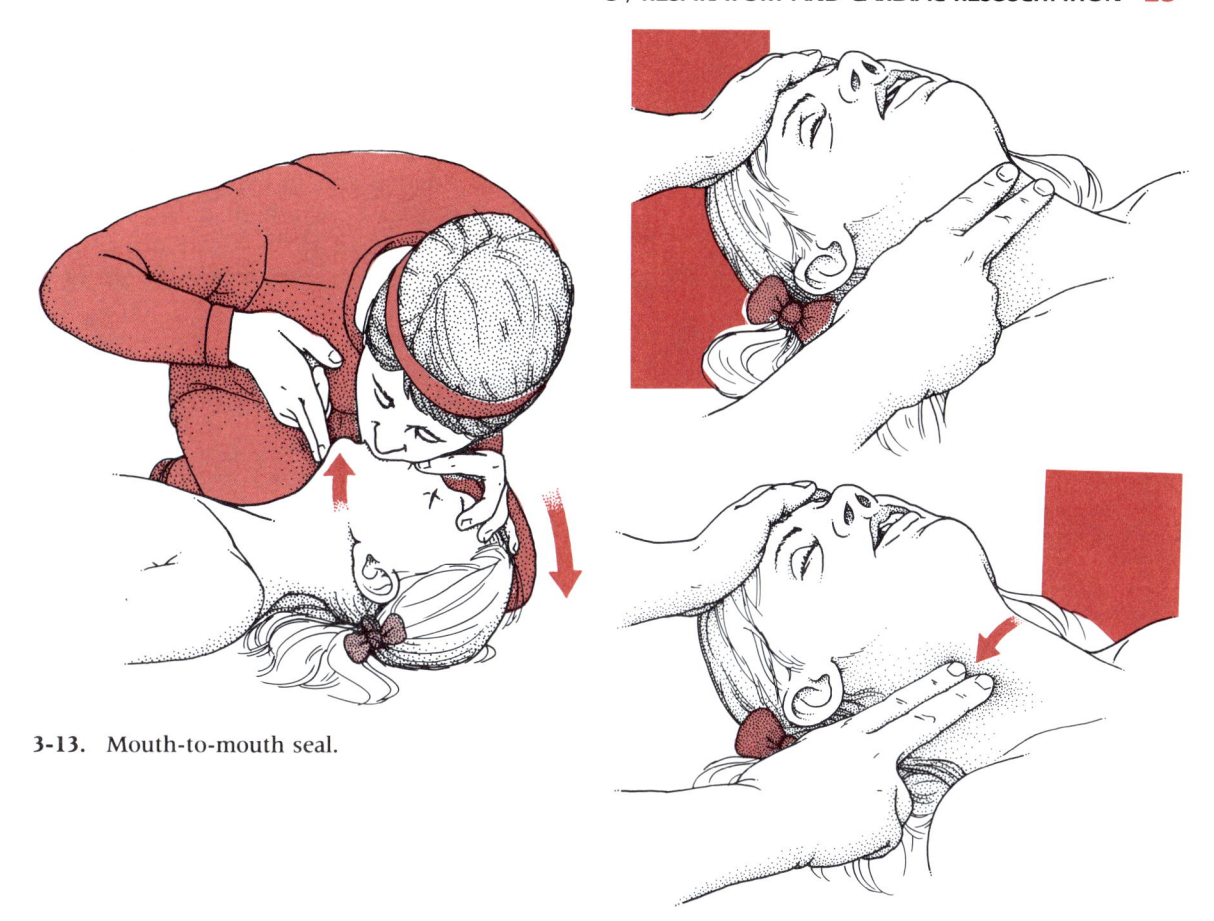

3 / RESPIRATORY AND CARDIAC RESUSCITATION 25

3-13. Mouth-to-mouth seal.

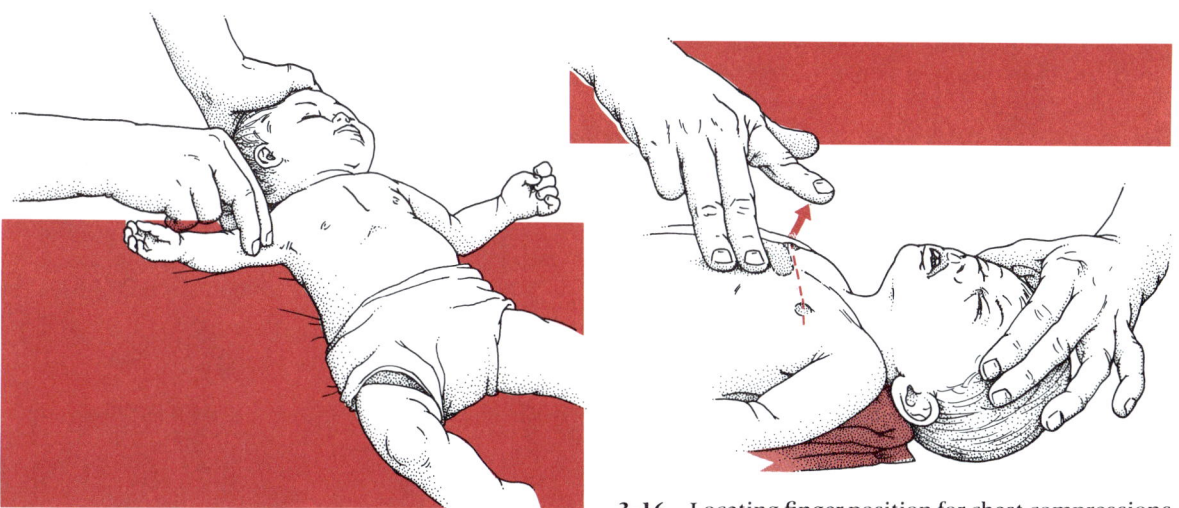

3-14. Locating and palpating brachial pulse.

3-15. Locating and palpating carotid artery pulse.

3-16. Locating finger position for chest compressions in infant.

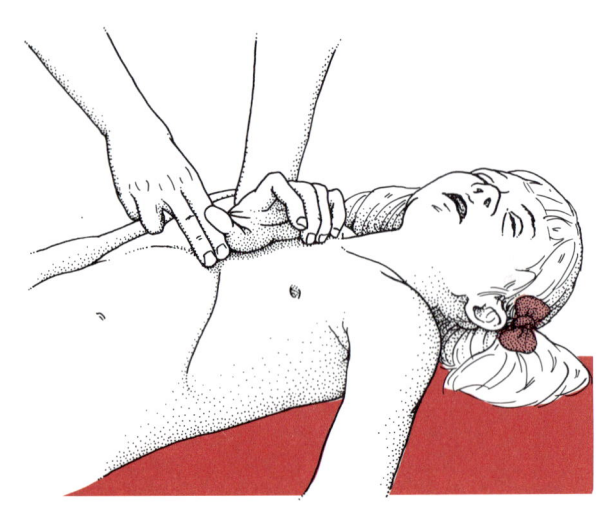

26 FIRST AID ESSENTIALS

3-17. Locating hand position for chest compressions in child.

minute or 5 in 3 seconds). The count will go quickly—one, two, three, four, five, PUFF.

For a child. Locate the lower edges of the rib cage to the "notch" where the ribs meet the breastbone in the center of the lower part of the chest. Place the middle finger on the notch, then the index finger next to it. (*See* Figure 3-17.)

Place the heel of your other hand on the breastbone next to the index finger you used to find the "notch." Keep fingers off the chest. The chest is compressed with one hand to the depth of 1 to 1½ inches at a rate of 80 to 100 times per minute (5 per 3–4 seconds). Give one breath every five compressions. If the child is large or older than about eight years, the method described for adults should be used. Compressions should be smooth, not jerky.

CHILD AND INFANT CHOKING

For a child over one year:

1. *Victim Standing or Sitting (Conscious).* Stand behind the victim and wrap your arms around the victim's waist. Make a fist with one hand. Place the fist's thumb side against the victim's abdomen, slightly above the navel and well below the tip of the breastbone. Grasp your fist with the other hand. Press the fist into the victim's abdomen with a quick, upward thrust. (*See* Figure 3-18.)

2. *Victim Lying (Conscious or Unconscious).* Place the victim on his or her back with the face up. Straddle the victim's thighs. Place the heel of one hand against the victim's abdomen, slightly above the navel and well below the tip of the breastbone. Place the other hand directly on top of the first hand. Press into the abdomen with a quick, upward thrust. (*See* Figure 3-19.)

For a child less than one year old:

1. Place the baby on your forearm, face down and with his head down low. Rest your forearm on your thigh for support.

2. Using the heel of your hand, hit the baby four times on the back, high between the shoulder blades. (*See* Figure 3-20.)

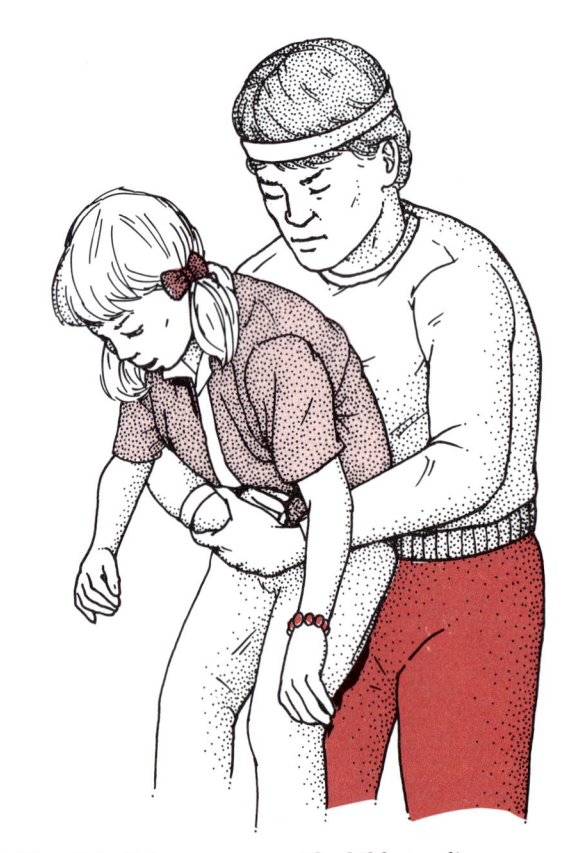

3-18. Heimlich maneuver with child standing.

3 / RESPIRATORY AND CARDIAC RESUSCITATION   **27**

3-19. Heimlich maneuver with child lying.

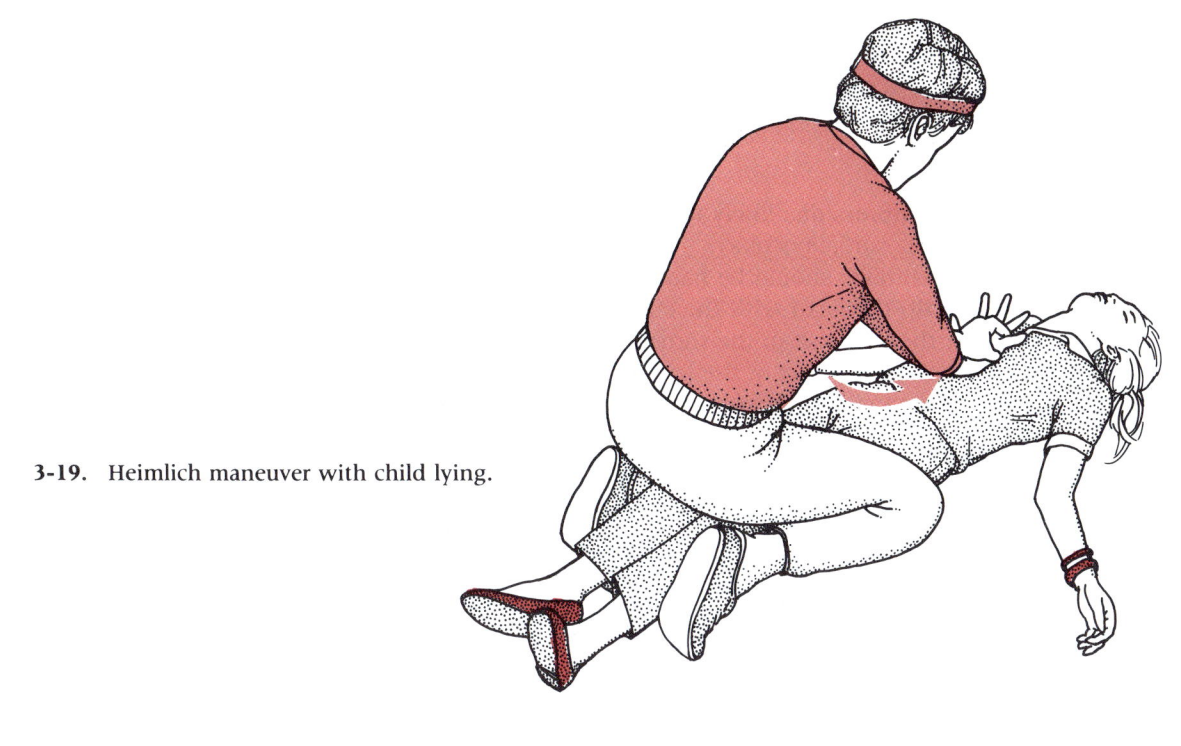

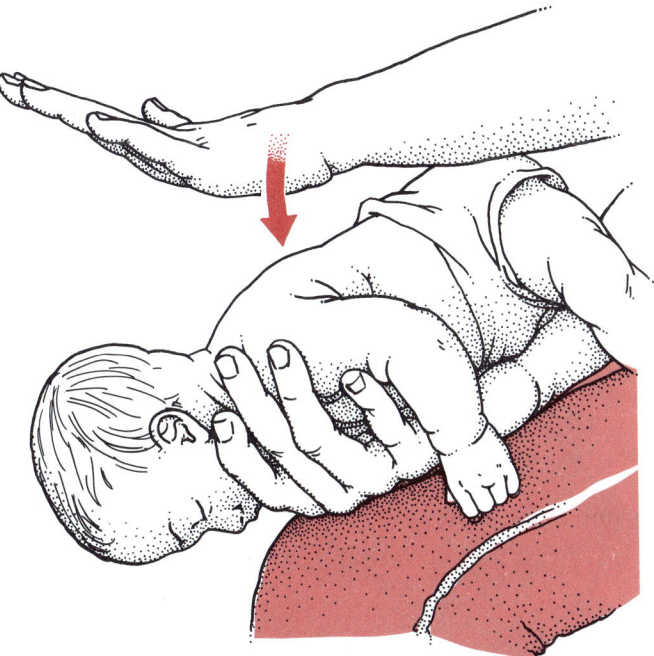

3-20. Back blow in infant.

3. If he/she is not yet breathing, support the head and neck and place him/her on the thigh with the head lower than the trunk and give four chest thrusts. These chest thrusts are performed in the same location as external chest compressions but at a slower rate.

Repeat this sequence of back blows and chest compressions until the airway opens or medical help arrives.

Avoid blind finger sweeps in infants and children since the foreign object may be pushed back into the airway, causing further blockage. Remove foreign object from the mouth *only if it can be seen.*

SELF-CHECK QUESTIONS

Activity 1: Adult Resuscitation

Multiple Choice

1. ☐ Are chest compressions likely to work if the victim is on a soft surface?
   A. Yes, a soft surface is okay.
   B. No, the surface should be hard.
2. ☐ When you tip the head with the chin lift, where do you place your fingertips?
   A. Under the soft part of the throat near the chin.
   B. Under the bony part of the jaw near the chin.
3. ☐ Which is the safer way to open the airway of a person who may have neck or back injuries?
   A. Push the jaw forward from the corners.
   B. Tip the head very gently, part way back.
4. ☐ How should you check for stopped breathing?
   A. Look at the chest; listen and feel for air coming out of the mouth.
   B. Look at the pupils of the eyes.
   C. Check the pulse.
5. ☐ When you give breaths to an adult, the breaths should be:
   A. Large and full.
   B. Small and gentle.
6. ☐ Before deciding whether to give CPR, check the victim's pulse for:
   A. 1–3 seconds
   B. 3–5 seconds
   C. 5–10 seconds
   D. 1–20 seconds
7. ☐ How do you find where to push on the chest for chest compressions?
   A. Push on the xiphoid.
   B. Measure up one finger-width from the middle finger on the xiphoid notch.
8. ☐ Give chest compressions:
   A. With a quick jerk.
   B. Smoothly and regularly.
9. ☐ Push on a victim's chest:
   A. At an angle.
   B. Straight down.
10. ☐ Compress an adult's chest at least:
    A. ¼ to ½ inch.
    B. 1½ to 2 inches.
11. ☐ In one-rescuer CPR, give chest compressions to an adult at the rate of:
    A. 100 per minute
    B. 80 per minute
    C. 60 per minute
    D. 40 per minute

12. ☐ What is the pattern of compressions and breaths in one-rescuer CPR for an adult victim?
    A. 15 compressions, 2 breaths
    B. 15 compressions, 1 breath
    C. 5 compressions, 2 breaths
    D. 5 compressions, 1 breath
13. ☐ Pushing on the xiphoid increases the:
    A. Amount of blood circulation.
    B. Chance of internal injuries.

Activity 2: Adult Choking

Multiple Choice

1. ☐ An adult victim is coughing forcefully. Should you give back blows and thrusts?
    A. Yes
    B. No
2. ☐ A person is coughing weakly and making wheezing noises. You should:
    A. Give abdominal thrust.
    B. Let the person alone and watch closely.
3. ☐ A victim who seems to be choking CAN speak. Should you give abdominal thrusts?
    A. Yes
    B. No
4. ☐ A conscious person is coughing forcefully trying to dislodge an object. Then the person stops coughing and cannot speak. You should:
    A. Give abdominal thrusts.
    B. Let the person alone and watch closely.
5. ☐ When you give abdominal thrusts to a conscious victim, what part of your fist do you place against the victim?
    A. The palm side
    B. The little finger side
    C. The thumb side
6. ☐ Give abdominal thrusts quickly:
    A. Inward and upward
    B. Straight back
7. ☐ Where do you place your fist to give abdominal thrusts?
    A. Over the breastbone
    B. Slightly above the navel
    C. Below the navel
8. ☐ To give abdominal thrusts to a victim who is lying down, place the heel of one hand:
    A. Slightly above the navel
    B. On the edge of the breastbone
    C. Below the navel
9. ☐ For a victim who is very fat or in advanced pregnancy, it is better to give:
    A. Abdominal thrusts
    B. Chest thrusts

Activity 3: Child and Infant Resuscitation

Multiple Choice

1. ☐ How should you check for stopped breathing?
   - A. Look at the chest; listen and feel for air coming out of the mouth.
   - B. Look at the pupils of the eyes.
   - C. Check the pulse.
2. ☐ How can you tell if your amount of breath is enough?
   - A. Stomach will form a pouch.
   - B. Chest will rise.
   - C. Your air backs up against incoming air.
3. ☐ Check a baby's pulse at the:
   - A. Middle of the upper arm
   - B. Wrist
   - C. Neck
4. ☐ When giving chest compressions to a baby, use:
   - A. 2 or 3 fingers
   - B. The heel of one hand
5. ☐ Push on the chest of a child or baby one finger-width:
   - A. Above nipple line
   - B. Below nipple line
   - C. Above xiphoid notch
6. ☐ How far do you compress a baby's chest?
   - A. 1½ to 2 inches
   - B. ½ to 1 inch
7. ☐ Give a baby chest compressions at the rate of:
   - A. 100 per minute
   - B. 80 per minute
   - C. 60 per minute
8. ☐ Give babies and children:
   - A. 15 compressions, 2 breaths
   - B. 5 compressions, 2 breaths
   - C. 15 compressions, 1 breath
   - D. 5 compressions, 1 breath
9. ☐ When giving chest compressions to a child, use:
   - A. 2 or 3 fingers or heel of one hand
   - B. The heel of one hand and the other hand on top.

Activity 4: Child and Infant Choking

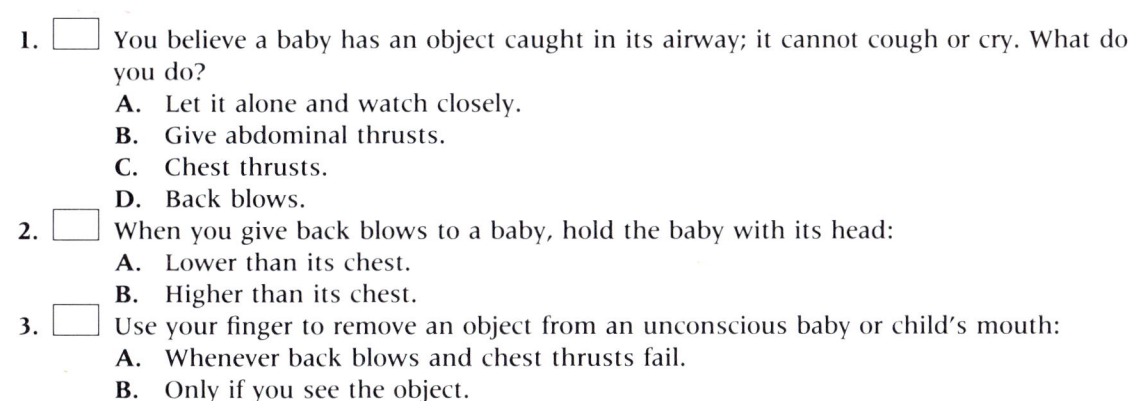

Multiple Choice

1. ☐ You believe a baby has an object caught in its airway; it cannot cough or cry. What do you do?
   A. Let it alone and watch closely.
   B. Give abdominal thrusts.
   C. Chest thrusts.
   D. Back blows.
2. ☐ When you give back blows to a baby, hold the baby with its head:
   A. Lower than its chest.
   B. Higher than its chest.
3. ☐ Use your finger to remove an object from an unconscious baby or child's mouth:
   A. Whenever back blows and chest thrusts fail.
   B. Only if you see the object.

BLS Summary Performance Sheet
Cardiopulmonary Resuscitation (CPR)

	Objectives	Actions		
		Adult (over 8 yrs.)	**Child** (1 to 8 yrs.)	**Infant** (under 1 yr.)
A. Airway	1. Assessment: Determine unresponsiveness.	Tap or gently shake shoulder.		
		Say, "Are you okay?"		Observe
	2. Get help.	Call out "Help!"		
	3. Position the victim.	Turn on back as a unit, supporting head and neck if necessary. (4–10 seconds)		
	4. Open the airway.	Head-tilt/chin-lift		
B. Breathing	5. Assessment: Determine breathlessness.	Maintain open airway. Place ear over mouth, observing chest. Look, listen, feel for breathing. (3–5 seconds)		
	6. Give 2 rescue breaths.	Maintain open airway.		
		Seal mouth to mouth		mouth to nose/mouth
		Give 2 rescue breaths, 1 to 1½ seconds each. Observe chest rise. Allow lung deflation between breaths.		
	7. Option for obstructed airway	a. Reposition victim's head. Try again to give rescue breaths.		
		b. Activate the EMS system.		
		c. Give 6–10 subdiaphragmatic abdominal thrusts (the Heimlich maneuver).		Give 4 back blows.
		^		Give 4 chest thrusts.
		d. Tongue–jaw lift and finger sweep	Tongue–jaw lift, but finger sweep only if you see a foreign object.	
		If unsuccessful, repeat a, c, and d until successful.		
C. Circulation	8. Assessment: Determine pulselessness.	Feel for carotid pulse with one hand; maintain head-tilt with the other. (5–10 seconds)		Feel for brachial pulse; keep head-tilt.
	9. Activate EMS system.	If someone responded to call for help, send them to activate the EMS system.		
	Begin chest compressions: 10. Landmark check	Run middle finger along bottom edge of rib cage to notch at center (tip of sternum).		Imagine a line drawn between the nipples.
	11. Hand position	Place index finger next to finger on notch:		Place 2–3 fingers on sternum, 1 finger's width below line. Depress ½–1 in.
		Two hands next to index finger. Depress 1½–2 in.	Heel of one hand next to index finger. Depress 1–1½ in.	^
	12. Compression rate	80–100 per minute		At least 100 per minute
CPR Cycles	13. Compressions to breaths.	2 breaths to every 15 compressions.	1 breath to every 5 compressions.	
	14. Number of cycles.	4 (52–73 seconds)	10 (60–87 seconds)	10 (45 seconds or less)
	15. Reassessment.	Feel for carotid pulse. (5 seconds)		Feel for brachial pulse.
		If no pulse, resume CPR, starting with 2 breaths.	If no pulse, resume CPR, starting with 1 breath.	
Option for pulse return	If no breathing, give rescue breaths.	1 breath every 5 seconds	1 breath every 4 seconds	1 breath every 3 seconds

BLS Performance Sheet
Adult One-Rescuer CPR

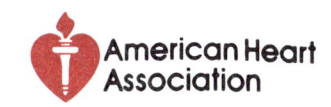

American Heart Association

Name _____ Date _____

Step	Objective	Critical Performance	S	U
1. AIRWAY	Assessment: Determine unresponsiveness.	Tap or gently shake shoulder.		
		Shout "Are you OK?"		
	Call for help.	Call out "Help!"		
	Position the victim.	Turn on back as unit, if necessary, supporting head and neck (4–10 sec).		
	Open the airway.	Use head-tilt/chin-lift maneuver.		
2. BREATHING	Assessment: Determine breathlessness.	Maintain open airway.		
		Ear over mouth, observe chest: look, listen, feel for breathing (3–5 sec).		
	Ventilate twice.	Maintain open airway.		
		Seal mouth and nose properly.		
		Ventilate 2 times at 1–1.5 sec/inspiration.		
		Observe chest rise (adequate ventilation volume.)		
		Allow deflation between breaths.		
3. CIRCULATION	Assessment: Determine pulselessness.	Feel for carotid pulse on near side of victim (5–10 sec).		
		Maintain head-tilt with other hand.		
	Activate EMS system.	If someone responded to call for help, send him/her to activate EMS system.		
		Total time, Step 1–Activate EMS system: 15–35 sec.		
	Begin chest compressions.	Rescuer kneels by victim's shoulders.		
		Landmark check prior to hand placement.		
		Proper hand position throughout.		
		Rescuer's shoulders over victim's sternum.		
		Equal compression-relaxation.		
		Compress 1½ to 2 inches.		
		Keep hands on sternum during upstroke.		
		Complete chest relaxation on upstroke.		
		Say any helpful mnemonic.		
		Compression rate: 80–100/min (15 per 9–11 sec).		
4. Compression/Ventilation Cycles	Do 4 cycles of 15 compressions and 2 ventilations.	Proper compression/ventilation ratio: 15 compressions to 2 ventilations per cycle.		
		Observe chest rise: 1–1.5 sec/inspiration; 4 cycles/52–73 sec.		
5. Reassessment*	Determine pulselessness.	Feel for carotid pulse (5 sec).† If there is no pulse, go to Step 6.		
6. Continue CPR	Ventilate twice.	Ventilate 2 times.		
		Observe chest rise: 1–1.5 sec/inspiration.		
	Resume compression/ventilation cycles.	Feel for carotid pulse every few minutes.		

* If 2nd rescuer arrives to replace 1st rescuer: (a) 2nd rescuer identifies self by saying "I know CPR. Can I help?" (b) 2nd rescuer then does pulse check in Step 5 and continues with Step 6. (During practice and testing only one rescuer actually ventilates the manikin. The 2nd rescuer simulates ventilation.) (c) 1st rescuer assesses the adequacy of 2nd rescuer's CPR by observing chest rise during ventilations and by checking the pulse during chest compressions.

† If pulse is present, open airway and check for spontaneous breathing (a) If breathing is present, maintain open airway and monitor pulse and breathing. (b) If breathing is absent, perform rescue breathing at 12 times/min and monitor pulse.

Instructor _____ Check: Satisfactory _____ Unsatisfactory _____

33

BLS Performance Sheet

Child One-Rescuer CPR*

American Heart Association

Name _____ Date _____

Step	Objective	Critical Performance	S	U
1. AIRWAY	Assessment: Determine unresponsiveness.	Tap or gently shake shoulder.		
		Shout "Are you OK?"		
	Call for help.	Call out "Help!"		
	Position the victim.	Turn on back as unit, if necessary, supporting head and neck (4–10 sec).		
	Open the airway.	Use head-tilt/chin-lift maneuver.		
2. BREATHING	Assessment: Determine breathlessness.	Maintain open airway.		
		Ear over mouth, observe chest: look, listen, feel for breathing (3–5 sec).		
	Ventilate twice.	Maintain open airway.		
		Seal mouth and nose properly.		
		Ventilate 2 times at 1–1.5 sec/inspiration.		
		Observe chest rise.		
		Allow deflation between breaths.		
3. CIRCULATION	Assessment: Determine pulselessness.	Feel for carotid pulse on near side of victim (5–10 sec).		
		Maintain head-tilt with other hand.		
	Activate EMS system.	If someone responded to call for help, send him/her to activate EMS system.		
		Total time, Step 1—Activate EMS system: 15–35 sec.		
	Begin chest compressions.	Rescuer kneels by victim's shoulders.		
		Landmark check prior to initial hand placement.§		
		Proper hand position throughout.		
		Rescuer's shoulders over victim's sternum.		
		Equal compression-relaxation.		
		Compress 1 to 1½ inches.		
		Keep hand on sternum during upstroke.		
		Complete chest relaxation on upstroke.		
		Say any helpful mnemonic.		
		Compression rate: 80–100/min (5 per 3–4 sec).		
4. Compression/Ventilation Cycles	Do 10 cycles of 5 compressions and 1 ventilation.	Proper compression/ventilation ratio: 5 compressions to 1 slow ventilation per cycle.		
		Observe chest rise: 1–1.5 sec/inspiration (10 cycles/60–87 sec).		
5. Reassessment†	Determine pulselessness.	Feel for carotid pulse (5 sec).‡ If there is no pulse, go to Step 6.		
6. Continue CPR	Ventilate once.	Ventilate one time.		
		Observe chest rise: 1–1.5 sec/inspiration.		
	Resume compression/ventilation cycles	Feel for carotid pulse every few minutes.		

* If child is above age of approximately 8 years, the method for adults should be used.

† 2nd rescuer arrives to replace 1st rescuer: (a) 2nd rescuer identifies self by saying "I know CPR. Can I help?" (b) 2nd rescuer then does pulse check in Step 5 and continues with Step 6. (During practice and testing only one rescuer actually ventilates the manikin. The 2nd rescuer simulates ventilation.) (c) 1st rescuer assesses the adequacy of 2nd rescuer's CPR by observing chest rise during ventilations and by checking the pulse during chest compressions.

‡ If pulse is present, open airway and check for spontaneous breathing. (a) If breathing is present, maintain open airway and monitor breathing and pulse. (b) If breathing is absent, perform rescue breathing at 15 times/min and monitor pulse.

§ Thereafter, check hand position visually.

Instructor _____ Check: Satisfactory _____ Unsatisfactory _____

34

BLS Performance Sheet

Infant CPR

American Heart Association

Name _____ Date _____

Step	Objective	Critical Performance	S	U
1. AIRWAY	Assessment: Determine unresponsiveness.	Tap or gently shake shoulder.		
	Call for help.	Call out "Help!"		
	Position the infant.	Turn on back as unit, supporting head and neck.		
		Place on firm, hard surface.		
	Open the airway.	Use head-tilt/chin-lift maneuver to sniffing or neutral position.		
		Do not overextend the head.		
2. BREATHING	Assessment: Determine breathlessness.	Maintain open airway.		
		Ear over mouth, observe chest: look, listen, feel for breathing (3–5 sec).		
	Ventilate twice.	Maintain open airway.		
		Make tight seal on infant's mouth and nose with rescuer's mouth.		
		Ventilate 2 times at 1–1.5 sec/inspiration.		
		Observe chest rise.		
		Allow deflation between breaths.		
3. CIRCULATION	Assessment: Determine pulselessness.	Feel for brachial pulse (5–10 sec).		
		Maintain head-tilt with other hand.		
	Activate EMS system.	If someone responded to call for help, send him/her to activate EMS system.		
		Total time, Step 1—Activate EMS system: 15–35 sec.		
	Begin chest compressions.	Imagine line between nipples (intermammary line).		
		Place 2–3 fingers on sternum, 1 finger's width below intermammary line.		
		Equal compression–relaxation.		
		Compress vertically, ½ to 1 inches.		
		Keep fingers on sternum during upstroke.		
		Complete chest relaxation on upstroke.		
		Say any helpful mnemonic.		
		Compression rate: at least 100/min (5 in 3 sec or less).		
4. Compression/Ventilation Cycles	Do 10 cycles of 5 compressions and 1 ventilation.	Proper compression/ventilation ratio: 5 compressions to 1 slow ventilation per cycle.		
		Pause for ventilation.		
		Observe chest rise: 1–1.5 sec/inspiration; 10 cycles/45 sec or less.		
5. Reassessment	Determine pulselessness.	Feel for brachial pulse (5 sec).* If there is no pulse, go to Step 6.		
6. Continue CPR	Ventilate once.	Ventilate 1 time.		
		Observe chest rise: 1–1.5 sec/inspiration.		
	Resume compression/ventilation cycles.	Feel for brachial pulse every few minutes.		

* If pulse is present, open airway and check for spontaneous breathing and pulse. (b) If breathing is absent, perform rescue breathing at 20 (a) If breathing is present, maintain open airway and monitor breathing times/min and monitor pulse.

Instructor _____ Check: Satisfactory _____ Unsatisfactory _____

BLS Performance Sheet
Adult FBAO Management: Conscious

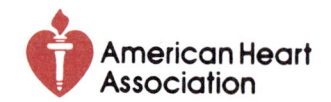

American Heart Association

Name _____ Date _____

Step	Objective	Critical Performance	S	U
1. Assessment	Determine airway obstruction.	Ask "Are you choking?"		
		Determine if victim can cough or speak.		
2. Heimlich Maneuver	Perform abdominal thrusts.	Stand behind the victim.		
		Wrap arms around victim's waist.		
		Make a fist with one hand and place the thumb side against victim's abdomen in the midline slightly above the navel and well below the tip of the xiphoid.		
		Grasp fist with the other hand.		
		Press into the victim's abdomen with quick upward thrusts.		
		Each thrust should be distinct and delivered with the intent of relieving the airway obstruction.		
		Repeat thrusts until either the foreign body is expelled or the victim becomes unconscious (see below).		

Victim with Obstructed Airway Becomes Unconscious (Optional Testing Sequence)

Step	Objective	Critical Performance	S	U
3. Positioning	Position the victim.	Turn on back as unit.		
		Place face up, arms by side.		
	Call for help.	Call out "Help!" or, if others respond, activate EMS system.		
4. Foreign Body Check	Perform finger sweep.*	Keep victim's face up.		
		Use tongue–jaw lift to open mouth.		
		Sweep deeply into mouth to remove foreign body.		
5. Breathing Attempt	Ventilate.	Open airway with head-tilt/chin-lift.		
		Seal mouth and nose properly.		
		Attempt to ventilate.		
6. Heimlich Maneuver	(Airway is obstructed.) Perform abdominal thrusts.	Straddle victim's thighs.		
		Place heel of one hand against victim's abdomen, in the midline slightly above the navel and well below the tip of the xiphoid.		
		Place second hand directly on top of first hand.		
		Press into the abdomen with quick upward thrusts.		
		Perform 6–10 abdominal thrusts.		
7. Foreign Body Check	(Airway remains obstructed.) Perform finger sweep.*	Keep victim's face up.		
		Use tongue–jaw lift to open mouth.		
		Sweep deeply into mouth to remove foreign body.		
8. Breathing Attempt	Ventilate.	Open airway with head-tilt/chin-lift.		
		Seal mouth and nose properly.		
		Attempt to ventilate.		
9. Sequencing	(Airway remains obstructed.) Repeat sequence.	Repeat Steps 6–8 until successful.†		

* During practice and testing, simulate finger sweeps.

† After airway obstruction is cleared, ventilate twice and proceed with CPR as indicated.

Instructor _____ Check: Satisfactory _____ Unsatisfactory _____

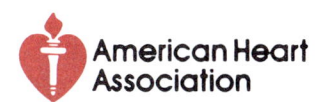

BLS Performance Sheet
Child FBAO Management: Conscious*

American Heart Association

Name _____ Date _____

Step	Objective	Critical Performance	S	U
1. Assessment	Determine airway obstruction.*	Ask "Are you choking?"		
		Determine if victim can cough or speak.		
2. Heimlich Maneuver	Perform abdominal thrusts (only if victim's cough is ineffective and there is increasing respiratory difficulty).	Stand behind the victim.		
		Wrap arms around victim's waist.		
		Make a fist with one hand and place the thumb side against victim's abdomen, in the midline slightly above the navel and well below the tip of the xiphoid.		
		Grasp fist with the other hand.		
		Press into the victim's abdomen with quick upward thrusts.		
		Each thrust should be distinct and delivered with the intent of relieving the airway obstruction.		
		Repeat thrusts until either the foreign body is expelled or the victim becomes unconscious (see below).		

Victim with Obstructed Airway Becomes Unconscious (Optional Testing Sequence)

Step	Objective	Critical Performance	S	U
3. Positioning	Position the victim.	Turn on back as unit.		
		Place face up, arms by side.		
	Call for help.	Call out "Help!" or if others respond, activate EMS system.		
4. Foreign Body Check	Manual removal of foreign body if one is found. DO NOT perform blind finger sweep.	Keep victim's face up.		
		Use tongue–jaw lift to open mouth.		
		Look into mouth; remove foreign body ONLY IF VISUALIZED.		
5. Breathing Attempt	Ventilate.	Open airway with head-tilt/chin-lift.		
		Seal mouth and nose properly.		
		Attempt to ventilate.		
6. Heimlich Maneuver	(Airway is obstructed.) Perform abdominal thrusts.	Kneel at victim's feet if on the floor, or stand at victim's feet if on a table.		
		Place heel of one hand against victim's abdomen, in the midline slightly above navel and well below tip of xiphoid.		
		Place second hand directly on top of first hand.		
		Press into the abdomen with quick upward thrusts.		
		Perform 6–10 abdominal thrusts.		
7. Foreign Body Check	(Airway remains obstructed.) Manual removal of foreign body if one is found. DO NOT perform blind finger sweep.	Keep victim's face up.		
		Use tongue–jaw lift to open mouth.		
		Look into mouth; remove foreign body ONLY IF VISUALIZED.		
8. Breathing Attempt	Ventilate.	Open airway with head-tilt/chin-lift.		
		Seal mouth and nose properly.		
		Reattempt to ventilate.		
9. Sequencing	(Airway remains obstructed.) Repeat sequence.	Repeat Steps 6–8 until successful.†		

* This procedure should be initiated in a conscious child only if the airway obstruction is due to a witnessed or strongly suspected aspiration and if respiratory difficulty is increasing and the cough is ineffective. If obstruction is caused by airway swelling due to infection such as epiglottitis or croup, these procedures may be harmful; the child should be rushed to the nearest ALS facility, allowing the child to maintain the position of maximum comfort.

† After airway obstruction is cleared, ventilate twice and proceed with CPR as indicated.

Instructor _____ Check: Satisfactory _____ Unsatisfactory _____

BLS Performance Sheet

Infant FBAO Management: Conscious*

American Heart Association

Name _____ Date _____

Step	Objective	Critical Performance	S	U
1. Assessment	Determine airway obstruction.*	Observe breathing difficulties.*		
2. Back Blows	Deliver 4 back blows.	Supporting head and neck with one hand, straddle infant face down, head lower than trunk, over your forearm supported on your thigh.		
		Deliver 4 back blows, forcefully, between the shoulder blades with the heel of the hand (3–5 sec).		
3. Chest Thrusts	Deliver 4 chest thrusts.	While supporting the head, sandwich infant between your hands and turn on back, with head lower than trunk.		
		Deliver 4 thrusts in the midsternal region in the same manner as external chest compressions, but at a slower rate (3–5 sec).		
4. Sequencing	Repeat sequence.	Repeat Steps 2 and 3 until either the foreign body is expelled or the infant becomes unconscious (see below).		

Infant with Obstructed Airway Becomes Unconscious (Optional Testing Sequence)

Step	Objective	Critical Performance	S	U
5. Call for Help.	Call for help.	Call out "Help!" or, if others respond, activate EMS system.		
6. Foreign Body Check	Manual removal of foreign body if one is found (tongue–jaw lift, NOT blind finger sweep).	Keep victim's face up.		
		Place thumb in infant's mouth, over tongue. Lift tongue and jaw forward with fingers wrapped around lower jaw.		
		Look into mouth; remove foreign body ONLY IF VISUALIZED.		
7. Breathing Attempt	Ventilate.	Open airway with head-tilt/chin-lift.		
		Seal mouth and nose properly.		
		Attempt to ventilate.		
8. Back Blows	(Airway is obstructed.) Deliver 4 back blows.	Supporting head and neck with one hand, straddle infant face down, head lower than trunk, over your forearm supported on your thigh.		
		Deliver 4 back blows, forcefully, between the shoulder blades with the heel of the hand (3–5 sec).		
9. Chest Thrusts	Deliver 4 chest thrusts.	While supporting the head and neck, sandwich infant between your hands and turn on back, with head lower than trunk.		
		Deliver 4 thrusts in the midsternal region in the same manner as external chest compressions, but at a slower rate (3–5 sec).		
10. Foreign Body Check	(Airway remains obstructed.) Manual removal of foreign body if one is found.	Keep victim's face up.		
		Do tongue–jaw lift, but NOT blind finger sweep.		
		Look into mouth, remove foreign body ONLY IF VISUALIZED.		
11. Breathing Attempt	Ventilate.	Open airway with head-tilt/chin-lift.		
		Seal mouth and nose properly.		
		Reattempt to ventilate.		
12. Sequencing	(Airway remains obstructed.) Repeat sequence.	Repeat Steps 8–11 until successful.†		

* This procedure should be initiated in a conscious infant only if the airway obstruction is due to a witnessed or strongly suspected aspiration and if respiratory difficulty is increasing and the cough is ineffective. If the obstruction is caused by airway swelling due to infections, such as epiglottitis or croup, these procedures may be harmful; the infant should be rushed to the nearest ALS facility, allowing the infant to maintain the position of maximum comfort.

† After airway obstruction is cleared, ventilate twice and proceed with CPR as indicated.

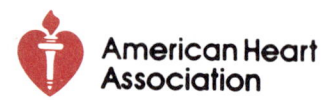

Instructor _____ Check: Satisfactory _____ Unsatisfactory _____

BLS Performance Sheet
Adult FBAO Management: Unconscious

American Heart Association

Name _____ Date _____

Step	Objective	Critical Performance	S	U
1. Assessment	Determine unresponsiveness.	Tap or gently shake shoulder. Shout "Are you OK?"		
	Call for help.	Call out "Help!"		
	Position the victim.	Turn on back as unit, if necessary, supporting head and neck (4–10 sec).		
	Open the airway.	Use head-tilt/chin-lift maneuver.		
	Determine breathlessness.	Maintain open airway.		
		Ear over mouth, observe chest: look, listen, feel for breathing (3–5 sec).		
2. Breathing Attempt	Ventilate.	Maintain open airway.		
		Seal mouth and nose properly.		
		Attempt to ventilate.		
	(Airway is obstructed.) Ventilate.	Reposition victim's head.		
		Seal mouth and nose properly.		
		Reattempt to ventilate.		
	(Airway remains obstructed.) Activate EMS system.	If someone responded to call for help, send him/her to activate EMS system.		
3. Heimlich Maneuver	Perform abdominal thrusts.	Straddle victim's thighs.		
		Place heel of one hand against victim's abdomen in the midline slightly above the navel and well below the tip of the xiphoid.		
		Place second hand directly on top of first hand.		
		Press into the abdomen with quick upward thrusts.		
		Each thrust should be distinct and delivered with the intent of relieving the airway obstruction.		
		Perform 6–10 abdominal thrusts.		
4. Foreign Body Check	Perform finger sweep.*	Keep victim's face up.		
		Use tongue–jaw lift to open mouth.		
		Sweep deeply into mouth to remove foreign body.		
5. Breathing Attempt	Ventilate.	Open airway with head-tilt/chin-lift maneuver.		
		Seal mouth and nose properly.		
		Reattempt to ventilate.		
6. Sequencing	Repeat sequence.	Repeat Steps 3–5 until successful.†		

* During practice and testing simulate finger sweeps.

† After airway obstruction is cleared, ventilate twice and proceed with CPR as indicated.

Instructor _____ Check: Satisfactory _____ Unsatisfactory _____

BLS Performance Sheet

Child FBAO Management: Unconscious

American Heart Association

Name _____ Date _____

Step	Objective	Critical Performance	S	U
1. Assessment	Determine unresponsiveness.	Tap or gently shake shoulder.		
		Shout "Are you OK?"		
	Call for help.	Call out "Help!"		
	Position the victim.	Turn on back as unit, if necessary, supporting head and neck (4–10 sec).		
	Open the airway.	Use head-tilt/chin-lift maneuver.		
	Determine breathlessness.	Maintain open airway.		
		Ear over mouth, observe chest: look, listen, feel for breathing (3–5 sec).		
2. Breathing Attempt	Ventilate.	Maintain open airway.		
		Seal mouth and nose properly.		
		Attempt to ventilate.		
	(Airway is obstructed.) Ventilate.	Reposition victim's head.		
		Seal mouth and nose properly.		
		Reattempt to ventilate.		
	(Airway remains obstructed.) Activate EMS system.	If someone responded to call for help, send him/her to activate EMS system.		
3. Heimlich Maneuver	Perform abdominal thrusts.	Kneel at victim's feet if on the floor, or stand at victim's feet if on a table.		
		Place heel of one hand against victim's abdomen in the midline slightly above navel and well below tip of xiphoid.		
		Place second hand directly on top of first hand.		
		Press into the abdomen with quick upward thrusts.		
		Each thrust should be distinct and delivered with the intent of relieving the airway.		
		Perform 6–10 abdominal thrusts.		
4. Foreign Body Check	(Airway remains obstructed.) Manual removal of foreign body if one is found. DO NOT perform blind finger sweep.	Keep victim's face up.		
		Use tongue–jaw lift to open mouth.		
		Look into mouth; remove foreign body ONLY IF VISUALIZED.		
5. Breathing Attempt	Ventilate.	Open airway with head-tilt/chin-lift maneuver.		
		Seal mouth and nose properly.		
		Reattempt to ventilate.		
6. Sequencing	Repeat sequence.	Repeat Steps 3–5 until successful.*		

* After airway obstruction is cleared, ventilate twice and proceed with CPR as indicated.

Instructor _____ Check: Satisfactory _____ Unsatisfactory _____

BLS Performance Sheet

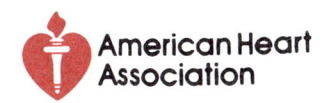

Infant FBAO Management: Unconscious

American Heart Association

Name _____ Date _____

Step	Objective	Critical Performance	S	U
1. Assessment	Determine unresponsiveness.	Tap or gently shake shoulder.		
	Call for help.	Call out "Help!"		
	Position the infant.	Turn on back as unit, if necessary, supporting head and neck.		
		Place on firm, hard surface.		
	Open the airway.	Use head-tilt/chin-lift maneuver to sniffing or neutral position.		
		Do not overextend the head.		
	Determine breathlessness.	Maintain open airway.		
		Ear over mouth, observe chest: look, listen, feel for breathing (3–5 sec).		
2. Breathing Attempt	Ventilate.	Maintain open airway.		
		Make tight seal on mouth and nose of infant with rescuer's mouth.		
		Attempt to ventilate.		
	(Airway is obstructed.) Ventilate.	Reposition infant's head.		
		Seal mouth and nose properly.		
		Reattempt to ventilate.		
	(Airway remains obstructed.) Activate EMS system	If someone responded to call for help, send him/her to activate EMS system.		
3. Back Blows	Deliver 4 back blows.	Supporting head and neck with one hand, straddle infant face down, head lower than trunk, over your forearm supported on your thigh.		
		Deliver 4 back blows, forcefully, between the shoulder blades with the heel of the hand (3–5 sec).		
4. Chest Thrusts	Deliver 4 chest thrusts.	While supporting the head and neck, sandwich infant between your hands and turn on back, with head lower than trunk.		
		Deliver 4 thrusts in the midsternal region in the same manner as external chest compressions, but at a slower rate (3–5 sec).		
5. Foreign Body Check	(Airway remains obstructed.) Manual removal of foreign body if one is found (tongue–jaw lift, NOT blind finger sweep).	Keep victim's face up.		
		Place thumb in infant's mouth, over tongue. Lift tongue and jaw forward with fingers wrapped around lower jaw.		
		Look into mouth; remove foreign body ONLY IF VISUALIZED.		
6. Breathing Attempt	Ventilate.	Open airway with head-tilt/chin-lift.		
		Seal mouth and nose properly.		
		Reattempt to ventilate.		
7. Sequencing	Repeat sequence.	Repeat Steps 3–6 until successful.*		

* After airway obstruction is cleared, ventilate twice and proceed with CPR as indicated.

Instructor _____ Check: Satisfactory _____ Unsatisfactory _____

4

Shock

- Shock Due to Injury (Hypovolemic)
- Anaphylactic Shock (Allergic Reaction)
- Fainting

Every injury has some degree of shock. It can develop immediately following an injury or later.

Shock occurs when the body's tissues or organs are inadequately supplied with oxygenated blood. Three factors are necessary to maintain normal flow and distribution: (1) a functioning heart, (2) adequate amount of blood, and (3) an intact circulatory system. Abnormalities in any one of these can produce shock.

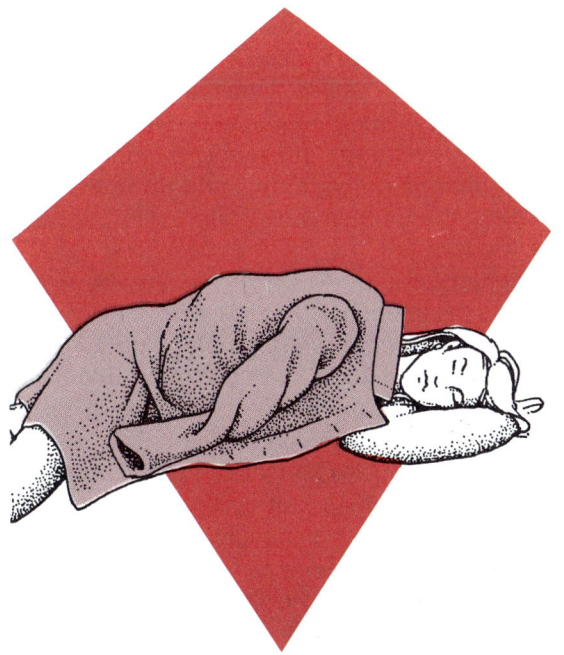

No matter what the cause of shock, the consequences are the same—inadequate circulation of oxygenated blood.

SHOCK DUE TO INJURY (HYPOVOLEMIC)

Hypovolemic shock is a life threatening situation in which the body's vital functions are seriously threatened by insufficient blood, or oxygen in the blood, reaching the body tissues.

Some degree of shock can be attributed to every injury. Therefore, a first aider should treat for shock in all serious injuries. A first aider cannot reverse shock once it develops, but he or she can prevent it from worsening.

Signs and symptoms of shock include: pale or bluish and cool skin; moist and clammy skin; overall weakness; vomiting; dull, sunken look to the eyes; pupils widely dilated; and unusual thirst. (*See* Figure 4-1.)

Unfortunately there is little that a first aider can do. First aid for hypovolemic shock includes:

1. Maintain an open airway.
2. Control all obvious bleeding.
3. Elevate the lower extremities about twelve inches unless the injury makes this impossible or when it is not advisable, such as chest injuries, unconsciousness, etc. This allows the blood in the legs to be returned to the heart more readily. Excessive elevation (over 12 inches) of

44 FIRST AID ESSENTIALS

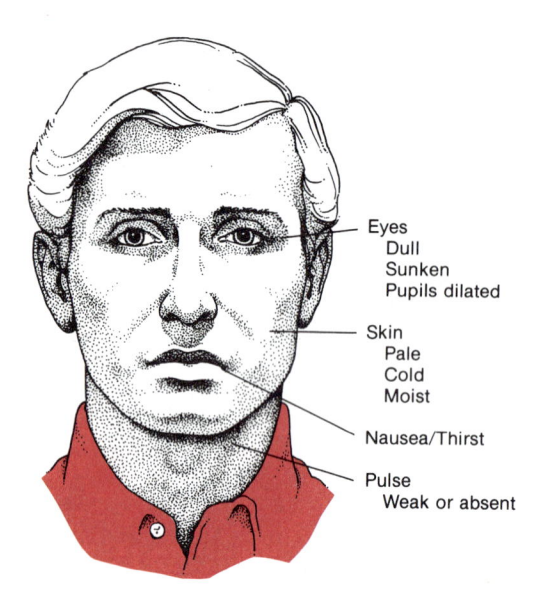

Eyes
  Dull
  Sunken
  Pupils dilated

Skin
  Pale
  Cold
  Moist

Nausea/Thirst

Pulse
  Weak or absent

4-1. Signs and symptoms of shock

the legs adversely affects the victim's breathing. Do not lift the foot of a stretcher or bed since breathing becomes more difficult.

4. Prevent the loss of body heat by putting blankets under and over the victim. Do not attempt to warm the victim.

5. Generally, keep the victim on his or her back. However, some victims in shock may require another position. (See Figure 4-2.) For example, those with head or chest injury or stroke should have their heads and upper bodies elevated. This will reduce pressure on the brain. Those with lung disease or a heart attack should also be in a semi-sitting position. These victims can breathe better. An unconscious or vomiting victim should lie on his or her side.

6. Do not give the victim anything to eat or drink. Eating or drinking may cause the victim to become nauseated and vomit.

7. Handle victims gently.

ANAPHYLACTIC SHOCK (ALLERGIC REACTION)

Although the incidence of severe allergic reactions to various substances is very low, when it happens, it can be a life-threatening emergency. Substances that most often cause allergic reactions may be grouped as follows:

1. *Insect stings.* Stings of the bee, wasp, yellow jacket, or hornet can cause very rapid and severe anaphylactic reactions.

2. *Injections.* The injections from various medications (e.g., tetanus antitoxin or drugs such as penicillin) may cause severe reactions.

3. *Ingestion.* Eating foods such as fish, shellfish, or berries or taking medications or drugs such as oral penicillin can cause slower but equally severe reactions to someone who is sensitive to any of them.

4. *Inhalation.* The inhalation of dusts, pollens, or materials to which an individual is especially sensitive may cause rapid and severe reactions.

If the sting is from a honeybee, carefully remove the stinger by gently scraping with a knife blade or fingernail. Removing the stinger reduces the amount of venom entering the body. Do not squeeze the stinger while removing it because you could be injecting more venom.

Quickly assess the victim's skin around the sting. If it is red and inflamed, an allergic reaction is occurring and there is danger of developing anaphylactic shock. Other signs of anaphylactic shock include: weakness, coughing and/or wheezing, breathing difficulty, severe itching or hives, nausea and vomiting, and dizziness.

Maintain an open airway and restore breathing if necessary.

Immediately ask the victim if he has an anaphylaxis kit (commonly known as an emergency bee sting kit). These are available only by prescription. If the individual does, inject the epinephrine, and then massage the injection site vigorously to speed the distribution of epinephrine throughout the victim's body. The injection should relieve the reaction; but if the kit is not available, the victim's anaphylaxis will worsen rapidly. Refer to Chapter 7 for more details on insect stings.

Continue to assess the victim's airway and ask if he is having trouble breathing or if he feels as though his throat is closing up. Apply a constric-

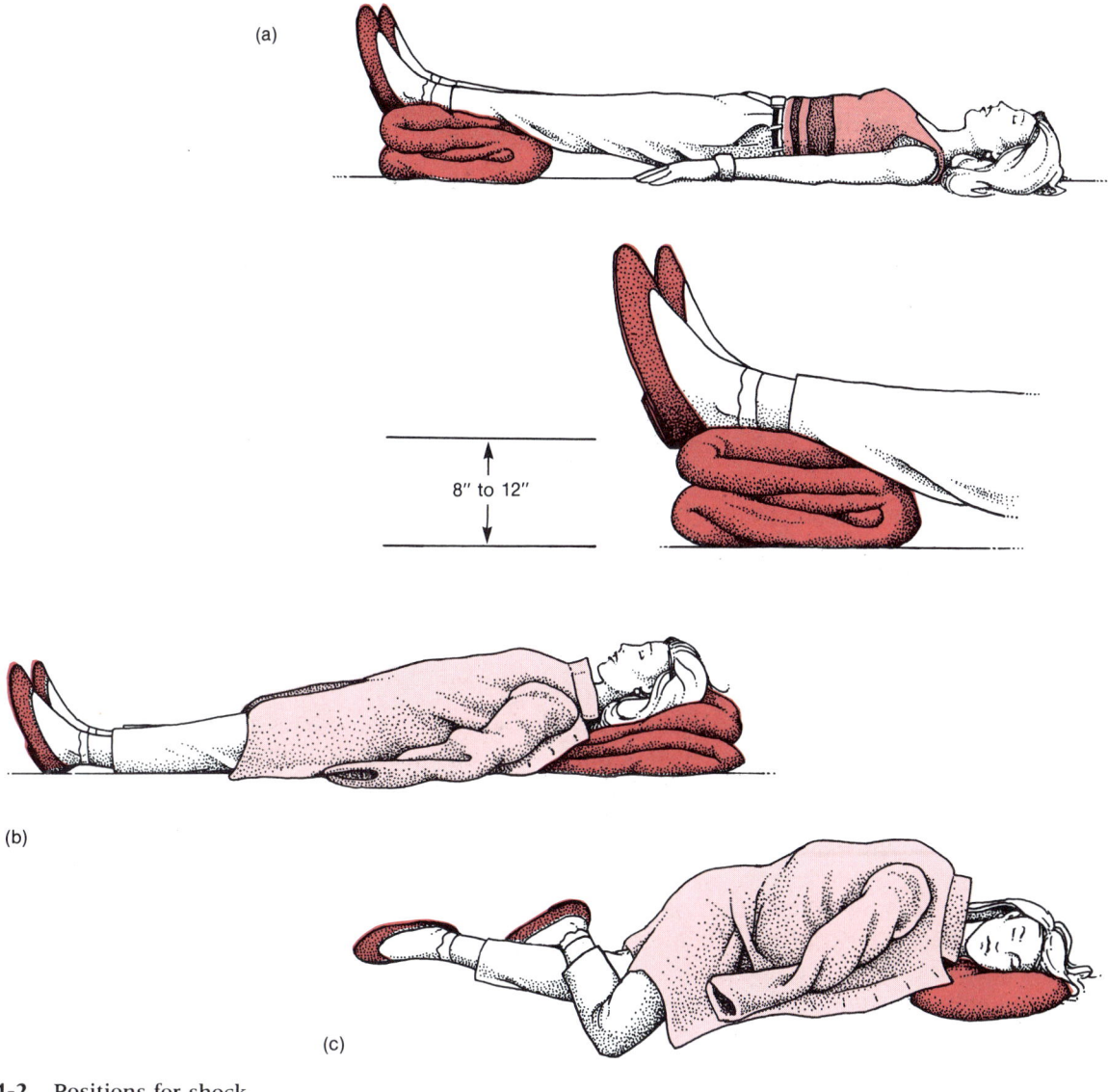

4-2. Positions for shock
(a) Elevate the feet and legs 8–12 inches for most situations.
(b) If the individual is having respiratory difficulty, the head and shoulders should be elevated.
(c) If the individual is unconscious, place the person on the side.

tion as though his throat is closing up. Apply a constriction band just above the sting site, if on an arm or leg. Seek medical attention promptly, preferably at the nearest hospital emergency room.

The victim may have breathing difficulty as bronchospasm and swelling of the larynx develop. If the victim stops breathing, open the airway and begin resuscitation. Trained

46 FIRST AID ESSENTIALS

medical personnel could perform a cricothyrotomy or tracheotomy. First aiders should *not* perform these medical maneuvers. Remember, the only really effective treatment for severe allergic reactions is an immediate injection of epinephrine.

FAINTING

Fainting may result from many different causes, the most common being a psychic disturbance of an unpleasant nature, which sets off a chain of effects not unlike those seen in shock. Some persons faint from merely seeing blood or from seeing or hearing unpleasant things. Also, there is a type of fainting that occurs in those who are required to spend a long time in an upright position with little movement as, for instance, a soldier who is being held at attention for a considerable period of time. In such a case there is a loss of circulating blood volume, due to accumulation of blood in the legs. Fainting is a loss of consciousness. Staying conscious is dependent on normal brain function. To function normally, the brain needs a large supply of oxygen. When the oxygen supply to the brain is interrupted, fainting may occur.

There are numerous other causes of fainting, including epilepsy, heart disorder, and cerebrovascular disease. Many are not serious, but an alert first aider should be especially concerned if the fainting victim:

- Is over forty years old.
- Has had repeated attacks of unconsciousness.
- Does not awaken within four or five minutes.
- Loses consciousness while sitting or lying down.
- Faints for no apparent reason.

Signs of Fainting

Fainting may occur suddenly or may be preceded by warning signs, including any or all of the following:

- Dizziness and the victim tells of "spots" before his eyes
- Nausea
- Paleness
- Sweating

First Aid

Important things not to do include:

- *Do not* pour water on the person's face.
- *Do not* give the person anything to drink until he or she has fully recovered.
- *Do not* use stimulants such as smelling salts or ammonia capsules.
- *Do not* slap the person's face.

When a person looks as though on the verge of fainting:

- Prevent him or her from falling.
- Lie the victim on his or her back and elevate the legs eight to twelve inches.

After fainting has occurred or if fainting is anticipated:

- Lie the victim down and elevate the legs eight to twelve inches.
- If vomiting begins, turn the person on his or her side to keep the airway open and clear.
- Loosen clothing around the person's neck (such as a tight necktie or collar).
- Wet a cloth with cool water and wipe the person's forehead and face.

Most cases of fainting are not serious and the victim regains consciousness quickly. However, seek medical attention if recovery is not complete within five minutes. If the victim has fallen, assess for injuries.

Allergic Reaction

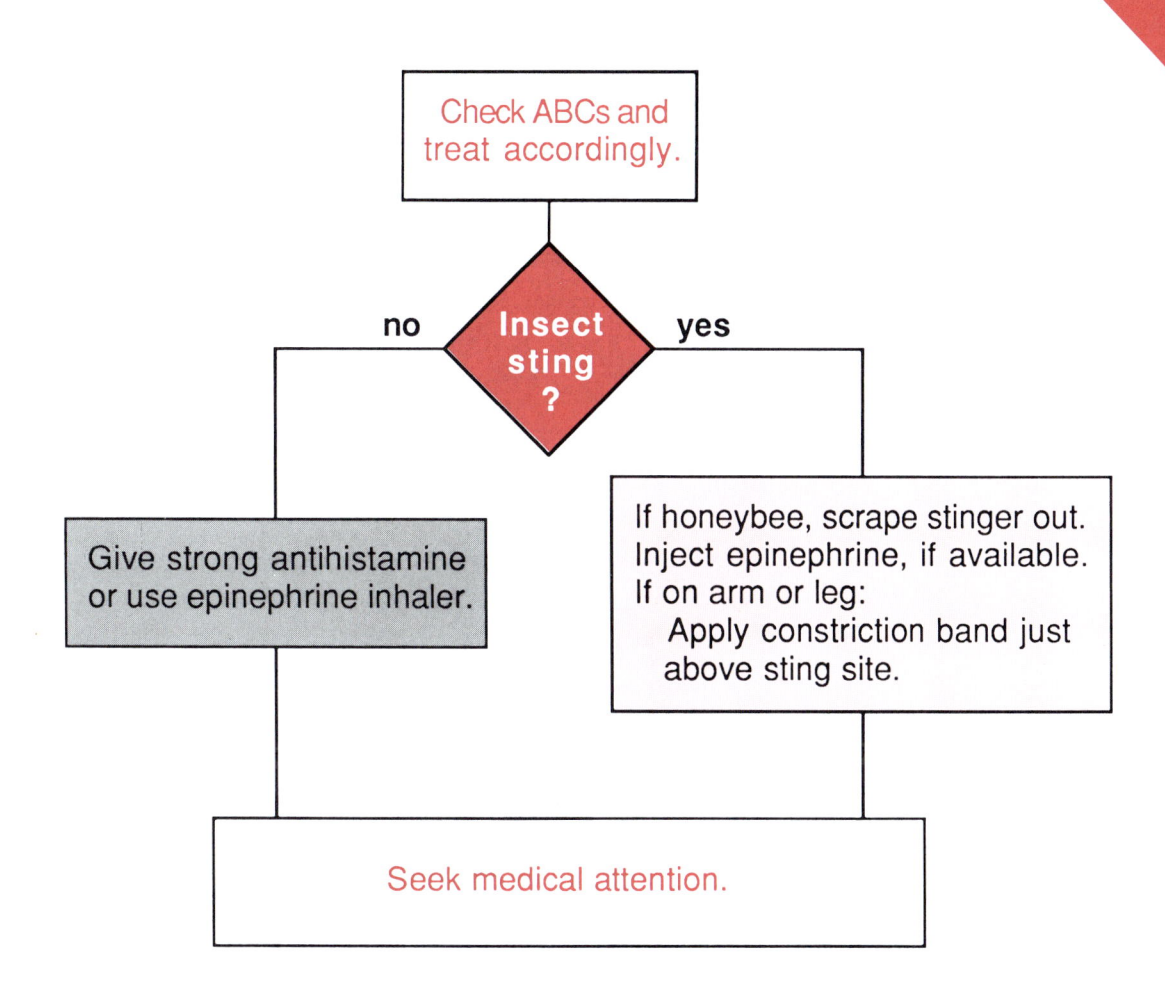

```
Check ABCs and
treat accordingly.
        │
    Insect sting?
   no ◆ yes
   │        │
   │    If honeybee, scrape stinger out.
   │    Inject epinephrine, if available.
   │    If on arm or leg:
   │        Apply constriction band just
   │        above sting site.
   │        │
Give strong antihistamine
or use epinephrine inhaler.
        │
Seek medical attention.
```

Hypovolemic Shock

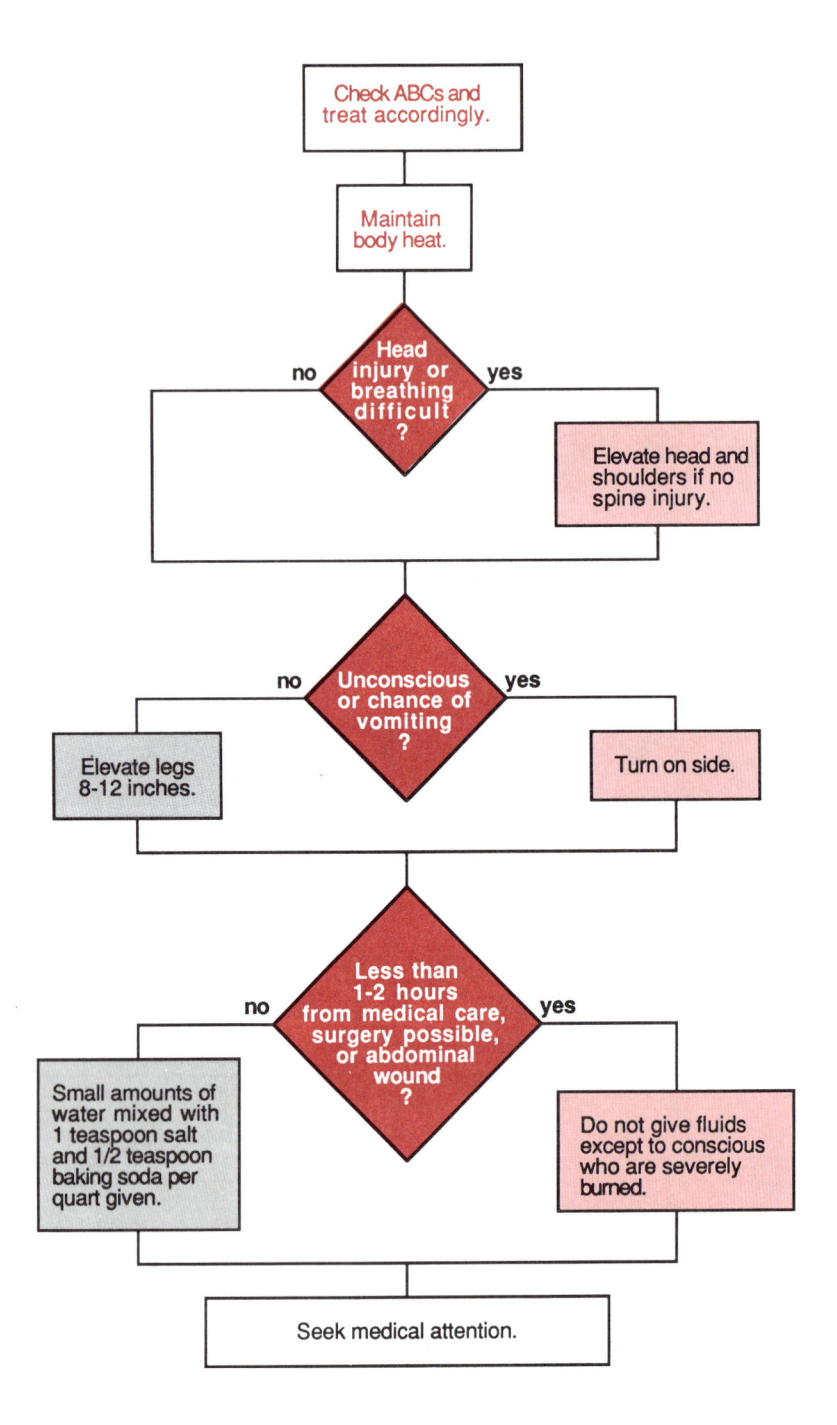

```
                    ┌─────────────────┐
                    │ Check ABCs and  │
                    │ treat accordingly.│
                    └────────┬────────┘
                             │
                    ┌────────┴────────┐
                    │ Maintain        │
                    │ body heat.      │
                    └────────┬────────┘
                             │
                         ╱ Head ╲
              no       ╱ injury or ╲    yes
         ┌──────────── breathing ────────────┐
         │            ╲ difficult ╱          │
         │              ╲   ?   ╱            │
         │                ╲   ╱              │
         │                                   ▼
         │                          ┌─────────────────┐
         │                          │ Elevate head and│
         │                          │ shoulders if no │
         │                          │ spine injury.   │
         │                          └────────┬────────┘
         │                                   │
         │        ╱ Unconscious ╲             │
         │  no  ╱  or chance of  ╲  yes       │
         ├─────  vomiting  ──────────────────┤
         │      ╲      ?       ╱              │
         ▼        ╲          ╱                ▼
  ┌──────────────┐                      ┌──────────────┐
  │ Elevate legs │                      │ Turn on side.│
  │ 8-12 inches. │                      └──────┬───────┘
  └──────┬───────┘                             │
         │                                     │
         │        ╱ Less than ╲                │
         │      ╱  1-2 hours   ╲               │
         │  no ╱ from medical care,╲ yes       │
         ├──── surgery possible, ─────────────┤
         │     ╲ or abdominal  ╱               │
         │       ╲   wound   ╱                 │
         ▼         ╲   ?   ╱                   ▼
┌──────────────────┐                  ┌──────────────────┐
│ Small amounts of │                  │ Do not give fluids│
│ water mixed with │                  │ except to conscious│
│ 1 teaspoon salt  │                  │ who are severely │
│ and 1/2 teaspoon │                  │ burned.          │
│ baking soda per  │                  └────────┬─────────┘
│ quart given.     │                           │
└────────┬─────────┘                           │
         │                                     │
         └──────────────┬──────────────────────┘
                        ▼
              ┌──────────────────────┐
              │ Seek medical attention.│
              └──────────────────────┘
```

Fainting

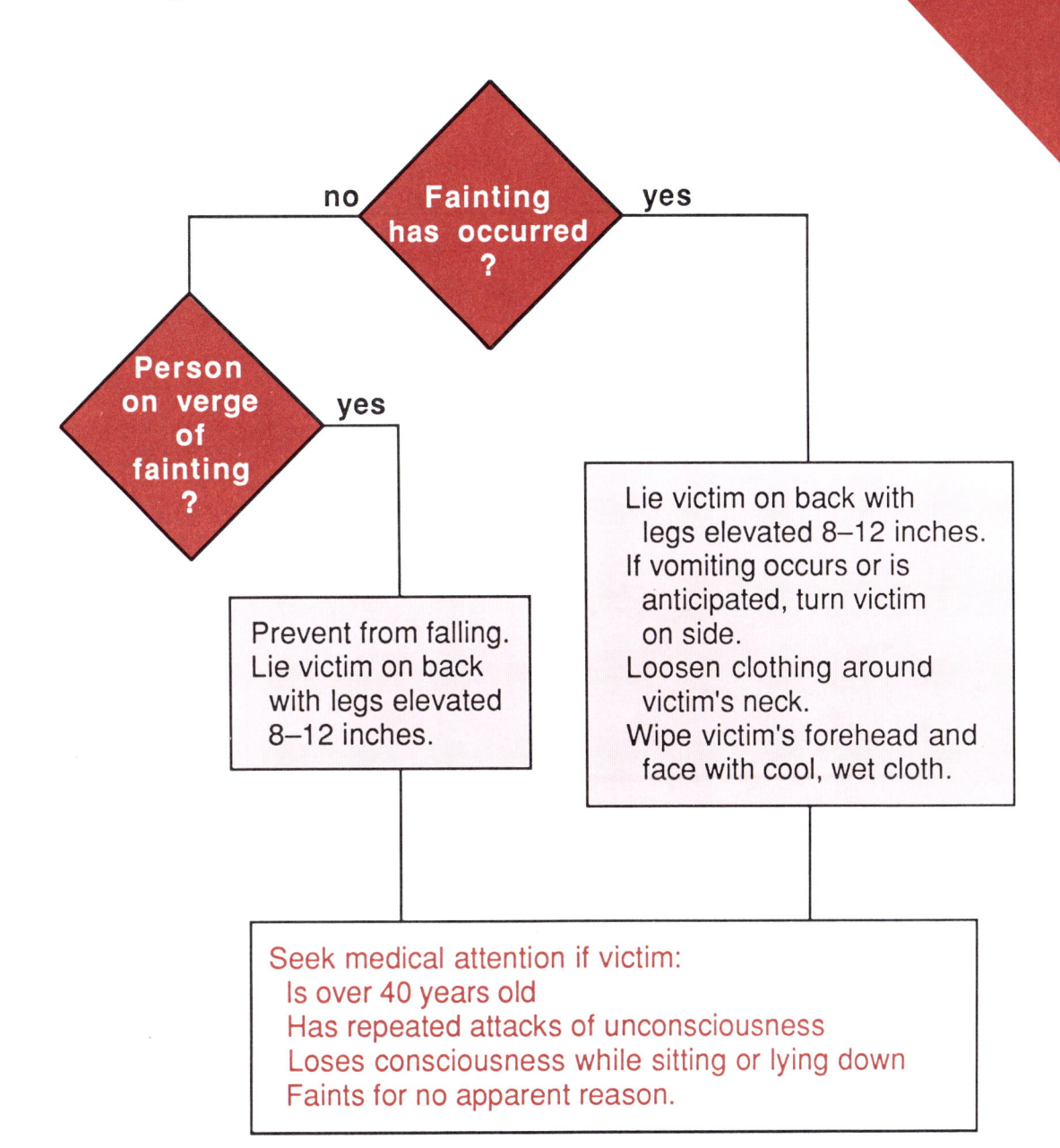

Fainting has occurred?
- **no** → **Person on verge of fainting?**
  - **yes** → Prevent from falling. Lie victim on back with legs elevated 8–12 inches.
- **yes** → Lie victim on back with legs elevated 8–12 inches. If vomiting occurs or is anticipated, turn victim on side. Loosen clothing around victim's neck. Wipe victim's forehead and face with cool, wet cloth.

Seek medical attention if victim:
 Is over 40 years old
 Has repeated attacks of unconsciousness
 Loses consciousness while sitting or lying down
 Faints for no apparent reason.

SELF-CHECK QUESTIONS

Activity 1: Hypovolemic Shock

A. Mark each statement true (T) or false (F).

1. ☐ Shock results when parts of the body do not receive enough blood.
2. ☐ Shock is a concern only in life-threatening injuries.
3. ☐ People's lives can be threatened by shock.

B. Choose the correct completions for the following statement:
When a person experiences shock, usually the

	Choice 1		*Choice 2*
1. ☐	skin is pale/bluish	OR ☐	red.
2. ☐	skin is dry	OR ☐	moist.
3. ☐	skin is hot	OR ☐	cool.
4. ☐	pupils are widely dilated	OR ☐	constricted.
5. ☐	victim feels hungry	OR ☐	nausea.

C. A victim begins showing signs of shock. Check which of the following you would do:

1. ☐ Attempt to warm the victim.
2. ☐ Give fluids to the victim.
3. ☐ Handle the victim gently.
4. ☐ Help a conscious victim walk around to aid blood flow to the heart.
5. ☐ Place a conscious victim on his back and elevate the feet and legs, if injuries will not be aggravated.
6. ☐ Elevate head-injured-victim's head.

D. Match each condition or injury with the particular position for a conscious victim.

Condition of Injury   *Best Position*

1. ☐ Crushed chest injury   1. On victim's side
2. ☐ Vomiting   2. Victim flat on back with legs elevated 8–12 inches
3. ☐ Unconscious   3. Semi-sitting and supported
4. ☐ Heart attack   4. Semi-sitting and inclined to the injured side
5. ☐ Head injury
6. ☐ Stroke
7. ☐ Amputated fingers

Activity 2: Anaphylactic Shock

A. Choose which can cause anaphylactic (allergic reaction) shock in sensitive people:
1. ☐ Sting by honeybee
2. ☐ Eating fish
3. ☐ Taking aspirin
4. ☐ Injection of penicillin
5. ☐ Breathing pollens

B. Choose the statements for signs, and symptoms of anaphylactic shock:
1. ☐ Red and inflamed skin around a sting site
2. ☐ Coughing and/or wheezing
3. ☐ Breathing difficulty
4. ☐ Severe itching or hives
5. ☐ Nausea and vomiting
6. ☐ Bleeding from the nose
7. ☐ Extreme thirst

C. Mark each statement true (T) or false (F) regarding anaphylactic (allergic reaction) shock:
1. ☐ A respiratory emergency can develop after a bee sting.
2. ☐ A bee's stinger should be scraped off the victim's skin.
3. ☐ Though the victim appears in distress, these reactions are *not* life threatening.
4. ☐ First aiders can perform a tracheotomy if breathing difficulty appears.
5. ☐ The only really effective treatment for severe allergic reaction is an immediate injection of epinephrine.

Activity 3: Fainting

A. Mark each statement true (T) or false (F).
  1. ☐ Lack of oxygen to the brain causes fainting.
  2. ☐ Recovery within 5 minutes usually occurs after a fainting episode.
  3. ☐ Seeing blood or seeing unpleasant things may cause some to faint.
  4. ☐ A person may report feeling dizzy or seeing "spots" just before fainting.
  5. ☐ When a person's face becomes red and dry, fainting may occur.

B. What should you do for a person turning pale and saying he feels dizzy?

   Yes   No
  1. ☐   ☐   Prevent him from falling.
  2. ☐   ☐   Place a cold towel on his forehead.
  3. ☐   ☐   Loosen clothing around the person's neck.
  4. ☐   ☐   Place him in a semi-sitting position.

C. What should you do for a person suddenly collapsing and falling to the floor?

   Choice 1   *Choice 2*
  1. ☐ Pour water on his face   OR   ☐ Wipe his face with cool, wet cloth.
  2. ☐ Loosen clothing around   OR   ☐ Do not bother about loosening clothing.
       victim's neck
  3. ☐ Elevate feet and legs   OR   ☐ Place victim in a semi-sitting position.
  4. ☐ Use smelling salts or   OR   ☐ Do *not* use smelling salts or ammonia inhalants.
       ammonia inhalants.
  5. ☐ Seek medical help if victim   OR   ☐ Seek medical help for all fainting episodes.
       does not recover within
       5 minutes

5

Bleeding

- Types of External Bleeding
- Types of Wounds
- Wounds Requiring Medical Attention
- Infection
- Tetanus
- Amputation
- Animal Bites

Of all the injuries seen by first aiders, bleeding may not only be the most visible but may also be the most often cared for.

The total blood volume in an average-sized individual is between five and six quarts. Although the average healthy adult can easily tolerate losses of a pint (the amount usually taken from blood donors), rapid loss of one quart or more of the total blood volume by bleeding often leads to irreversible shock and to death. A child's losing one pint is extremely dangerous.

TYPES OF EXTERNAL BLEEDING

External bleeding classifications include:

Arterial: Blood from an artery spurts, and it is bright red in color because it is rich in oxygen. All blood exposed to air turns red, so the color cannot be relied upon to indicate origin. Arterial bleeding is less likely to clot than other types of bleeding. When completely severed, arteries often constrict and seal themselves off. However, if an artery is not completely severed but is torn or has a hole in its wall, it will probably continue to bleed. The blood loss from the wound is often rapid and profuse, as blood spurts from the wound. Unless a very large artery has been severed, it is unlikely that a person will bleed to death before control measures can be put into effect.

Unlike bleeding from other vessels, arterial bleeding, unless it is from only a small artery, will not clot because a blood clot can form only when there is a slow flow or no flow at all. Therefore, arterial bleeding is dangerous, and some external means of control must be used to stop the flow.

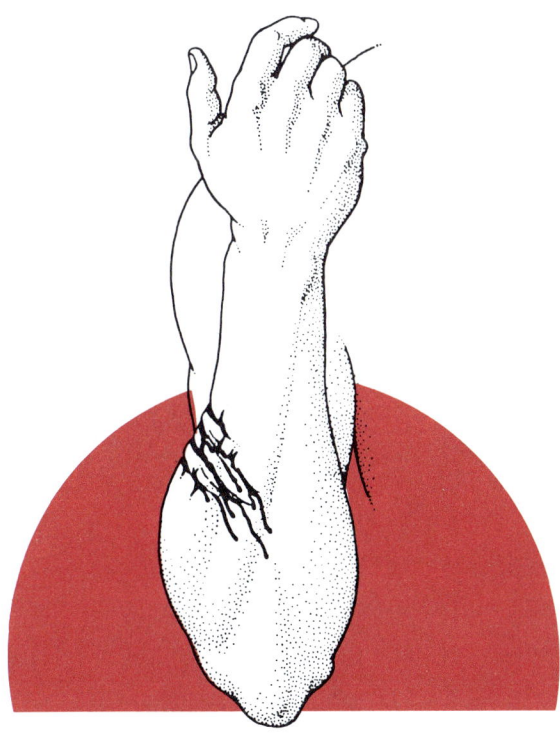

53

Some vessels are so large and carry such pressure that, even if a clot did form, it would be forced out. This might happen, too, if inept handling of a wound disturbed a clot or if pressure were released too soon. Therefore, once arterial bleeding is stopped, control must be maintained long enough for the injured person to be safely transported to an adequate medical facility.

Venous: Bleeding from a vein is steady and is dark bluish-red color. This type of bleeding may be profuse, but it is easier to control than arterial bleeding.

With venous bleeding, particularly from a large vein, do not overlook the danger of an air bubble or air embolism. This can happen because the blood in the larger veins is being sucked back toward the heart; hence, when a large vein is cut, air may actually be sucked into the opening in the vein. The air bubble can be large enough to interfere with the ability of the heart to pump the blood because of the air block that is formed. Therefore, venous bleeding must be controlled quickly.

Veins are usually located closer to the body surface than are arteries. Most veins collapse when they are cut; however, bleeding from deep veins can be as profuse and as hard to control as arterial bleeding.

Capillary: Blood oozes from a capillary and is similar in color to venous blood. Capillary bleeding is usually not serious and is easily controlled. It is characterized by a general ooze from the tissues, the blood dripping steadily from the wound or gradually forming a puddle in it. This type of bleeding is not immediately dangerous. Quite frequently, this type of bleeding will more or less control itself by clotting spontaneously.

In hemophilia, the tendency to bleed, as well as the inability of the blood to clot, may be so great as to threaten life. Bleeding in a person with this condition is especially difficult to control because the problem is in the failure of the blood clotting mechanism itself, and there is as yet no known specific cure. Hospitalization is required. As an emergency care measure, firm compression on the bleeding site should be applied.

Controlling External Bleeding

The first aider's major concern with open wounds is to control bleeding. This can be accomplished in almost all cases by:

Direct pressure: Direct pressure with the hand over the wound using a dressing or gauze pad stops most bleeding. If the bleeding does not stop, apply additional pressure with your hand or pressure bandage. (*See* Figures 5-1 and 5-2.)

If sterile gauze is not available, use any clean fabric—handkerchief, bed sheet, sanitary napkin, and so on—never remove a dressing once it is in place because bleeding may start again. Apply another dressing on top of the blood-soaked one and hold them both in place.

If bleeding remains uncontrolled, try to grasp the blood vessel between your fingers or compress it between one finger and a bony part of the victim's body. However, do not waste valuable time attempting this. Direct pressure is usually the quickest and most efficient means of controlling external bleeding.

Elevation: Elevation may help control bleeding of an extremity. Application of direct pressure, however, on the wound site is still needed. When elevation of an extremity is used, gravity helps to reduce blood pressure and thus slows bleeding. (*See* Figure 5-3.)

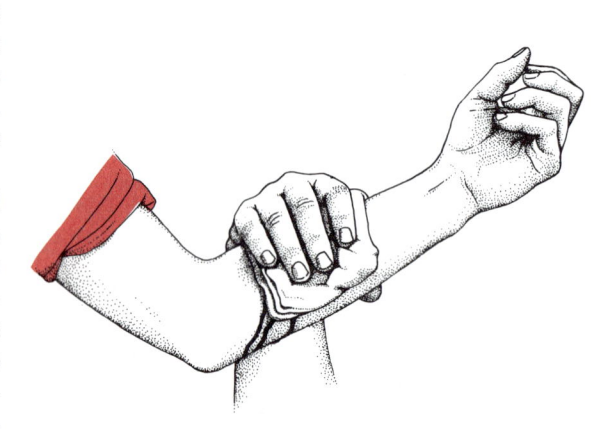

5-1. Applying direct pressure to a wound

5-2. Applying a pressure bandage

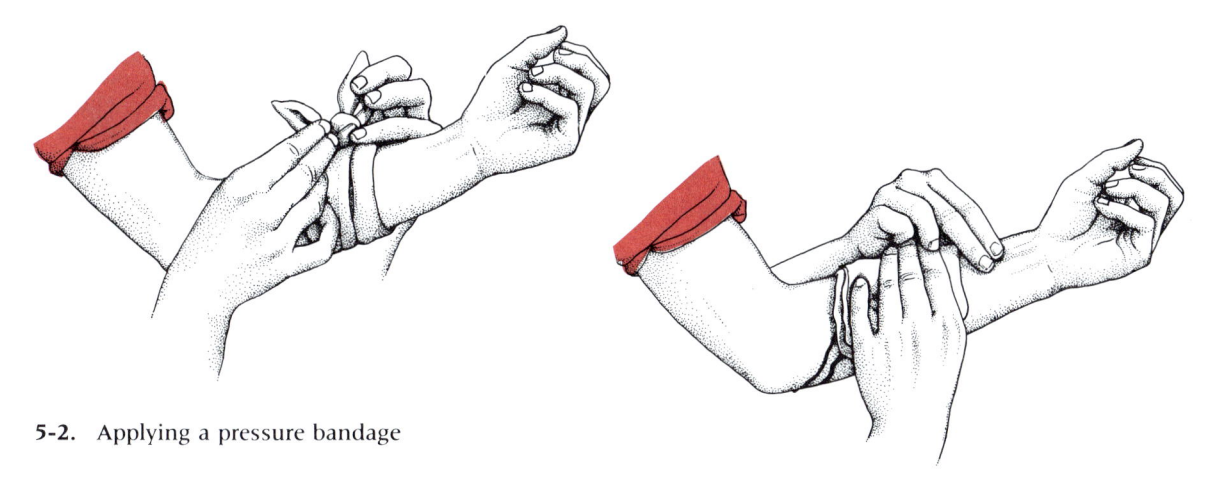

Pressure points: If direct pressure is not controlling severe bleeding in the arm or leg, pressure points may be used. Such pressure can be applied most effectively at the point where an artery is relatively near the surface and where it passes close to a bony structure against which it can be compressed. These points are known as pressure points. There are twenty-two such points, eleven on each side. Of these eleven, two are usually used to control most cases of external bleeding. The two easiest and most commonly used are the brachial point in the arm and the femoral point in the groin. (*See* Figure 5-4.)

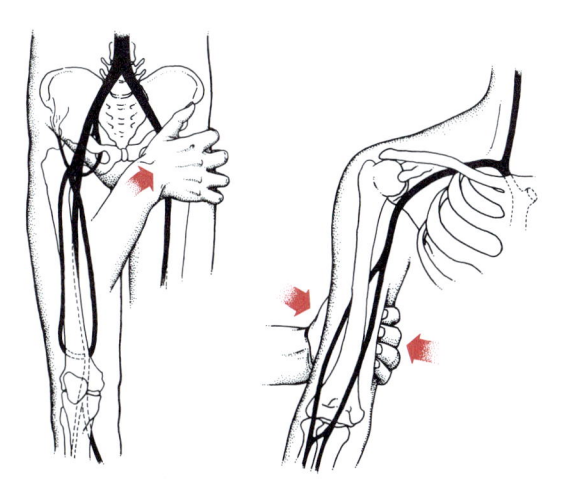

5-3. Applying direct pressure to a wound and elevating the wound above the victim's heart

5-4. Proper hand positions for applying brachial and femoral pressure

Use pressure points only after direct pressure and elevation have failed to control the bleeding. Pressure points may help slow blood flow enough to make direct pressure more effective.

Tourniquet: A tourniquet is used only in a severe emergency when other means will not stop bleeding in an extremity. A tourniquet can damage nerves and blood vessels and can result in the loss of an arm or leg. Apply it close to the bleeding site in order to preserve more of the arm or leg for fitting an artificial limb. Use strong, wide, flat materials—never rope or wire.

Once you apply a tourniquet, do not loosen it. If a tourniquet is loosened, clots may be dislodged resulting in enough blood loss to cause severe shock and death. By leaving the tourniquet in place, more limbs may possibly be lost, but more lives will be saved.

Use a tourniquet only as a last resort to control a life-threatening bleeding that cannot be stopped by any other means. Besides, tourniquets are rarely, if ever, necessary.

TYPES OF WOUNDS

Soft-tissue injuries involve the skin and usually are classified as closed or open. In a closed injury, such as a bruise or contusion, there is

56 FIRST AID ESSENTIALS

5-5. Types of wounds
(a) abrasion
(b) laceration
(c) incision
(d) puncture
(e) avulsion
(f) amputation

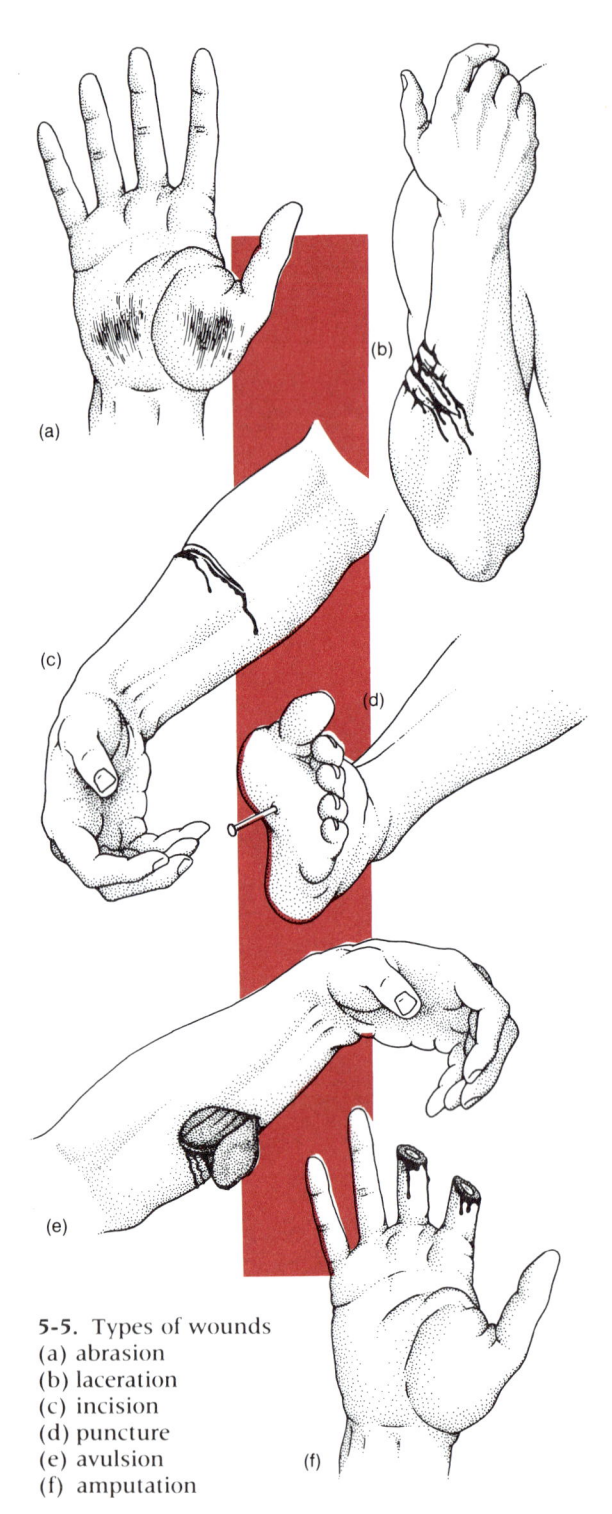

damage to the soft tissue beneath the skin but no actual break in the skin. Contusions are marked by local pain and swelling. If small blood vessels beneath the skin have been broken, there will be a black and blue mark as well. If large vessels have been torn beneath the contused area, a hematoma, or collection of blood beneath the skin, will be evident as a lump with bluish discoloration. Closed wounds should be treated with pressure and cold applications to minimize swelling but otherwise require no specific treatment. Closed injuries can be serious and are often overlooked.

An open wound is one in which there is disruption of the skin and, therefore, is susceptible to external bleeding and contamination. Open wounds may be of several types.

An abrasion, as shown in Figure 5-5, is a superficial wound caused by rubbing or scraping resulting in partial loss of the skin surface.

A laceration, as illustrated in Figure 5-5, is a cut made by a sharp instrument, such as a knife or razor blade, that produces a jagged incision through the skin surface and underlying structures. A laceration can be the source of significant bleeding if the sharp instrument also has disrupted the wall of a blood vessel, especially an artery. Thus, significant bleeding can result from lacerations in regions of the body where major arteries lie close to the surface, such as in the wrists.

A puncture wound, also shown in Figure 5-5, is a stab from a pointed object, such as a nail, ice pick, or knife. Special treatment of the puncture wound is required when the object causing the injury remains impaled in the wound. A discussion of this type of wound is provided in the section concerning impaled objects.

An incision is an open wound caused by sharp objects such as knives, razor blades, and sharp glass or metal edges. (*See* Figure 5-5.) The wound is smooth edged and bleeds freely. The amount of bleeding depends upon the depth, location, and size of the wound. There may be severe damage to muscles, nerves, and tendons if the wound is deep.

TABLE 5-1. Types of Open Wounds

Type	Cause(s)	Signs and Symptoms	First Aid
Abrasion (scrape)	Rubbing or scraping	Only skin surface affected	Remove all debris.
		Little bleeding	Wash away from wound with soap and water.
Incision (cut)	Sharp objects	Smooth edges of wound	Control bleeding.
		Severe bleeding	Wash wound.
Laceration (tearing)	Blunt object tearing skin	Veins and arteries can be affected	Control bleeding.
		Severe bleeding	Wash wound.
		Danger of infection	
Puncture (stab)	Sharp pointed object pierces skin	Wound is narrow and deep into veins and arteries	Do not remove impaled objects.
		Embedded objects	
		Danger of infection	
Avulsion (torn off)	Machinery, Explosives	Tissue torn off or left hanging	Control bleeding.
		Severe bleeding	Take avulsed part to medical facility.

An avulsion is the tearing of a patch of skin or other tissue that if not totally torn from the body creates a loose, hanging flap. (*See* Figure 5-5.) Avulsions can involve such parts as eyeballs, ears, fingers, or hands.

Amputations involve the cutting or tearing off of a body part such as fingers, toes, hands, feet, arms or leg. (*See* Figure 5-5.) A discussion of severed or amputated parts is provided in the section concerning amputations.

Table 5-1 summarizes information on open wounds.

Minor Wounds

Cuts resulting in minor wounds are commonplace. In fact, the most frequently seen injury is a minor wound. During an average day, everyone can expect to see a bandage covering a minor wound. Every home, especially those with small children, should have an ample supply of bandages.

Minor wounds involve only the superficial layers of the skin and are not associated with severe bleeding. Most of these injuries can be handled safely without professional medical help. When caring for minor cuts and wounds, take the following steps:

1. When possible, wash hands in a vigorous scrubbing action using soap and water.

2. Allow the wound to bleed slightly. Apply direct pressure to the wound with a clean cloth. Continue pressure for three minutes. (Clotting may take six to seven minutes.)

3. Using a sterile gauze pad or a clean cloth saturated with soap and water, gently wash dirt away from the wound edges. Hydrogen peroxide (3% solution) helps to bubble away old blood and clots—not to disinfect the wound or destroy anaerobic bacteria as is often thought. Foreign bodies—such as dirt or gravel—must be removed to avoid infection and a tattoo look after the skin is healed.

58 FIRST AID ESSENTIALS

4. Flush the wound liberally with large quantities of water.

5. Those who feel they must use an antiseptic should use isopropyl (rubbing) alcohol. It should be applied, if at all, on the intact skin around the wound, not in the wound. First aid antiseptic salves, sprays, and solutions probably do no good, and they may even retard healing.

6. Cover the wound with a sterile gauze dressing and bandage. A Band-aid™-type dressing is commonly used on small cuts. The dressing should not be airtight because it might trap moisture given off by the skin and encourage the growth of bacteria. If the wound is more of a scrape than a cut, one of the plastic "non-stickable" coverings may be helpful because they do not stick to the wound.

7. Small (less than one inch) lacerations heal faster and with less scarring if the wound edges are brought together by one or more pieces of tape. These are commonly known as "butterfly" bandages and can be made or purchased. (*See* Figure 5-6.)

8. If the wound bleeds after a bandage is applied and the bandage becomes stuck, it is best to leave it on as long as the wound is healing normally. Pulling the scab loose to change the dressing can only retard healing and increase the chances of infection. If a bandage must be removed, soak it in warm water or hydrogen peroxide to help soften the scab and make removal easier.

Dressings for a wound are most needed usually in the first twenty-four hours after an injury. During this time the scab has not yet formed and the wound is especially susceptible to infection.

Dressings serve a number of functions, including:

1. Protecting the wound from outside contamination.
2. Shielding the wound from further injury.
3. Preventing the spread of germs, blood, and other wound materials to surrounding areas.
4. Preventing the wound from getting either too wet or too dry.

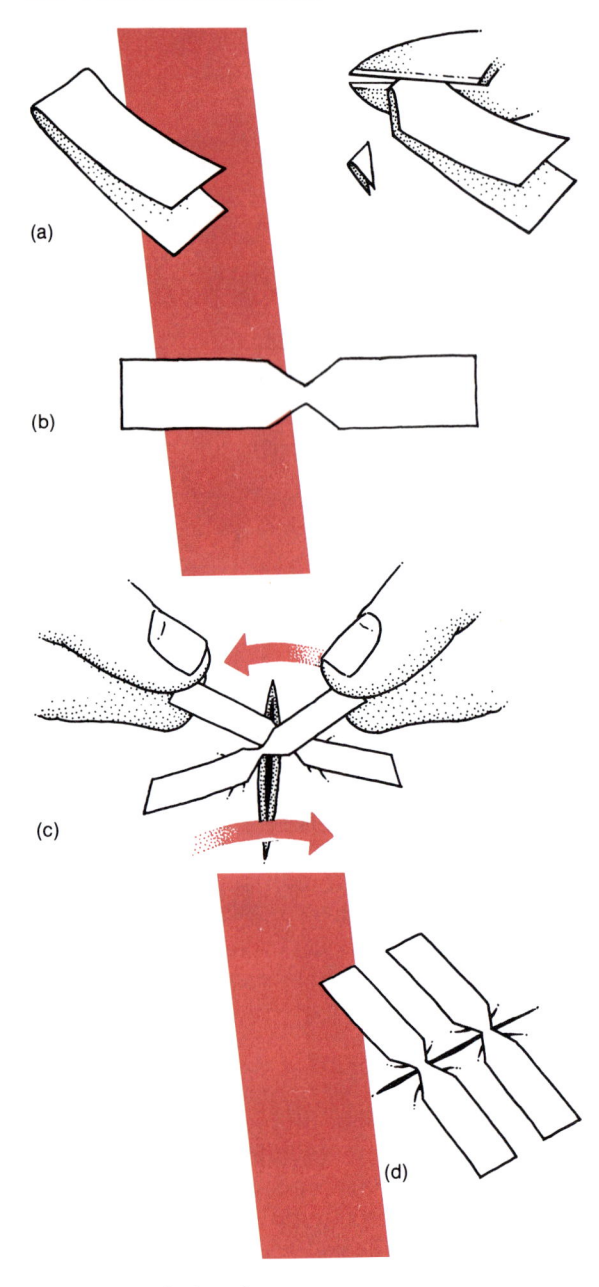

5-6. Butterfly bandage
(a) Fold a piece of tape and cut off both corners at the fold.
(b) The straightened tape reveals the "butterfly."
(c) Pull two butterfly bandages together to close and hold the wound edges together.
(d) Butterfly bandages holding edges together. Cover the butterflies and wound with a sterile dressing.

5. Increasing the comfort of the victim while covering the wound site so the victim and others are not disturbed by its appearance.

WOUNDS REQUIRING MEDICAL ATTENTION

In today's world, many hazards cause a variety of wounds and bleeding. (Refer to Table 5-1.) These injuries generate a fair amount of anxiety and concern, especially regarding the question of whether or not to acquire professional medical care for the victim.

All of us will have the opportunity to decide about obtaining medical assistance for a wounded victim. To aid in this decision, consider the following types of wounds that require medical care:

1. Arterial bleeding.
2. Bleeding that cannot be controlled.
3. Any deep incision, laceration, or avulsion that:
    a. Goes into the muscle or bone
    b. Is located on a body part that bends and puts stress on the cut (elbows, knees, etc.)
    c. Tends to gape widely
    d. Is on the thumb or palm of hand (because nerves may be cut, later affecting the sense of touch).
4. Any puncture that is large or deep, is made by a dirty object, or does not bleed freely.
5. Large embedded objects.
6. Deeply embedded objects of any size.
7. Foreign matter left in a wound.
8. Human and animal bites.
9. Wounds where a scar would be noticeable. Stitched cuts usually heal with less scarring than unstitched ones.
10. Cuts to eyelids need sutures to prevent later drooping.
11. A slit lip needs stitches because it scars easily.
12. Any wound that a first aider is not certain how to care for.

Stitches

Stitches should be placed within six to eight hours of the injury. If the amount of contamination is small and the wound area is very vascular, the time may be extended to twelve hours.

It is good to stitch up cuts and wounds for several reasons:

1. Healing occurs more quickly.
2. Infection is less likely.
3. Scarring is lessened.

Most stitched wounds do well if the physician's advice is followed. The physician's instructions usually include:

- Keep the stitches clean and dry. Gently clean the wound area with a cotton-tipped applicator and hydrogen peroxide once or twice a day.
- Notify the physician promptly if the wound area becomes red or swollen or if pus begins to form because the wound has become infected.

Removal of most stitches follows these guidelines:

1. Face: three to five days
2. Scalp: six to eight days
3. Trunk: seven to ten days
4. Extremities: seven to ten days
5. Joints: twelve to sixteen days
6. Hands: seven to ten days
7. Feet: seven to ten days

Wounds not requiring stitches include:

1. Cut edges of the skin that tend to fall together.
2. Cuts less than one inch long that are not deep.

Gaping wounds may be closed by using the butterfly bandage only if all of the following are found:

1. The wound is less than eight to twelve hours old.
2. The wound is very clean; and
3. It is impossible to get a physician to stitch it the same day the wound occurred.

INFECTION

All wounds, large or small, present one common danger—infection. Serious wounds also present the danger of severe bleeding. Most people are alert to these hazards.

Microorganisms grow in abundance on the skin and especially the hands because our hands touch so many things. Once an infection begins, damage can be extensive, so prevention is the best way to avoid this problem.

Every cut, large or small, should be washed immediately with soap and water. If the wound is deep, it may be best to leave the cleaning to trained medical personnel, who will use an antiseptic agent, such as Betadine™, and will irrigate the wound with sterile saline solution. Early cleansing can reduce the number of germs in and around the wound so that the body's natural defenses can ward off infection.

Because infection is a danger in all wounds, a tetanus shot is often given following a wound made with a dirty object. Because there are germs everywhere, it is a good idea to have a tetanus shot every ten years.

It is important to know how to recognize and treat an infected wound. Most infected wounds swell and become reddened. They may give off a sensation of heat and develop a throbbing pain and a pus discharge.

An infection that is not treated soon enough could cause more serious symptoms affecting other areas of the body. For example, the person with an infection may develop a fever. Lymph nodes near the infection may swell. If the infection is in the hand, lymph nodes in the armpit may swell. If the infection is in the leg, lymph nodes in the groin may swell. If the infection is in the head, lymph nodes in the neck may swell. Then, one or more red streaks may develop leading from the wound toward the heart. This is a serious sign that the infection is spreading and could cause death.

In the early stages of an infection, a physician may allow home treatment of applying warm, wet compresses; elevating the injured part; and taking antibiotics.

Some wounds are more likely to become infected than others. Special care should be given a wound received from a bite—either human or animal. Wounds of the hands and feet are susceptible to infection. Any head wound, especially of the scalp, has a high likelihood of infection and should be treated by a physician. Puncture wounds that are difficult to clean have a high incidence of infection, as do wounds made by dirty objects.

Many people have been led to believe that applying a medication such as an antiseptic or first aid antibiotic is important for preventing infections and promoting healing.

According to *Consumers Union*, using an antiseptic is usually superfluous. An antiseptic agent that can kill germs is also capable of killing living cells. Dead tissue in a wound provides an excellent medium in which bacteria can multiply.

Another problem with many antiseptics is that their efficacy or safety is unproved. Only two of the many products used as skin antiseptics were judged safe and effective according to the U.S. Food and Drug Administration. The two were ethyl alcohol (60% to 95% by volume) and isopropyl alcohol (50% to 91% by volume). The rest were not considered safe or effective.

The FDA also said that the familiar and commonly used antiseptics are not very good. For example, Mercurochrome™ makes a red dye mark on the skin but it does little else and kills few germs. Merthiolate™ does slow bacterial growth, but it does not kill bacteria, which then can grow again when the antiseptic wears off. It can be damaging to the skin and many people are allergic to it. Iodine kills bacteria, but its safety for use on the skin remains unproved.

If you feel you must use an antiseptic, choose isopropyl alcohol (rubbing alcohol) because it is cheaper than ethyl alcohol, but apply it only on the intact skin around a wound, not in the wound.

After cleaning a small wound, you should protect it from trauma and infection to allow normal healing. There are two ways of protecting a small wound:

1. Dressings and bandages
2. Skin-wound protectants with or without antibiotics

Most wounds need only cleaning and a dressing placed over the wound. If a skin protectant other than a dressing is desired, wash the wound first, then apply a small ribbon of the ointment on the wound, and then cover the ointment and the wound with a sterile dressing. The antibiotic can be replaced up to three times daily.

Many skin-wound protectants are available. This list is not all inclusive, but the following are recommended:

- Americaine™ and Vaseline Carbolated Petroleum Jelly™, which do not contain antibiotics
- Bacitracin™, Neomycin™, and Neosporin™, which do contain antibiotics

Remember that others are also deemed safe and effective according to *Consumers Union*.

TETANUS

Tetanus is caused by a toxin produced by a bacterium. The bacterium forms a spore that can survive in a variety of environments for years. It has been found in soil and air samples throughout the world, on human skin, and in human and animal feces.

The bacterium by itself does not cause tetanus. But when it enters a wound that contains little oxygen (e.g., a puncture wound), it can produce a toxin, which is a powerful poison. The toxin travels through the nervous system to the brain and spinal cord. It then causes contractions of certain muscle groups (particularly in the jaw). There is no known antidote to the toxin once it enters the nervous system. In the industrialized world, because of good medical care, almost half of the victims survive the disease.

Tetanus is a killer. The World Health Organization reports 50,000 deaths each year from tetanus, but some authorities estimate that the disease may kill as many as one million people per year. About one hundred deaths a year are reported in the United States.

Prevention

Even though no specific therapy for tetanus exists, vaccination can completely prevent the disease. Vaccination is a way to prepare your body's immune system to defend against a specific disease by introducing in advance a small amount of the infectious agent and its products.

Everyone needs a series of vaccinations to prepare the immune system to defend adequately against the toxin. Then a booster shot once every ten years is sufficient to jog the immune system's memory.

People who get wounds a long time after their last vaccination (i.e., ten years) or those who did not receive all the recommended vaccinations early in life may not be able to defend adequately against the tetanus toxin. In such cases, physicians administer solutions of tetanus antibodies that are collected from other people's blood.

Always clean wounds thoroughly with soap and water to eliminate tetanus and other bacteria that may contaminate wounds.

Tetanus is not contagious. With vaccination, it is preventable at low cost and at very low risk. Therefore, no one should get tetanus. However, tetanus remains an important health problem because the tetanus organism is found throughout the world.

AMPUTATION

As microsurgical procedure and instrumentation have improved, successful reimplantation of amputated body parts, especially of the extremities, has become common.

Blood loss in cases of complete amputations is often surprisingly quite minimal. Blood vessels at the injured ends tend to retract into the traumatized body parts and to contract in diameter as nature's mechanism of preventing life-threatening bleeding.

Bleeding control efforts should start with direct pressure along with elevation. Tissue, vessel, and nerve damage that could result from the application of a tourniquet will be avoided if these techniques are used.

The amputated part should be transported with great care. In most cases, the severed part should be recovered at the accident scene. But, in multi-casualty cases, in reduced lighting conditions, or when untrained people transport the injured, someone may be requested to locate and transport the missing body part to the hospital's emergency department after the victim's departure.

Studies have indicated that severed parts that have been without oxygen as a result of the loss of blood supply for more than six hours without cooling have little chance of survival; twenty-four hours is probably the maximum time allowable for an adequately cooled part (32–39°F). The severed part must not be packed in ice, however, as reimplantation of frozen parts is usually unsuccessful.

In caring for severed body parts, follow these procedures (*see* Figure 5-7):

1. Use a clean gauze. If gauze is unavailable, use a clean towel, washcloth, etc.
2. Wrap the amputated part with gauze or towel. Do not immerse the body part in water or ice. Controversy exists about using a wet or moist dressing on an amputated part since either can cause water logging and tissue softening.
3. If a plastic bag or container is available, put the wrapped, severed part in it.
4. Place the bag or container with the amputated part on a bed of ice, but do not submerge it.
5. Transport the part immediately to the emergency department.

If the injured part is still partially attached to the stump by a tendon or small skin "bridge," the treatment is essentially the same. The part can still be wrapped and ice placed on it after it is repositioned in the normal position. Do not sever the "bridge" attaching the part.

ANIMAL BITES

More than one million people are bitten by dogs each year. Such bites are responsible for 1% of all

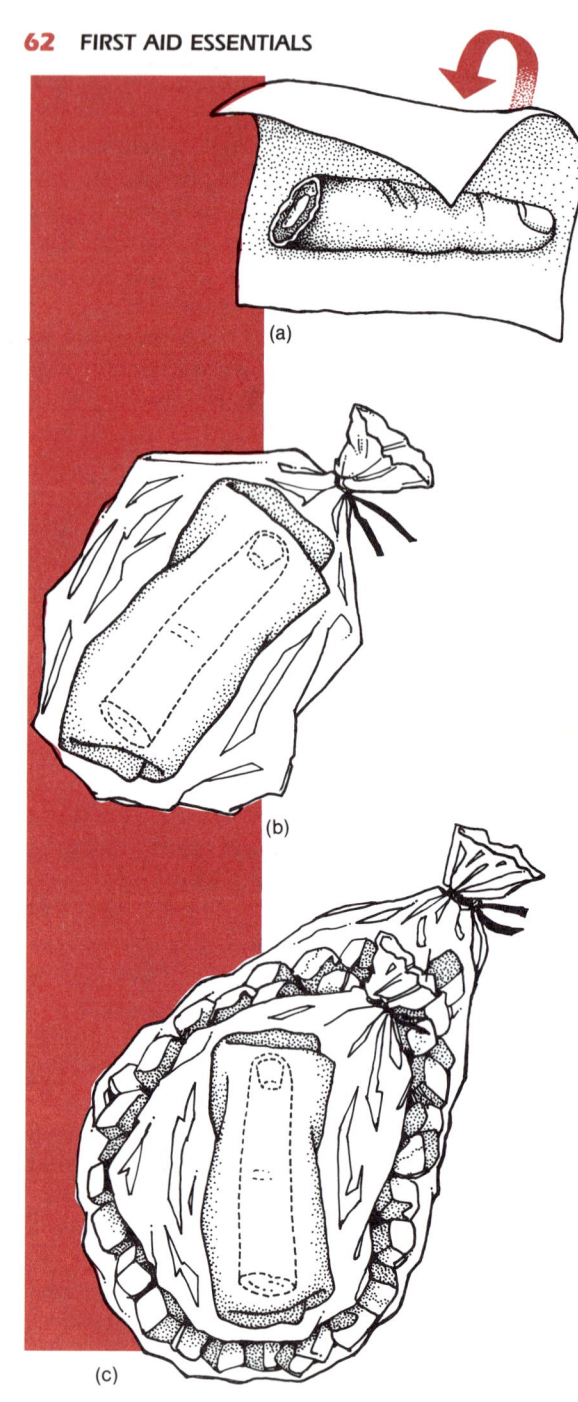

5-7 Care of amputated part
(a) Wrap the part completely in a gauze or towel.
(b) Place in a plastic bag or other type of water-proof container.
(c) Place bag or container inside larger bag or container filled with ice.

emergency room visits. About one bite in ten will need stitches, but all bites need complete cleaning, which may not be possible by a first aider.

From a first aid standpoint, the main concerns in animal bites are bleeding and infection. There may be considerable bleeding because many dogs' jaws are powerful enough to puncture sheet metal. The crushing nature of a bite often deposits bacteria deep beneath the surface of the skin, where it is hard to clean.

A dog's mouth may carry more than sixty different species of bacteria, some of which are very dangerous to humans. Cat bites are equally contaminated and dangerous.

The location of a bite is a critical factor in producing infection as well as in determining whether it needs professional medical treatment. Often the better the blood supply to the bitten area, the safer the bite because it is less likely to get infected. (Only 4% of facial bites studied became infected, whereas 33% of the hand bites did.) Puncture wounds have the greatest chance of developing infection as compared to lacerations.

All bites of the face, neck, and head should be professionally treated for two reasons: the closeness of the brain and the fact that they often must be irrigated and stitched to prevent scarring.

First Aid

Wash the wound with soap and water and rinse it thoroughly under running water. Washing should take at least five to ten minutes.

Then control bleeding with direct pressure and elevation. Puncture wounds can be encouraged to bleed. This helps remove bacteria deposited deep in the tissues. Most bites should be treated in a hospital emergency department or physician's office because of the danger of infection and the need for a tetanus shot.

Rabies

Rabies is an almost universally fatal disease in man and animal. Prevention remains the most significant factor in controlling the illness.

Rabies is caused by a virus found in warm-blooded animals. The rabies virus is spread from one animal to another usually through a bite that involves saliva from the affected animal.

Sources of rabies: Cases of rabies in animals remains high. Wild carnivores account for about 90% of the cases, and domestic pets representing the other 10%. Of all types of animals capable of carrying rabies, seven species were responsible for 97% of the documented cases. Of the wild animals, skunks were responsible for 62% of the reported cases; bats, 11.9%; raccoons, 6.7%; cattle, 6.4%; and foxes, 2.7%. Of the domestic animals, cats were responsible for 4% of the cases and dogs were responsible for 3%.

The prevalence of rabies in cats is interesting. This may be true because cats are frequent household pets, are not subject to prelicense vaccination laws as are dogs, and are not actively restricted by leash laws or other control measures. Stray cats roam frequently and are adopted into a household without much consideration for their immunization status.

Dogs are the other common source of rabies from domestic animals. Even though the incidence of the disease appears to be decreasing in this group, dog bites still constitute an estimated 1% of all hospital emergency department visits.

Treatment: If an animal does bite, try to capture it for observation without further endangering the captors. Every attempt should be made to avoid destroying the animal. If it is killed, the head and brain should be protected from damage so that they can be examined for rabies. If killed, it is best to transport the animal intact to prevent exposure to potentially infected secretions or tissues. If necessary, the animal's remains can be refrigerated. (Avoid freezing.)

Bites breaking the skin should be vigorously cleansed and washed with large amounts of soap and water. Medical care is of utmost importance, not only for repairing the wound, but also for consultation regarding further treatment.

Many people are still under the misconception that treatment for rabies involves a long, painful series of injections. Until 1980, it did take a series of twenty-three injections. A new vaccine has been found to be safer, less painful, and more effective than the old type. It takes only a series of five injections.

Bites from domestic animals that are not warm blooded, such as birds, snakes, and other reptiles do not carry the danger of rabies. But these, too, may become infected. Such bites should be washed well and watched for signs of infection.

Although rabies is an infrequent disease in humans, greater efforts are needed to control potential carriers, including domestic pets. All adults, especially those with children and those with cats or dogs, should be well versed in the basic facts regarding rabies. If a wild animal bites a human, the only certain way to rule out rabies is to examine the animal's brain. If the animal cannot be found or the brain cannot be examined, the human who was bitten may have to take rabies injections.

Bleeding Control

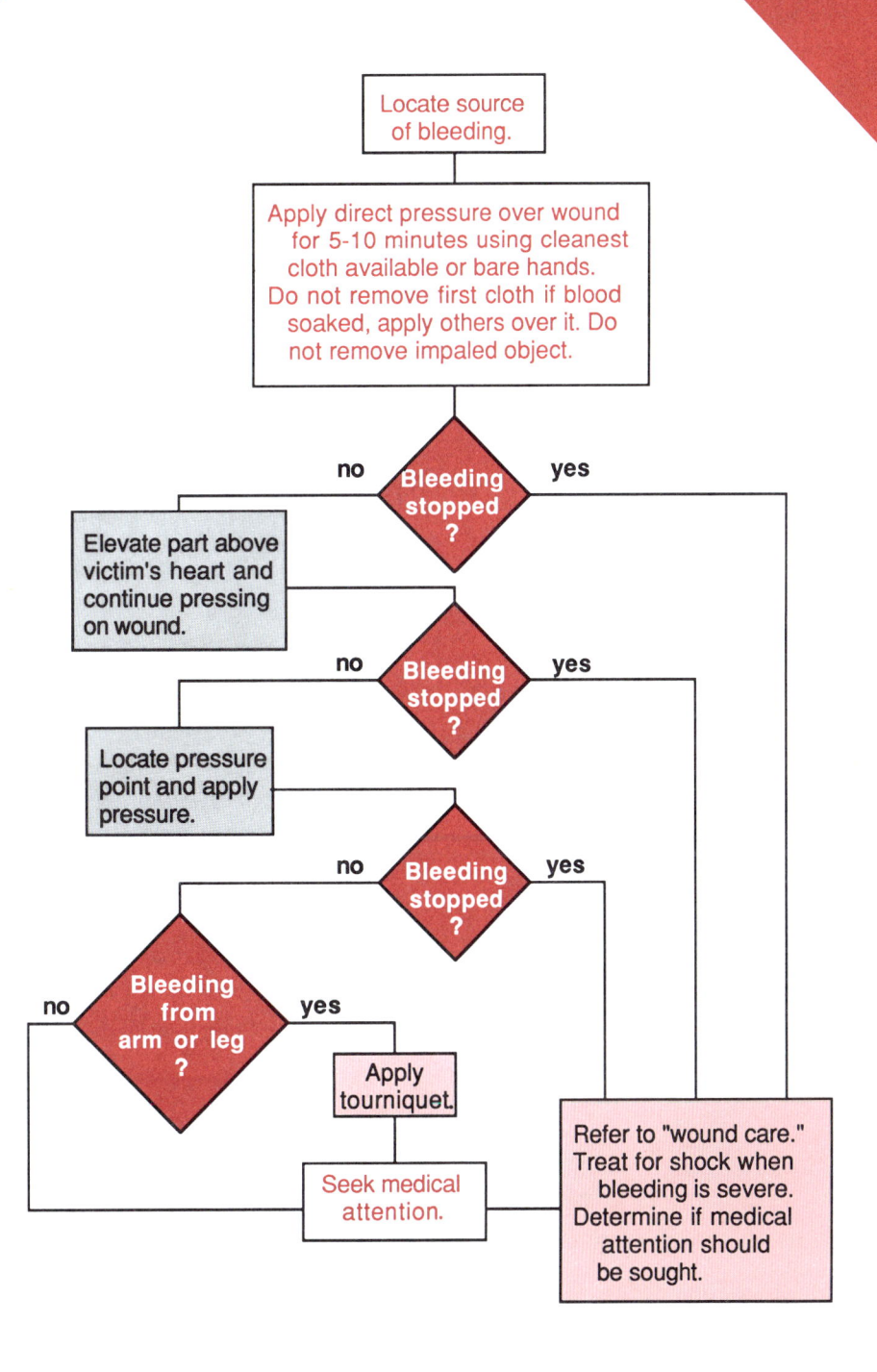

```
                    ┌──────────────┐
                    │Locate source │
                    │ of bleeding. │
                    └──────┬───────┘
                           │
         ┌─────────────────▼──────────────────┐
         │ Apply direct pressure over wound   │
         │ for 5-10 minutes using cleanest    │
         │ cloth available or bare hands.     │
         │ Do not remove first cloth if blood │
         │ soaked, apply others over it. Do   │
         │ not remove impaled object.         │
         └─────────────────┬──────────────────┘
                           │
              no       ◇ Bleeding ◇      yes
         ┌─────────────  stopped?  ─────────────┐
         │                                       │
   ┌─────▼──────────┐                            │
   │Elevate part    │                            │
   │above victim's  │                            │
   │heart and       │                            │
   │continue        │                            │
   │pressing on     │                            │
   │wound.          │                            │
   └─────┬──────────┘                            │
         │                                       │
              no       ◇ Bleeding ◇      yes     │
         ┌─────────────  stopped?  ─────────────┤
         │                                       │
   ┌─────▼──────────┐                            │
   │Locate pressure │                            │
   │point and apply │                            │
   │pressure.       │                            │
   └─────┬──────────┘                            │
         │                                       │
              no       ◇ Bleeding ◇      yes     │
         ┌─────────────  stopped?  ─────────────┤
         │                                       │
    no ◇ Bleeding ◇ yes                          │
   ┌── from arm ───┐                             │
   │   or leg?     │                             │
   │               ▼                             │
   │         ┌──────────┐                        │
   │         │  Apply   │                        │
   │         │tourniquet│                        │
   │         └────┬─────┘                        │
   │              │                              │
   │         ┌────▼──────┐                       │
   └────────►│Seek medical│                      │
             │ attention. │                      │
             └────────────┘                      │
                                                 ▼
                              ┌──────────────────────┐
                              │Refer to "wound care."│
                              │Treat for shock when  │
                              │bleeding is severe.   │
                              │Determine if medical  │
                              │attention should      │
                              │be sought.            │
                              └──────────────────────┘
```

65

Amputation

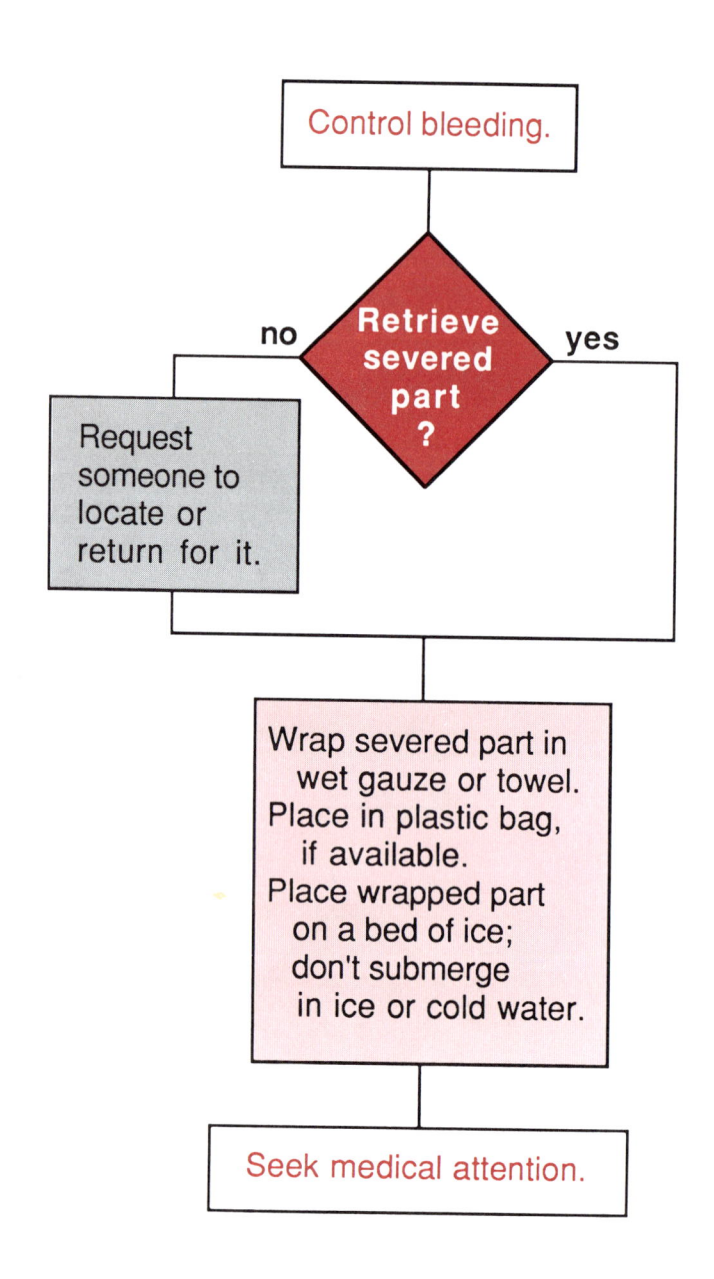

- Control bleeding.
- Retrieve severed part?
  - no → Request someone to locate or return for it.
  - yes → Wrap severed part in wet gauze or towel. Place in plastic bag, if available. Place wrapped part on a bed of ice; don't submerge in ice or cold water.
- Seek medical attention.

Animal Bites

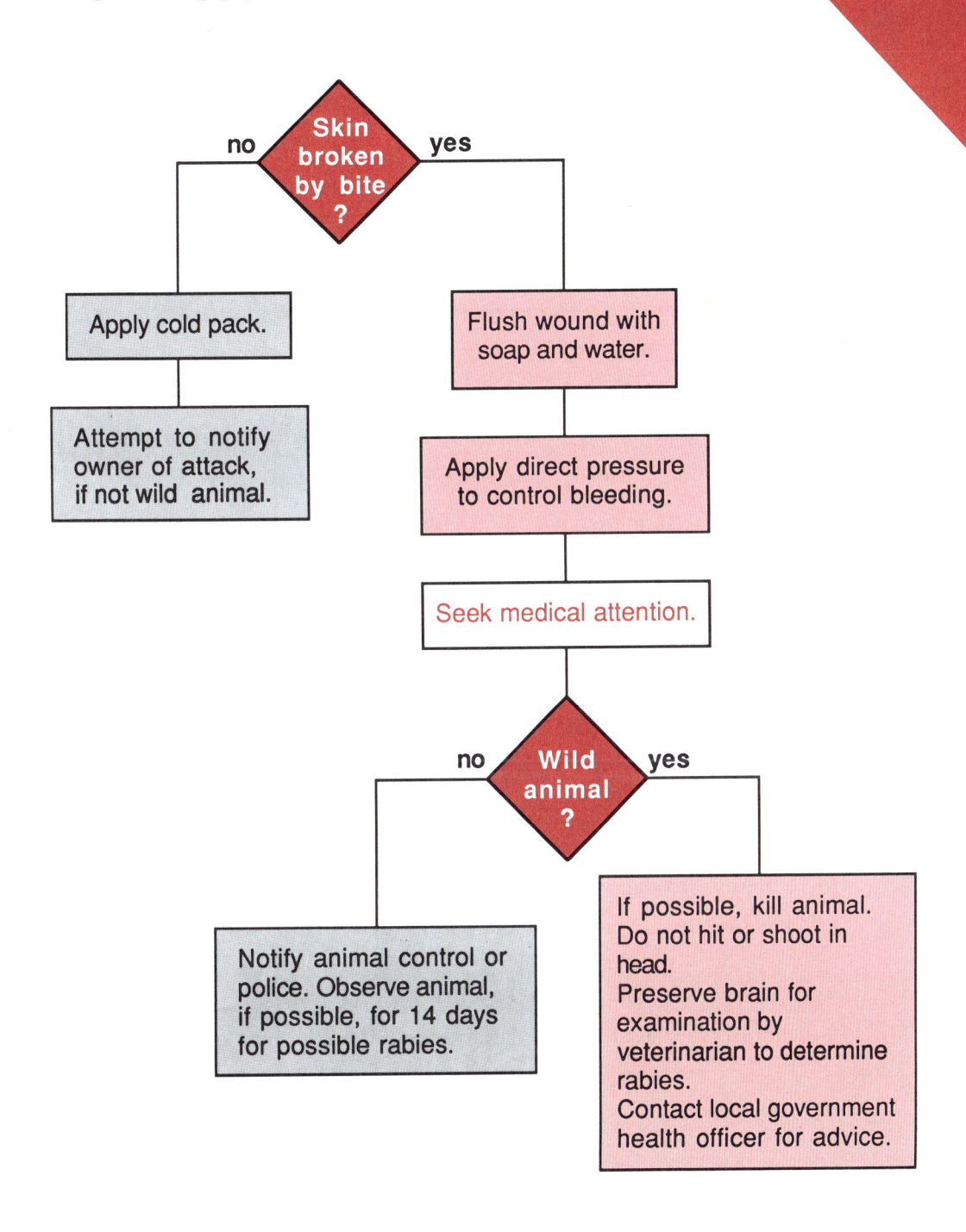

Skin broken by bite?

- **no** → Apply cold pack. → Attempt to notify owner of attack, if not wild animal.
- **yes** → Flush wound with soap and water. → Apply direct pressure to control bleeding. → Seek medical attention.

Wild animal?

- **no** → Notify animal control or police. Observe animal, if possible, for 14 days for possible rabies.
- **yes** → If possible, kill animal. Do not hit or shoot in head. Preserve brain for examination by veterinarian to determine rabies. Contact local government health officer for advice.

SELF-CHECK QUESTIONS

Activity 1: External Bleeding and Wounds

A. Mark each statement true (T) or false (F).
  1. ☐ Loss of blood occurs only in open wounds.
  2. ☐ A bruise on the thigh is an example of an external wound.
  3. ☐ Closed wounds occur when blood vessels beneath the skin have been broken.
  4. ☐ Bleeding from veins is usually fast and in spurts.
  5. ☐ Losing more than a quart of blood for an adult is life threatening.
  6. ☐ Completely severed arteries bleed more freely than partially cut arteries.
  7. ☐ Arterial bleeding is usually more serious than venous bleeding.

B. A sharp blade cuts a wrist and blood is flowing freely from the wound. Which of the following actions should be taken to control bleeding in this situation?
  1. ☐ Control bleeding by tightly pressing on the wound.
  2. ☐ If arm is elevated to control bleeding, direct pressure is no longer needed.
  3. ☐ Use the femoral pressure point if direct pressure fails.

C. Mark each statement true (T) or false (F).
  1. ☐ When washing a wound with soap and water, wash toward the wound.
  2. ☐ Hydrogen peroxide kills bacteria (germs) in a wound.
  3. ☐ If using rubbing alcohol, apply it on the skin around the wound, not in the wound.
  4. ☐ A "butterfly" bandage can be used to bring small cut skin edges together.
  5. ☐ If a dressing must be removed and part of the scab sticks to it, soak it in warm water to soften the scab for easier removal.
  6. ☐ Cuts to eyelids and lips should be stitched by a physician.
  7. ☐ Stitches can be placed by a physician hours after the injury occurred.

Activity 2: Infection and Tetanus

A. Mark the signs of an infected wound.

   Yes   No
1. ☐   ☐   Throbbing pain and pus discharge
2. ☐   ☐   Swollen lymph nodes
3. ☐   ☐   Blue streak from wound toward heart
4. ☐   ☐   Wound appears dry and crusty

B. Prevent infection by:

   Yes   No
1. ☐   ☐   Immediately washing a wound with soap and water
2. ☐   ☐   Getting a tetanus booster shot every year
3. ☐   ☐   Using rubbing or ethyl alcohol applied directly on the wound
4. ☐   ☐   Using mercurochrome or merthiolate instead of soap and water
5. ☐   ☐   Using any one of several recommended skin-wound protectants

Activity 3: Amputation

A wheat harvest worker caught his hand in a combine drive shaft and had his hand torn off. He came running from the field with blood running and his hand missing.

Mark each statement true (T) or false (F).

1. ☐ Usually small blood loss occurs in amputation cases.
2. ☐ An amputated part has little chance of survival.
3. ☐ Pack an amputated part in ice.
4. ☐ Cut off partially attached part.
5. ☐ Locate any amputated part, regardless of size, and take to the medical facility.
6. ☐ Amputated parts older than six hours without proper cooling have little chance of survival.

Activity 4: Animal Bites

A postman suffered severe damage to his right shoulder and arm after a pit bull attacked him while delivering mail to the dog owner's front porch.

Mark each statement true (T) or false (F).

1. ☐ Most dog bites should be treated by a physician.
2. ☐ In most cases, wash the wound with soap and water before attempting to stop bleeding.
3. ☐ Washing the wound should take only one or two minutes.
4. ☐ Control bleeding with direct pressure.

6

Specific Body Area Injuries

- Head Injuries • Eye Injuries • Nosebleeds
- Dental Emergencies • Chest Injuries • Abdominal Injuries
- Foreign Objects • Hand and Finger Injuries • Blisters

HEAD INJURIES

Head injury is the primary cause of death in accidents. Three types of injury that can occur to the head include skull fracture, concussion, and contusion.

A *skull fracture* is a crack in the cranium (bony case surrounding the brain). This crack may be small and visible only by x-ray (linear), or it may have many cracks radiating from the area of contact (comminuted). Even more severe is the *depressed* skull fracture in which the bone is driven inward into the brain. A fourth type is the *basal* skull fracture, where the base of the skull is damaged.

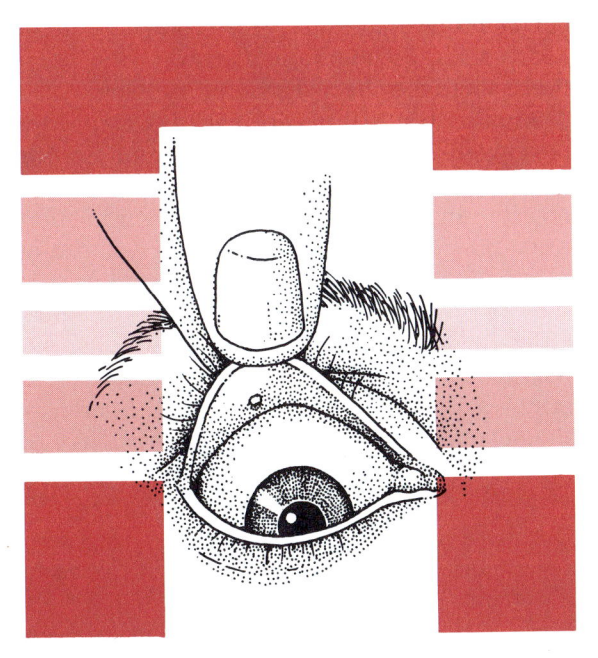

Signs and symptoms of a skull fracture include: pain at the point of injury, deformity of the skull, bleeding from ears and/or nose, cerebrospinal fluid leaking from ears or nose, discoloration under the eyes, and unequal pupils.

A second type of head injury is the *concussion*. The brain is surrounded by cerebrospinal fluid. When there is a blow to the head or the head flies forward and is then suddenly snapped back (whiplash), the brain may bang against the inside of the skull causing temporary loss of consciousness and a headache. Usually no permanent brain damage occurs. Sometimes, though, there may be short-term memory loss.

A more severe head injury is the *contusion*. It is caused by the same action as a concussion — the brain hitting the skull. It is a bruise of the brain — the blood vessels within the brain substance rupture and bleed. Inside the skull there is no way for the blood to escape, and there is no room for it to accumulate.

All head injuries have the potential for stopping breathing and heartbeat. Therefore, the first step in aiding this victim is to check for breathing. If the victim's awkward position is closing the airway, you are justified in moving him or her; but it is important to try to keep the head, neck, and spine in the same alignment. Once you have the victim in a workable position:

1. Open the airway by the jaw thrust maneuver. Do not hyperextend the neck. Give mouth-to-mouth resuscitation if needed.

2. If the victim is breathing, check his or her pulse next. Count it for a full 60 seconds. If it is less than 55 or more than 125, the victim may be in serious condition.

3. Now check for bleeding. Cover any bleeding head injury with a sterile dressing. If fluid is flowing from the ears, *do not* stop it. Otherwise, it could put pressure on the brain. If there is no evidence of a neck or back injury, try to place the victim in the coma position (on his or her side, knees up, head supported on one arm). Do not remove any object embedded in the skull.

4. Try to maintain the victim's body temperature with blankets if necessary, but do not overheat. In head injuries, it is common for the body temperature to rise, so monitor temperature as well as breathing and pulse while you wait for an ambulance.

When head injury victims are conscious, it is important to find out if they are thinking clearly. You may ask their name, address, location, and age, for example. If they cannot answer these questions, suspect brain injury and administer first aid accordingly. Observe pupil size—they should be equal and react to light. Note any limb weakness or paralysis. Touch feet and hands and ask the victim if there is a sensation. If the victim loses consciousness, all this information will be very important to medical personnel. The length of time of unconsciousness is also important.

Occasionally, the effect of a blow to the head may be delayed. Some time later the victim faints or develops a headache. Again, knowing the victim has sustained a blow to the head may explain these symptoms. Head injuries that produce these symptoms should be promptly checked by a physician.

Recognizing Concussion

It is not necessary to be hit on the head to receive a concussion, which is what most first aiders look for. It can occur simply from sudden deceleration of the head (e.g., in an automobile crash).

In the absence of unconsciousness (one of the best signs), a glassy-eyed look, uncoordination, inability to walk correctly, or obvious disorientation provide clues. The victim may complain of dizziness, lightheadedness, blurred vision, and disorientation.

Headaches may or may not follow head injury. If the victim complains of a headache immediately after a head injury, that is a significant symptom. On the other hand, it is common for people suffering a concussion to develop a headache a day or two later and sometimes even as long as a week following injury.

Mental Status Tests

It is important to ask the victim simple questions, such as subtracting numbers, what food was eaten for breakfast, and other short-term memory tests. Studies show that deficits in short-term memory are the first to occur after concussion.

Also ask what day it is, where he or she is, and personal questions such as birthday and home address. If the victim cannot answer these questions, there may be a significant problem.

Another test that may be useful is to give the person a list of five or six numbers and ask him or her to repeat them back in that order. Lists of objects can also be used as short-term memory tests. If a person fails on these tests, you can be sure he has been concussed.

If the victim loses consciousness momentarily, he or she should remain inactive. Anyone who remains unconscious for more than several minutes should be transported immediately to the hospital.

Degrees of Concussion

Concussion is sometimes described as having several different degrees. The value of categorizing them is in deciding how to manage the victim. Those categories are mild, moderate, and severe. (Refer to Table 6-1.)

TABLE 6-1 Concussion Guidelines

Type	Description	Guidelines
Mild	Momentary or no loss of consciousness.	Delay return to activity until medical evaluation has been made.
Moderate	Unconscious for less than five minutes.	Avoid vigorous activity for a few days or longer. Resume activity only when associated symptoms of headache, visual disturbances, etc. have been resolved.
Severe	Unconscious for more than five minutes.	Avoid rigorous activity for one month or longer. Clearance from a neurosurgeon is advised.

In a *mild* concussion, there is no loss of consciousness, but there is a disturbance of neurological function.

In the *moderate* concussion, there is a loss of consciousness for less than five minutes, usually with the inability to remember events after being injured.

In the *severe* concussion, there is a loss of consciousness for longer than five minutes, wandering eye movements, and a lack of purposeful responses.

A victim with a severe concussion must be seen immediately by a physician trained in managing head injuries and must be hospitalized. At the other end of the scale, the mild concussion does not require hospitalization but does require observation.

Head Injury Follow-Up

After a head injury, certain signs may indicate a need for medical attention. If any of the following signs appears within forty-eight hours of a head injury, you should seek medical attention:

1. *Headache.* A headache is to be expected. If it lasts more than one or two days or increases in severity, medical advice should be sought.

2. *Nausea, vomiting.* If nausea lasts more than two hours, you must seek medical advice. Vomiting once or twice, especially in children, after a severe head injury may be expected. Vomiting does not tell anything about the severity of the injury. However, if vomiting begins again hours after one or two episodes had ceased, consult a physician.

3. *Drowsiness.* If the victim wants to sleep, let him, but do wake him to check his state of consciousness and sense of orientation by asking his name, address, telephone number, and whether he can process information such as adding or multiplying numbers; if he cannot answer correctly or appears confused or disoriented, call the doctor. You will have to modify the questions for a small child.

Experts disagree on the time intervals for waking a sleeping victim to check consciousness. Some say every thirty minutes to an hour; others say every two to three hours. It would seem that on the night following a head injury, or during any nap, that the victim should be awakened at least every two hours to check for state of consciousness and the other signs in this list.

4. *Vision problems.* If the victim "sees double," if the eyes fail to move together, or if one pupil appears to be larger than the other, these are signs of possible trouble.

5. *Mobility.* The victim cannot use his arms or legs as well as previously or is unsteady in walking.

6. *Speech.* The victim slurs his speech or is unable to talk.

7. *Convulsions.*

EYE INJURIES

Correct treatment of an eye injury immediately following an accident can prevent loss of sight. However, because it is difficult to determine the extent of damage to the eye, medical help should be sought as soon as first aid is completed: call an ophthalmologist, your family physician or go to a nearby hospital emergency room immediately.

Specks In The Eye*

Never rub any speck or particle that is in the eye. Lift the upper lid over the lower lid allowing the lashes to brush the speck off the inside of the upper lid. Blink a few times and let the eye move the particle out. If the speck remains, keep the eye closed and seek medical help.

Blows To The Eye*

Apply an ice cold compress immediately for about 15 minutes to reduce pain and swelling. A black eye or blurred vision could signal internal eye damage. See your ophthalmologist immediately.

Cuts Of The Eye And Lid*

Bandage both eyes lightly and seek medical help immediately. Do not attempt to wash out the eye or remove an object stuck in the eye. Never apply hard pressure to the injured eye or eyelid. (See Figure 6-1.)

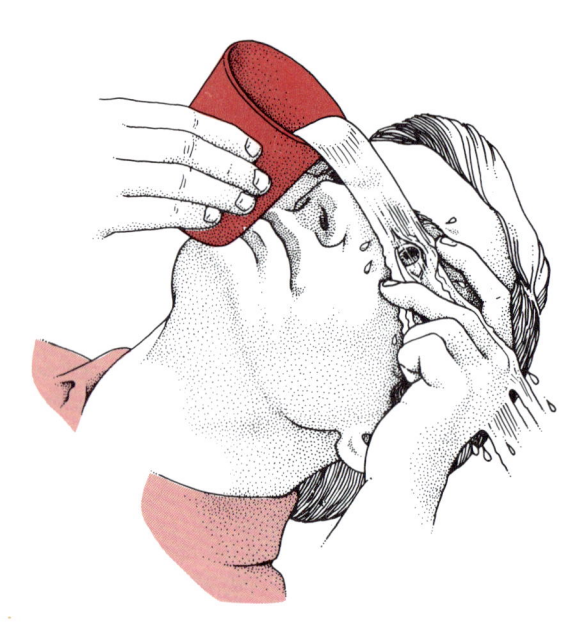

6-2. Immediately flush the eye in case of chemical burns.

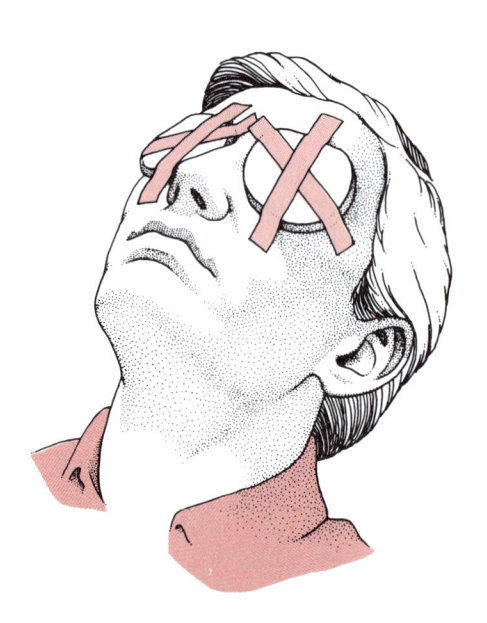

Chemical Burns*

Flood the eye with warm water immediately, using your fingers to keep the eye open as wide as possible. Hold head under a faucet or pour water into the eye from any clean container for at least 15 minutes, continuously and gently (See Figure 6-2.) Roll the eyeball as much as possible to wash out the eye. Do not use an eye cup. Do not bandage the eye. Seek medical help immediately after these steps are taken.

Avulsion Of The Eye

A blow to the face can avulse an eye from its socket. If such an injury occurs, do not attempt to push the eye back into the socket. Cover the extruded eye loosely with a sterile dressing that has been moistened with clean water. Then cover the eye with a paper cup, just like the same procedure for an impaled object in eye.

6-1. Cover both eyes to minimize eye movement (exception is chemical burns).

Foreign Objects in the Eye

(Refer to page 81.)

---

*American Academy of Ophthalmology, "Eye Injuries: Prevention and First Aid." Reprinted with permission.

Ultraviolet Eye Burns

Snow "blindness," exposure to sunlamps, and looking at a welding arc result in ultraviolet eye injuries. Initial symptoms appear after one to six hours after exposure. Victims report severe pain.

Rest in a darkened room with cold compresses on the eyes. Eye patches may be necessary. An analgesic for pain may be needed. Seek medical attention.

Contact Lenses

Determine if the victim is wearing contact lenses by asking him, checking on a driver's license, or looking for them on the eyeball by shining a light on the eye from the side. Lenses should be removed immediately only in cases of chemical eye burns.

Proper precautions should always be taken to protect the eyes. Knowing what to do and/or what not to do in the event of an eye injury can save the precious gift of eyesight.

Though prompt, proper treatment of eye injuries can save vision, it is important to remember that first aid is just that. It is immediate treatment that is "first," until experienced medical help is available. When an accident involves the eye, it is always wise to be safe: seek medical help immediately if there is pain or any question of damage or impaired vision.

NOSEBLEEDS

Severe nosebleed is frightening to the victim, occurs at inopportune times, and often challenges the skill of the first aider. Minor nosebleeds are usually self-limited and seldom require medical attention, unless they become recurrent.

Types of Nosebleeds

Nosebleeds can be divided into anterior (front) and posterior (back) types—those that bleed through the nose and those that bleed backward into the mouth or down the back of the throat. Anterior bleeding is by far the most common, occuring nine times out of ten.

Nosebleeds are most common in children, and the great majority of these cases, approximately 90%, originate in the anterior septum of the nose.

In older persons, bleeding usually occurs in the posterior nose.

Stopping a Nosebleed

Most nosebleeds from the anterior nasal septum can be stopped by simple procedures (*see* Figure 6-3):

1. Reassure the victim that most nosebleeds are not serious. Keep him or her quiet. Though a large amount of blood may appear to have been lost, most nosebleeds are not likely to be serious.

2. The victim should be in a sitting position to reduce blood pressure. Keep the head in an upright position or tilted slightly forward so that the blood can run out the front of the nose, not down the back of the throat, causing either choking or nausea and vomiting dark clots. These clots may be aspirated into the lungs.

3. If a foreign object in the nose is suspected, look into the nose, but do not probe with finger or swab.

4. With thumb and forefinger, apply steady pressure to both nostrils for five minutes before releasing. Remind the victim to breathe through his mouth and to spit out any accumulated blood.

5. If bleeding persists, have the victim gently blow the nose to remove any clots and excess blood, and to minimize sneezing. This allows new clots to form. This is a new concept for most first aiders. Then press the nostrils again for five minutes.

6. Some experts recommend soaking a cotton ball in hydrogen peroxide, a nasal decongestant (nose drops or spray), or plain water; wring out the excess; and gently insert the cotton ball inside the bleeding nostril. Criticism against this step is the lack of time and/or materials. When five minutes are up, slowly and gently remove the cotton.

76 FIRST AID ESSENTIALS

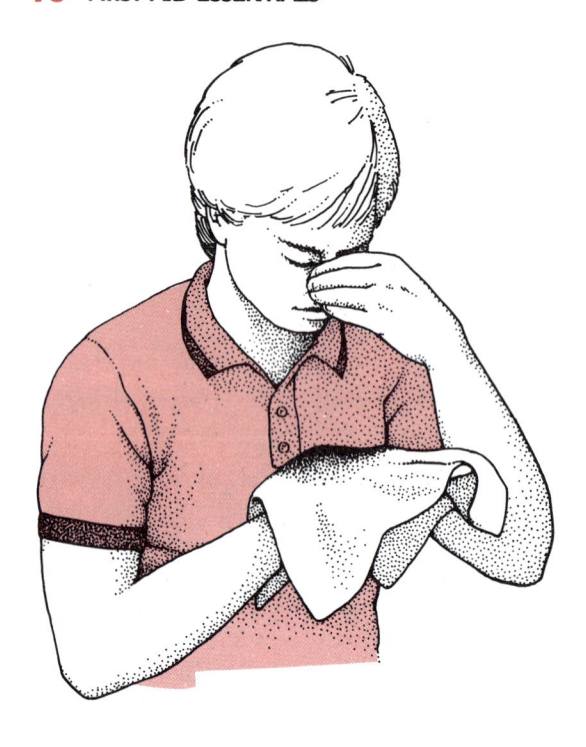

7. Place a roll of gauze between the upper lip and gum and press against it with your fingers.

8. Some experts recommend applying a cold compress over the nose.

9. If the victim is unconscious, place the victim on his side to prevent aspiration of blood and attempt the procedures in this list.

Seek Medical Care

You should seek medical attention if any of the following occurs:

1. The procedures do not stop the bleeding after a second attempt.
2. The signs and symptoms indicate a posterior source of bleeding.
3. The victim has hypertension.
4. The victim is taking anticoagulants (blood thinners) or large doses of aspirin.
5. The bleeding occurred after an injury to the nose.

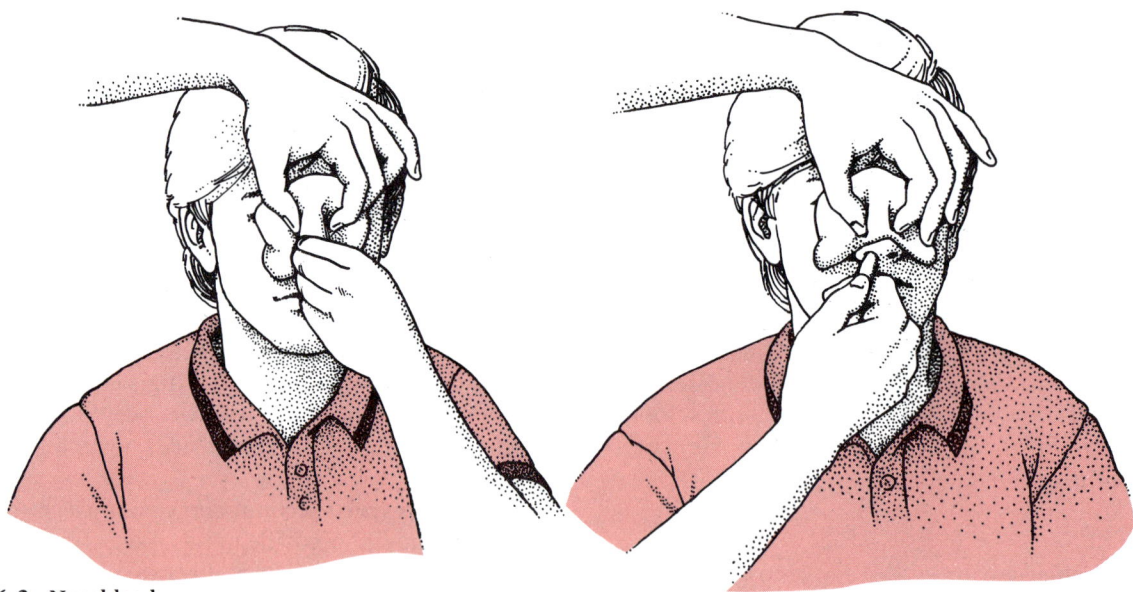

6-3. Nosebleeds
(a) Have the person sit leaning slightly forward to prevent blood from running down his throat. Have the person pinch his nose firmly for at least five full minutes.
(b) While the person is pinching, apply a cold compress to the nose and surrounding area.

(c) If pinching does not work, gently pack the nostril. Be sure that the end hangs out to aid in removing later. Then pinch the nose, with the gauze in it, for another five minutes.

Treatment of posterior bleeding is best left to a physician. It may involve cauterization with chemicals or electric needle. A physican may pack the nose with sterile gauze or insert and inflate a small balloon to create pressure on the ruptured part. As a last resort the doctor may tie off the bleeding vessel.

Care After A Nosebleed

After a nosebleed has stopped, you should suggest that the victim:

1. Sneeze through an open mouth, if there is a need to sneeze.
2. Not stoop or exert physically.
3. When lying down, elevate the head with two pillows.
4. Keep the nostrils moist by applying a little petroleum jelly just inside the nostril for a week and increase the humidity in the bedroom during the winter months with a cold-mist humidifier.
5. Avoid picking or rubbing the nose. If a child has an uncontrollable habit, trim his fingernails frequently.
6. Avoid hot drinks and alcohol beverages for a week.
7. Not smoke or take aspirin for a week.

Most victims with nosebleeds never need medical care. Most nosebleeds are self-limited and the victim can control the bleeding himself.

DENTAL EMERGENCIES*

First aiders often deal with dental emergencies. The following first aid procedures are guidelines for providing temporary relief for dental emergencies, but it is imperative to consult with a dentist as soon as possible (*See* Table 6-2).

Objects Wedged Between Teeth

Attempt to remove the object with dental floss. Guide the floss in carefully so the gum tissue is not injured. Do not use a sharp or pointed tool to remove the object. If unsuccessful, take the victim to a dentist.

Bitten Lip or Tongue

Apply direct pressure to the bleeding area with a clean cloth. If the lip is swollen, apply a cold compress. Take the victim to a hospital emergency room if the bleeding persists or if the bite is severe.

Knocked-Out Tooth

When a permanent tooth is completely knocked out in an accident, save it and take it, along with the victim, to the dentist immediately. With proper first aid procedures, the tooth can be given an opportunity for successful reimplantation (placing the tooth back in the socket). Do not attempt to clean the tooth because this destroys necessary connective fibers which assist in the reimplantation process. Do *not* put the tooth in mouthwash or alcohol or scrub it with abrasives or chemicals. And do *not* touch the root of the tooth.

Place the tooth in a cup of milk or cool water or wrap it loosely in a clean, wet cloth or gauze, Take the victim and tooth to a dentist immediately (within thirty minutes). Some experts recommend that the tooth be placed in the victim's mouth to keep it moist until dental treatment is available. This method though convenient presents the risk, especially in children, of being accidentally swallowed.

A partially extracted tooth can be pushed into place without rinsing the tooth. Then seek a dentist so the loose tooth can be stabilized. If in remote areas with no dentist nearby, replant a knocked-out tooth by first running cool water over it to clean away debris (do not scrub the tooth), and then by gently repositioning it into the socket, using adjacent teeth as a guide. Push the tooth so the top is even with the adjacent teeth. Successful replanting occurs best within thirty minutes of the accident. See a dentist as soon as possible.

---
*American Dental Association. Reprinted with permission.

TABLE 6-2. Dental Emergency Procedures

Toothache	Rinse the mouth vigorously with warm water to clean out debris. Use dental floss to remove any food that might be trapped between the teeth. (*Do not place aspirin on the aching tooth or gum tissues*.) See your dentist as soon as possible.
Orthodontic Problems (Braces and Retainers)	If a wire is causing irritation, cover end of the wire with a small cotton ball, beeswax, or a piece of gauze, until you can get to the dentist.
	If a wire is embedded in the cheek, tongue, or gum tissue, do not attempt to remove it. Go to your dentist immediately.
	If an appliance becomes loose or a piece of it breaks off, take the appliance and the piece and go to the dentist.
Knocked-Out Tooth	If the tooth is dirty, rinse it gently in running water. *Do not scrub it.*
	Gently insert and hold the tooth in its socket. If this is not possible, place the tooth in a container of milk or cool water.
	Go immediately to your dentist (within 30 minutes, if possible). Don't forget to bring the tooth.
Broken Tooth	Gently clean dirt or debris from the injured area with warm water. Place cold compresses on the face, in the area of the injured tooth, to minimize swelling.
	Go to the dentist immediately.
Bitten Tongue or Lip	Apply direct pressure to the bleeding area with a clean cloth. If swelling is present, apply cold compresses. If bleeding does not stop, go to a hospital emergency room.
Objects Wedged Between Teeth	Try to remove the object with dental floss. Guide the floss carefully to avoid cutting the gums. If not successful in removing the object, go to the dentist. Do not try to remove the object with a sharp or pointed instrument.
Possible Fractured Jaw	Immobilize the jaw by any means (handkerchief, necktie, towel). If swelling is present, apply cold compresses. Call your dentist or go immediately to a hospital emergency room.

Source: Copyright by the American Dental Association. Reprinted by permission.

Broken Tooth

Immediate attention is necessary when a child breaks a tooth or else it may need to be extracted. Attempt to clean any dirt, blood, and debris from the injured area with a sterile gauze pad and warm water.

Apply a cold compress on the face next to the injured tooth to minimize swelling. If a jaw fracture is suspected, immobilize the jaw by any available means — place a scarf, handkerchief, tie, or towel over and under the chin, and tie the ends on top of the victim's head. In either case, immediately take the victim to an oral surgeon or hospital emergency room.

Although temporary relief can be provided in most dental emergencies, by all means, when in doubt, consult a dentist as soon as possible.

Toothache

Rinse the mouth vigorously with warm water to clean out debris. Use dental floss to remove any food that might be trapped between the teeth. Do not place aspirin on the aching tooth or gum tissues.

If a cavity is present, insert a small cotton ball soaked in oil of cloves (eugenol). Do not cover a cavity with cotton if there is any pus discharge or facial swelling. See your dentist as soon as possible.

CHEST INJURIES

Chest injuries are a leading cause of accidental death. For example, of all traffic fatalities in the United States, 35% to 40% of the victims have chest injuries; and the majority of these deaths were due to chest injuries alone. Chest injuries may also be the result of gunshot woulds, stab wounds, falls, or blows.

Signs of Chest Injuries

The important signs of chest injuries are:

1. Pain at the injury site
2. Painful breathing
3. Difficult breathing
4. Cyanosis (blueness of the lips, fingernails), indicating oxygen deficiency
5. Coughing up bright red frothy blood, indicating a punctured lung
6. Failure of one or both sides of the chest to expand normally when inhaling

Types of Chest Injuries

Rib fractures: These are usually caused by direct blows or compression of the chest. The upper four ribs are rarely fractured because they are protected by the collarbone and shoulder blade. The lower two ribs are hard to fracture because they are attached only on one end and have freedom to move (known as "floating" ribs). The victim can usually point out the exact injury site. There may or may not be a rib deformity, contusion, or a laceration of the area. Deep breathing, coughing, or movement is usually quite painful.

Simple rib fractures should not be bound, strapped, or taped. Such wrapping predisposes the victim to pneumonia. Instead, the victim can hold a pillow against the injured area. Instruct him to take deep breaths to prevent pneumonia. With multiple fractures of the ribs, the victim may be more comfortable with the arm strapped to the chest with a sling and several swathes.

Flail chest: When three or more ribs are broken, each in two places, the segment of the chest wall will move independently of the rest of the chest wall when the victim attempts to breathe. Often the movement of the injured segment of the chest wall moves in the opposite direction to the rest of the chest wall. This is called paradoxical respiration.

The signs and symptoms of a flail chest include:

1. The same signs and symptoms of fractured ribs
2. The failure of a section of the chest wall to move with the rest of the chest wall when the victim is breathing.

The first aid for a flail chest is to immobilize the ribs to improve breathing. Place the victim in a semi-sitting position, inclined to the injured side to assist breathing.

Penetrating wounds: Stab and gunshot wounds are examples of penetrating chest wounds. Sucking chest wounds, rib fractures, or laceration of the heart or blood vessels of the chest may result. The wound must be closed quickly because it can result in air outside the lung entering the chest cavity. Do not remove or attempt to remove an impaled object penetrating the chest because bleeding and air in the chest cavity can result. Stabilize the foreign object, and seek medical attention for the injured victim.

If the victim starts to get worse after the penetrating wound has been sealed, lift the dressing off the wound to allow air to escape from the chest cavity—immediate improvement should be shown. Then, reapply the seal over the wound and be prepared to relieve the build-up of air in the chest cavity by the same method.

Summary: Almost all types of chest injuries require the same initial care. Breathing should be checked and taken care of if needed. Open chest wounds must be covered. Broken ribs are usually immobilized by a sling and swathe, rather than by adhesive taping. Bleeding from the chest wall should be controlled, preferably by direct pressure. Embedded or protruding foreign objects (e.g., knives) should be bandaged in place and left alone. Medical care should be sought.

ABDOMINAL INJURIES

Abdominal injuries may be closed or open, and they may involve hollow or solid organs.

Closed injuries are those in which the abdomen is damaged by a severe blow (e.g., hitting a steering wheel or the dashboard of a car or being tackled in football), but in which there is no open wound or bleeding to the outside. *Open* injuries are those in which a foreign body has entered the abdomen, and bleeding to the outside is occurring. Examples are stab or gunshot wounds.

The rupture of hollow organs (e.g., organs of the digestive system such as stomach or intestines) spills the contents into the peritoneal cavity causing inflammation. Rupture of solid organs (e.g., the liver) may result in severe bleeding.

Signs and Symptoms

The signs and symptoms of abdominal injury can include:

1. Victim is in pain, often starting as mild pain then rapidly become severe.
2. Victim has cramps in the abdominal area.
3. Victim will be still, usually with legs drawn up.
4. Breathing will be rapid and shallow.
5. Skin wounds and penetrations may be evident.
6. Victim may be nauseated and may vomit.
7. Organs may protrude.
8. There may be blood in the urine.
9. Victim tries to protect his abdomen.

Types of Abdominal Injuries

Blunt wounds: Severe bruises of the abdominal area can result from a blow to the abdomen. Within the abdomen, the liver, spleen, or intestine may be lacerated or ruptured. In fact, any internal organ could be affected.

Place the victim on one side in a comfortable position. Vomiting may occur. Combat shock by maintaining body warmth, giving no liquids unless hours from a medical facility, and keeping the victim lying on his side in case of vomiting. Seek medical attention for the victim.

Penetrating injuries: This type of injury presents a special problem. Assume that major damage has occurred. In these injuries, hollow organs are usually lacerated.

If a penetrating object is still in place, leave it and bandage it so that external bleeding is controlled and the object is stable. Do not withdraw it. If there is vomiting, place the victim on his side. Make the victim as comfortable as possible and seek medical attention.

Protruding organs: When an injury has resulted in the abdominal organs lying outside the abdominal cavity, do not try to replace them within the abdomen. Cover them with a moist, sterile dressing. It is important to cover extruding organs and to keep them moist and warm. Do not cover protruding organs with material that clings or loses its substance when wet (e.g., cotton). Time will be lost in surgery in removing the mess. (*See* Figure 6-4.)

Summary: For all abdominal injuries, suspect shock and work to prevent it. Be alert for vomitus and turn the victim on his side if it does occur. Afterwards, wipe the mouth out. Do not remove penetrating objects, but control bleeding and stabilize the object. Do not touch protruding organs, but cover them with a sterile dressing and keep the dressing moist. Do not give anything to eat or drink.

FOREIGN OBJECTS

Managing foreign objects in the body is relatively simple and straightforward as long as the first aider follows some basic treatment principles.

6 / SPECIFIC BODY AREA INJURIES 81

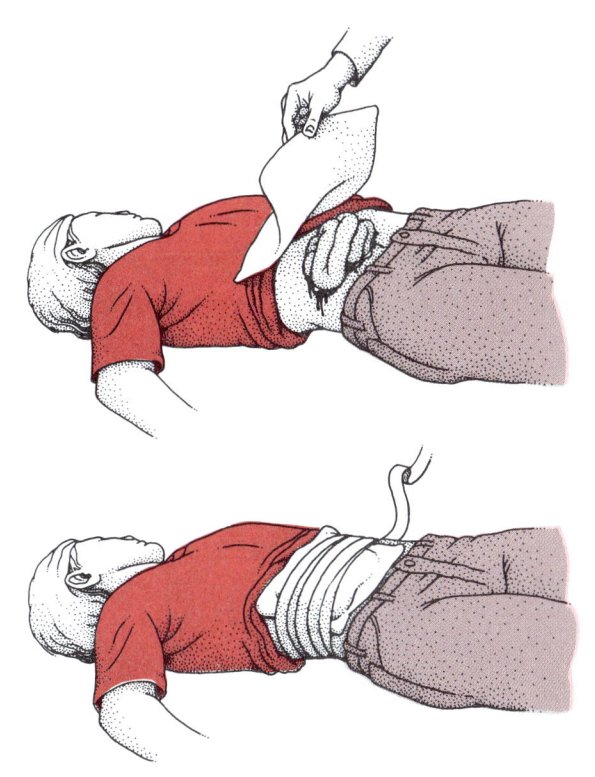

6-4. Protruding organs. Do not replace them. Cover them with a moist, sterile dressing.

The most basic principle of emergency care is to keep things simple. You usually do not need a lot of supplies and equipment to care for a victim with a foreign object embedded somewhere in his or her body. Another basic principle that needs repeating is to treat the *entire* victim. Do not let the obvious injury lure you to overlook other possibilities such as prevention and care of shock.

Eyes

The most common eye injury may be due to a foreign body that has been blown onto the outer surface of the eye. Common foreign bodies include eyelashes, sand, soot, cinders, chips of rust, paint, and metal shavings.

Most foreign bodies are flushed out of the eye by a large amount of tears produced by the irritation. However, sometimes the foreign body remains and must be removed either by a first aider or someone with greater medical expertise.

Foreign bodies on the eye are often difficult to see and must be looked for carefully. Usually such foreign bodies lodge under the upper lid. In this case, the first method to try is to gently rinse the eye by pouring clean water over the eye. If this method does not work, the foreign body is probably stuck under the upper lid and the lid will have to be everted to get the foreign body out. To evert a lid, ask the victim to look down while you grasp the eyelash of their upper lid between your thumb and index finger. Place a smooth narrow object horizontally along the outer surface of the eyelid, and then pull the eyelid gently forward and upward so that it folds back on itself over the smooth narrow object. (*See* Figure 6-5.)

When the foreign object is found, try to remove it with a dampened (not dry) sterile gauze. Do not, however, use another object (i.e., toothpick, match stick) to remove the foreign body if it is lying on the surface of the eyeball. If you are unsuccessful, you should patch both eyes and transport the victim to a medical facility.

Do not try to remove an impaled foreign object. It should be stabilized in place. One way to do this is to take a stack of 4-inch gauze pads and cut a hole in the center of the stack large enough to fit over the object. Then carefully pass the stack of gauze pads over the object, so that the dressing is resting gently against the surrounding skin. To prevent the impaled object from being caught or jarred, position a paper cup or similar item over the gauze pads so that the object is enclosed within it but not touching it. Fasten the paper cup in place. (*See* Figure 6-6.)

When patching the injured eye, the uninjured eye should also be patched. The reason for patching the uninjured eye is that normally both eyes move together. If the uninjured eye starts looking around to check out the scenery, the eye with the impaled object will move as well, and this can further damage the injured eye. When covering both eyes, take time to explain to the victim what you are doing and why the patch is necessary.

82 FIRST AID ESSENTIALS

Nose

Foreign bodies in the nose are a problem mainly among small children who seem to gain some satisfaction from putting peanuts, beans, raisins, and similar objects in their nostrils.

A foreign object in the nose can usually be removed by one of several methods:

1. Sneeze out the foreign object by sniffing pepper or tickling the opposite nostril.
2. Blow gently as the opposite nostril is compressed.
3. Use tweezers to pull out an object that is easily visible. Be careful not to push on it and lodge it farther in the nostril. Some experts do not suggest this procedure because the object may have penetrated the nasal tissues.
4. Consult a physician if the object cannot be expelled. Probing into a nostril may jam the foreign body deeper into the nose.

Ears

Various foreign bodies such as insects, seeds, match sticks, and cotton can become lodged in the ear canal. This type of emergency most often occurs with young children.

Do *not* try to kill a lodged insect by poking something in the ear. Insects are attracted to light, so it may be coaxed out with light. If outdoors, pull the earlobe gently to straighten the canal and turn the ear toward the sun. If indoors, turn off all the lights and shine a flashlight into the ear while pulling gently on the earlobe. The insect might crawl out toward the light.

6-5. Loose or invisible object in eye
(a) If tears or gentle flushing do not remove object, gently pull lower lid down. Remove an object by gently flushing with lukewarm water or a wet sterile gauze.
(b) If no object is seen inside lower lid, check the upper lid.
(c) Tell the person to look down. Pull gently downward on upper eyelashes. Lay a swab or match stick across the top of the lid.
(d) Fold the lid over the swab or match stick. Remove an object by gently flushing with lukewarm water or a wet sterile gauze.

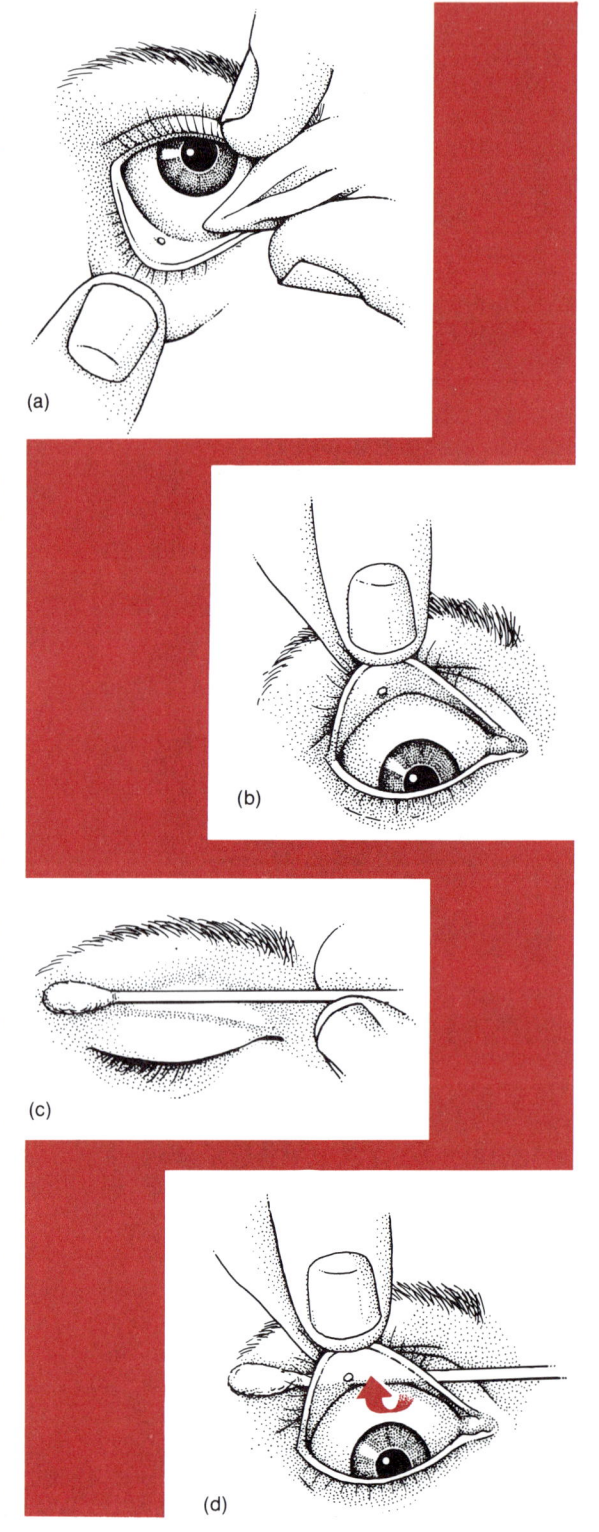

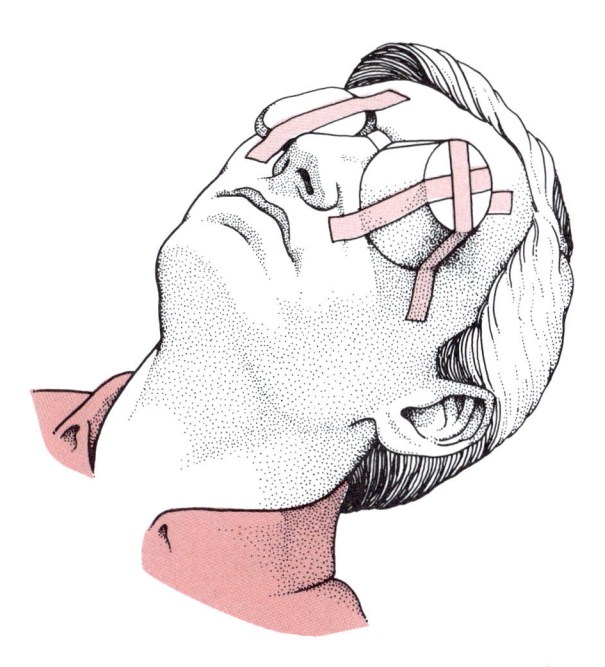

6-6. Use paper cup or make paper cone to cover the impaled object or an avulsed eye.

Cheek

An impaled object in the cheek should be removed quickly. As long as the object remains impaled in the cheek, it will be impossible to control blood flowing into the mouth and throat and, if dislodged, the object may pose a threat as an airway obstruction.

Removal of an impaled object in the cheek represents the only situation where it is permissible for a first aider to remove an impaled object. If the cheek is perforated, carefully remove the impaled object by pulling it out in the direction it entered the cheek. If it cannot be easily done, leave the object in place.

Once the object is removed, pack the space between the cheek and gums with gauze pads and apply pressure against the packing with a dressing held against the outside of the cheek. Periodically check the packing inside because it could induce gagging or block the airway.

Abdomen and Chest

When an object is impaled in the abdomen or chest, do not remove the object because serious bleeding and further damage may occur to nerves, blood vessels, or other tissue.

If there is external bleeding, control it by direct pressure on the surrounding tissue but not on the impaled object.

Place bulky dressings around the object to immobilize it. Do *not* shorten the impaled object unless is is too long. It must be stabilized in place to prevent motion.

Most cases of foreign objects usually require medical attention. Obvious exceptions are small splinters embedded under the skin.

Most impaled objects can be treated in a similar way as shown in Figure 6-7.

Fishhook Embedded

When only the point and not the barb of a fishhook penetrates the skin, you can easily remove a fishhook by backing the hook out. However, if the barb of the hook enters the skin, follow these procedures:

If the light method fails, inserting a little oil (mineral, baby, or olive oil) may cause the insect to float out when you turn the victim's ear down and allow the oil to run out. Do not use this method if you are not absolutely sure that the foreign body in the ear is an insect because, if it is a bean, popcorn, or other similar object, it may swell and be difficult to move.

Do *not* go into the ear canal with a pin, toothpick, or other slender object to remove foreign bodies. These items may force the object farther into the ear and damage the lining of the ear canal or eardrum.

Some experts recommend that foreign bodies can occasionally be jarred loose from an ear canal by gently pounding with the hand on the opposite side of the head with the affected ear held down. Other experts do not recommend this procedure.

If the object cannot be seen or cannot be easily removed, seek medical attention.

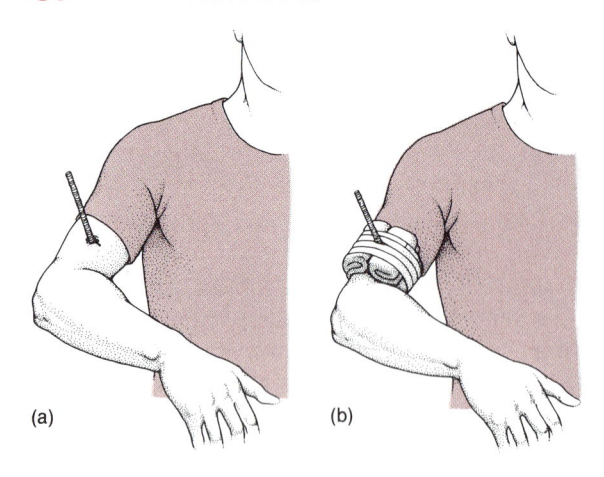

6-7. Impaled object
(a) Do not remove nor disturb.
(b) Control bleeding by applying direct pressure to the wound. Stabilize the impaled object.

1. If the medical care is near, transport the victim and have a physican remove the hook.

2. If in a remote area far from medical care, remove the hook by either the pliers method or the fishline method.

Pliers Method
You must have pliers with tempered jaws that will cut through a hook. Cut through an extra hook to ensure that the pliers are capable of cutting through a hook. If so, use cold or hard pressure to provide temporary anesthesia. Then push the embedded barb further in, in a shallow curve, until the point and barb come out through the skin. Cut the barb off and back the hook out the way it came in. After removing the hook, treat the wound. Most of the time the proper kind of pliers is lacking or the barb is buried too deeply to be pushed on through. (*See* Figure 6-8.)

Fishline Method
Loop a piece of fishline over the eye of the embedded hook and bring it down to the middle of the hook's curve. Immobilize the victim's hand (or wherever the hook is embedded). Use cold or hard pressure to provide temporary anesthesia. With your other hand, press down and back on the eye of the hook as you sharply jerk the hook

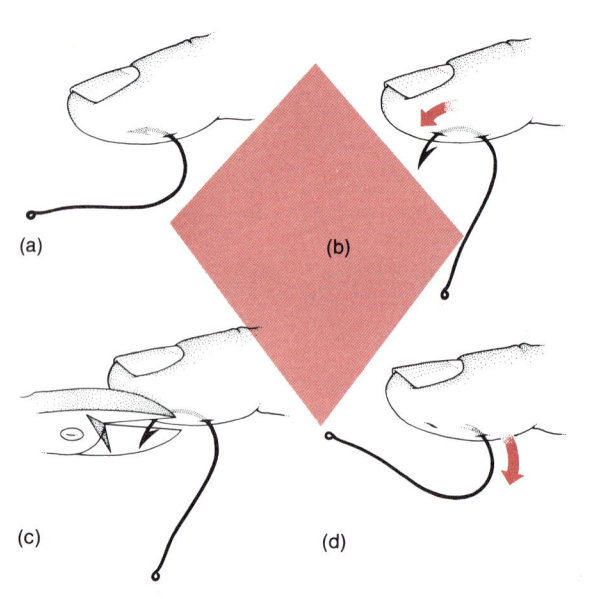

6-8. Pliers method

with the loop. The jerk movement should be parallel to the skin surface. The hook will neatly come out of the same hole it entered, causing little pain. After removing the hook, treat the wound. (*See* Figure 6-9.)

HAND AND FINGER INJURIES

The hand is a marvel of structural organization that, considering its complexity, is able to sustain considerable abuse. Nevertheless, hands may often be injured. Fractures, often the results of direct blows, are among the most serious injuries that occur to the hand and fingers and are discussed in Chapter Ten.

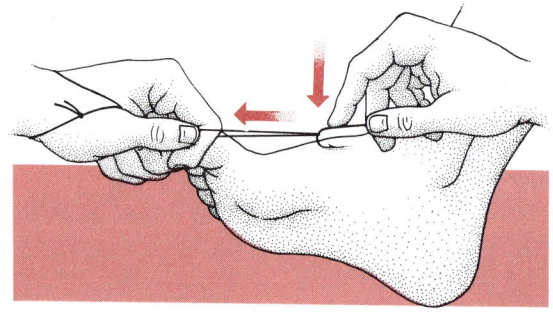

6-9. Fish line method

Fingernail Hematoma

Any direct blow to the fingertip or to the fingernail can cause the accumulation of blood directly beneath the nail. A purple discoloration is visible under the nail. This is a minor injury but is an extremely painful condition because of the accumulation of blood underneath the fingernail.

First aid: The victim should place the finger in ice water until the hemorrhage ceases. If painful, the pressure of blood should then be released from under the fingernail. The entrapped blood may be released in two different ways. One way is to use a sharp knife to drill by rotary action drill a hole through the fingernail. A second way, which is faster, is to heat a paper clip to a red-hot temperature and to lay the red-hot paper clip on the surface of the nail with moderate pressure. This melts a hole through the nail to the site of the blood. The nail has no nerves, thus there will be no pain. Be sure not to pierce the nail unless a blood blister is really present. (*See* Figure 6-10.)

Laceration

A laceration that involves the hand should not be considered a minor injury. It should be taken seriously because nerve and tendon damage can accompany lacerations. If there is any doubt as to the damage, consult an orthopedic or hand surgeon immediately. Standard treatment of bleeding should be applied before referral.

Splinters

If a splinter passes under the nail and breaks off flush, you may remove it by grasping the end of it with tweezers, after cutting a V-shaped notch in the nail to gain access to the splinter.

Finger Avulsion

The finger is the body part that becomes avulsed or amputated most often.

First aid: Successful reimplantation of amputated body parts has become common. Blood loss in cases of complete amputations is often surprisingly quite minimal. Direct pressure controls most bleeding. You should retrieve the amputated part and follow these procedures:

1. Wrap the amputated part with a gauze or cloth. Do not immerse the part in water.
2. If possible, put the wrapped part in a plastic bag or container.
3. Place the wrapped, amputated part on a bed of ice, but do not submerge.
4. Seek medical attention immediately.

If the part is still partially attached by a tendon or a piece of skin, the part can still be wrapped and ice placed on it after it is repositioned in the normal position.

Ring Removal

Most rings stuck on fingers are removed with a combination of lubrication and gentle tugging. But sometimes a finger is too swollen for the ring to be removed in the usual manner. Removal is simple with a ring cutter—if it is available. If not, try the following techniques:

1. Slide the ring off after lubricating the finger with grease, oil, butter, petroleum jelly, or some other slippery substance.

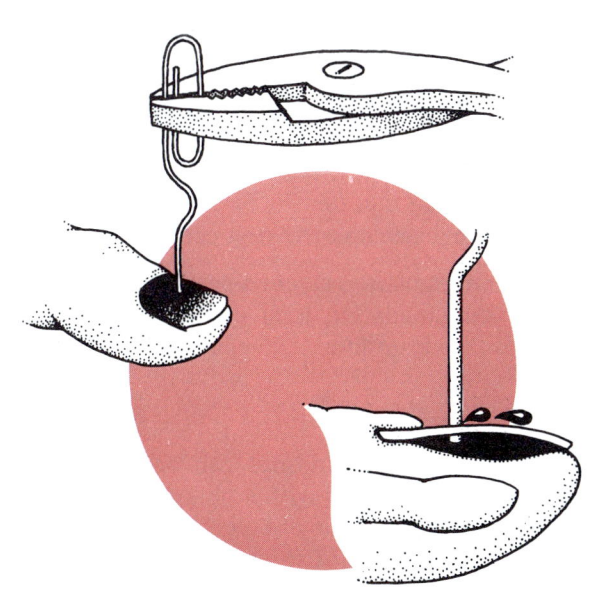

6-10. Making a hole in a fingernail

2. Immerse the finger in ice water for several minutes in an effort to reduce the swelling. Move the ring to a point on the finger where it is loose. Gently massage the finger from tip to hand; this may move the fluid from the swollen area. After a few minutes of massaging, lubricate the finger again and try to slip the ring off.

3. Slide three or four inches of thin string under the ring toward the hand. (*See* Figure 6-11.) The string may need to be pushed through with a match stick or toothpick. Then wrap the string tightly around the finger below the ring for about three-quarters of an inch, going toward the fingernail and away from the ring. Each wrap should be right next to the one before. While holding the wrapping snugly in place with the fingers of one hand, grasp the upper end of the string with the other hand. Pull the string downward over the ring. This starts an unwrapping process. If the finger is not too badly swollen, the ring may slide over the string that is still wrapped around the finger and continue to move as you continue to unwrap. It may be necessary to repeat the procedure several times to get the ring completely off the finger.

4. Start about three-quarters of an inch to one inch from the ring edge and smoothly wind string around the finger going toward the ring with one strand touching the next. Continue winding smoothly and tightly right up to the edge of the ring. The advantage of this method is that it tends to push the swelling toward the hand. Slip the end of the string under and through the ring. (You may have to push it through with a match stick or toothpick.) Slowly unwind the string on the hand side of the ring and the ring is gently twisted off the finger over the spiraled string.

5. Carefully cut the narrowest portion of the ring with a ring saw, jeweler's saw, ring cutter, or a fine hacksaw blade. If anything other than a ring saw is used, take care to protect exposed portions of the finger.

6. Inflate an ordinary balloon about three-quarters full. Tie the end. The slender tube-shaped balloons work best. Insert the victim's swollen finger into the end of the balloon so that the balloon rolls back evenly around the finger. In about fifteen minutes the finger should return to its normal size and the ring can be removed.

Ring strangulation can be a serious problem if it cuts off circulation long enough. Gangrene may result within four or five hours.

Bandaging

All hand and finger injuries can be effectively bandaged and dressed with a bulky hand dressing. The injured hand is formed into what is called the "position of function" (finger joints flexed moderately similar to the position in which one would most comfortably hold a

(a)

(b)

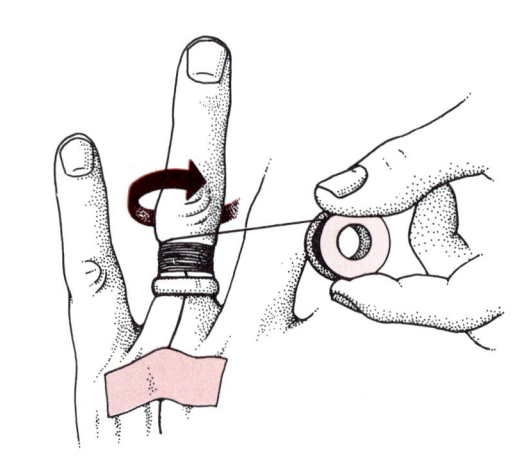

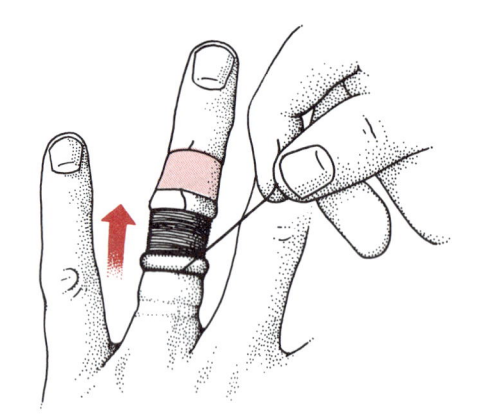

6-11. Ring removal with string

6 / SPECIFIC BODY AREA INJURIES

baseball). A roller bandage is then placed in the palm of the hand. A padded board splint is applied to the palm side of the hand and secured with a roller bandage. (*See* Figure 12-16.)

BLISTERS

Because many activities involve walking, running, jumping, and other such motions, it is not surprising that the feet have more than their fair share of skin injuries. Perhaps the most common skin injuries are blisters due to friction. Blisters are most often caused by ill-fitting shoes or wrinkled socks.

Blisters can be avoided by buying properly fitting shoes or boots, breaking the shoes/boots in prior to their extensive use, putting adhesive tape over the areas that are prone to blister, or wearing two pairs of socks. The inner pair should be of form-fitting, thin material, and the outer pair should be made of bulkier wool or a wool blend. A person can also apply Vaseline™ to cut down on the friction.

Once a blister has formed, you should prevent further injury by covering the blister with tape, moleskin, or a doughnut of gauze or felt cut in a doughnut shape. It is best to leave blisters unbroken, whenever possible. If the pain is unbearable, then the blister can be broken.

When a blister must be broken, first wash the area with soap and water. Then make a small hole at the base of the blister with a sterilized needle. Sterilize the needle by either soaking it in rubbing alcohol or holding it over the top of a match flame. (*See* Figure 6-12.)

Drain the fluid and apply a sterile dressing to protect the area from further irritation. In some cases, the blister may have to be drained up to three times in the first twenty-four hours. Roofs of blisters should remain intact.

If a blister has ruptured and its roof is gone, apply a sterile dressing. All ruptured blisters should be cleaned with soap and water to prevent infection.

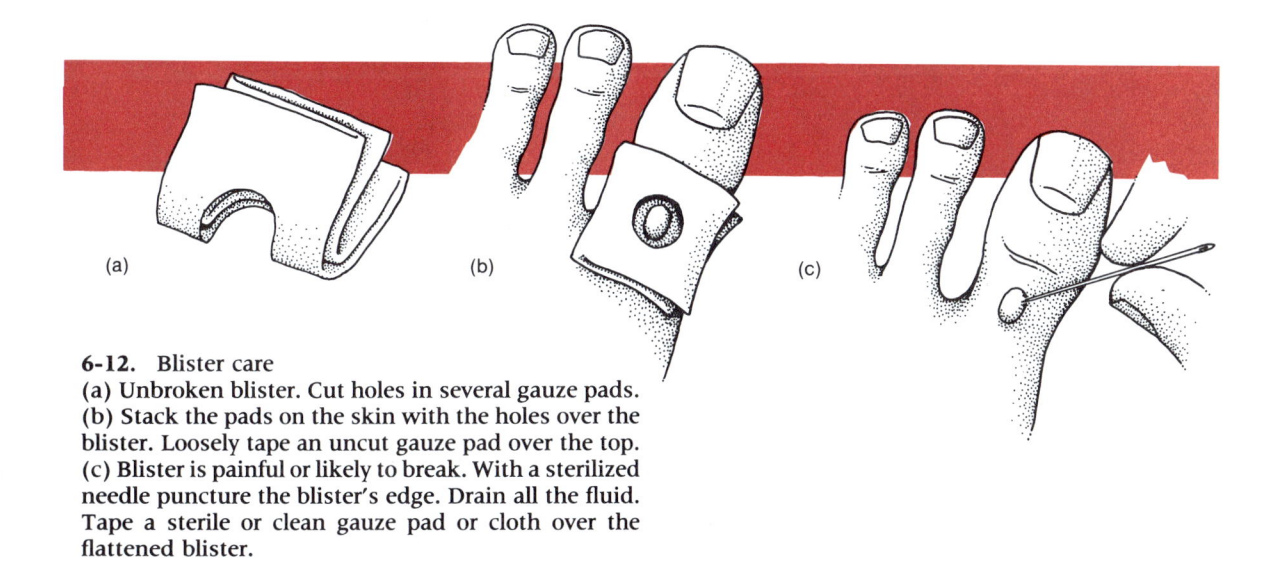

6-12. Blister care
(a) Unbroken blister. Cut holes in several gauze pads.
(b) Stack the pads on the skin with the holes over the blister. Loosely tape an uncut gauze pad over the top.
(c) Blister is painful or likely to break. With a sterilized needle puncture the blister's edge. Drain all the fluid. Tape a sterile or clean gauze pad or cloth over the flattened blister.

Head Injury

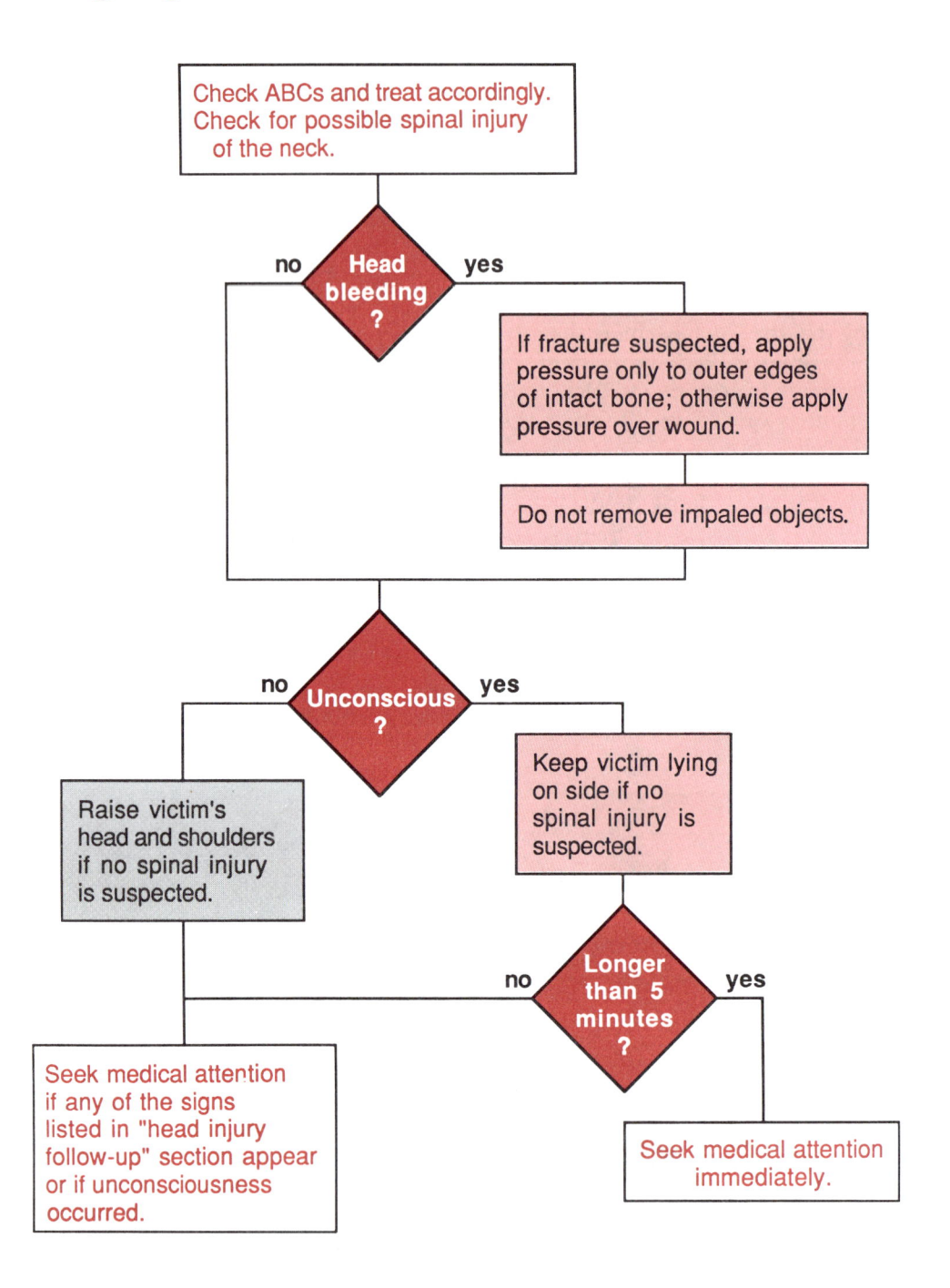

- Check ABCs and treat accordingly. Check for possible spinal injury of the neck.

Head bleeding?

- **yes**: If fracture suspected, apply pressure only to outer edges of intact bone; otherwise apply pressure over wound.
  - Do not remove impaled objects.

Unconscious?

- **no**: Raise victim's head and shoulders if no spinal injury is suspected.
  - Seek medical attention if any of the signs listed in "head injury follow-up" section appear or if unconsciousness occurred.

- **yes**: Keep victim lying on side if no spinal injury is suspected.

Longer than 5 minutes?

- **no**: Seek medical attention if any of the signs listed in "head injury follow-up" section appear or if unconsciousness occurred.
- **yes**: Seek medical attention immediately.

Eye Injuries

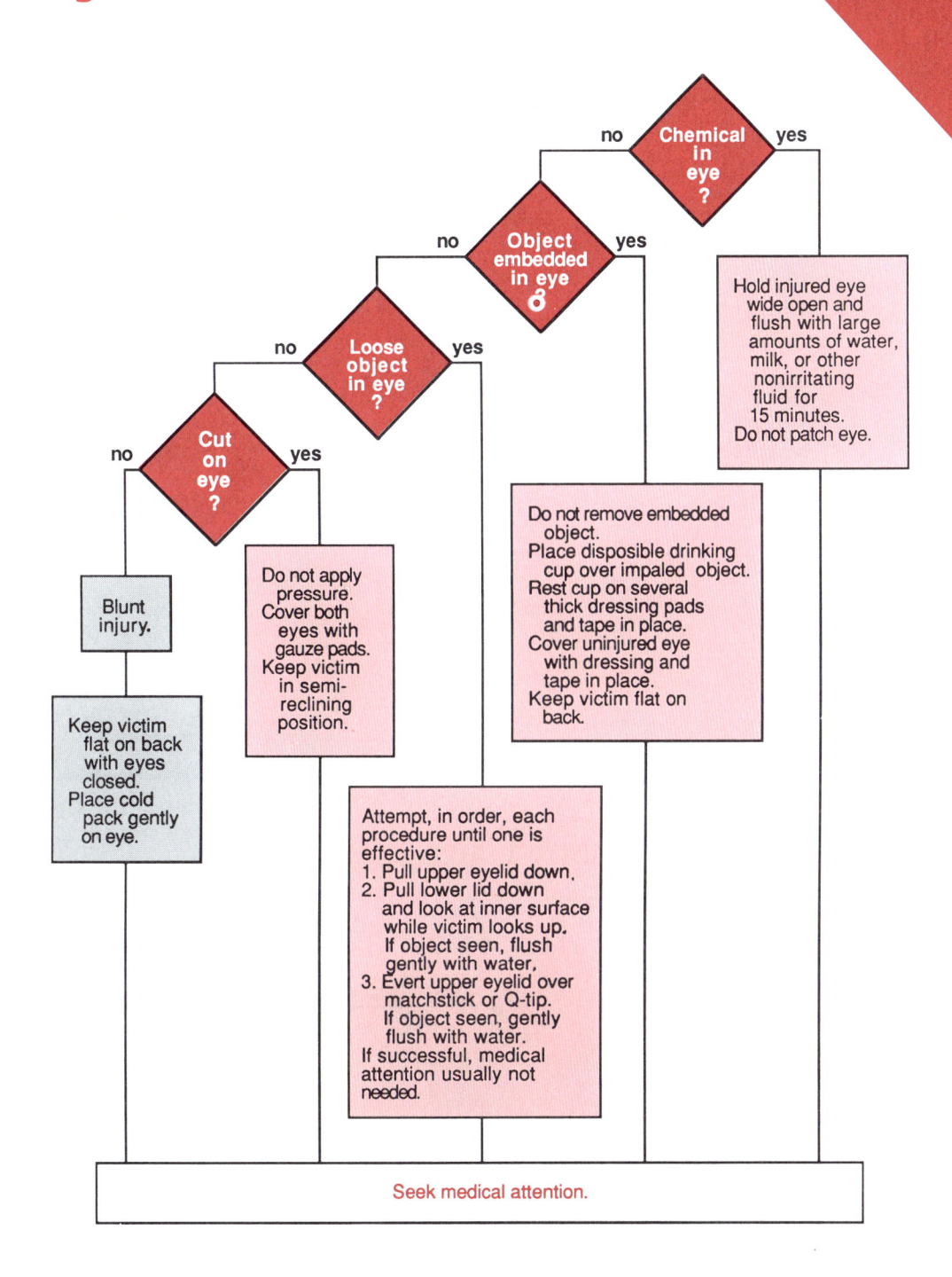

Chemical in eye?
- yes → Hold injured eye wide open and flush with large amounts of water, milk, or other nonirritating fluid for 15 minutes. Do not patch eye.
- no ↓

Object embedded in eye?
- yes → Do not remove embedded object. Place disposible drinking cup over impaled object. Rest cup on several thick dressing pads and tape in place. Cover uninjured eye with dressing and tape in place. Keep victim flat on back.
- no ↓

Loose object in eye?
- yes → Attempt, in order, each procedure until one is effective:
  1. Pull upper eyelid down.
  2. Pull lower lid down and look at inner surface while victim looks up. If object seen, flush gently with water.
  3. Evert upper eyelid over matchstick or Q-tip. If object seen, gently flush with water.

  If successful, medical attention usually not needed.
- no ↓

Cut on eye?
- yes → Do not apply pressure. Cover both eyes with gauze pads. Keep victim in semi-reclining position.
- no ↓

Blunt injury.

Keep victim flat on back with eyes closed. Place cold pack gently on eye.

Seek medical attention.

89

Nosebleeds

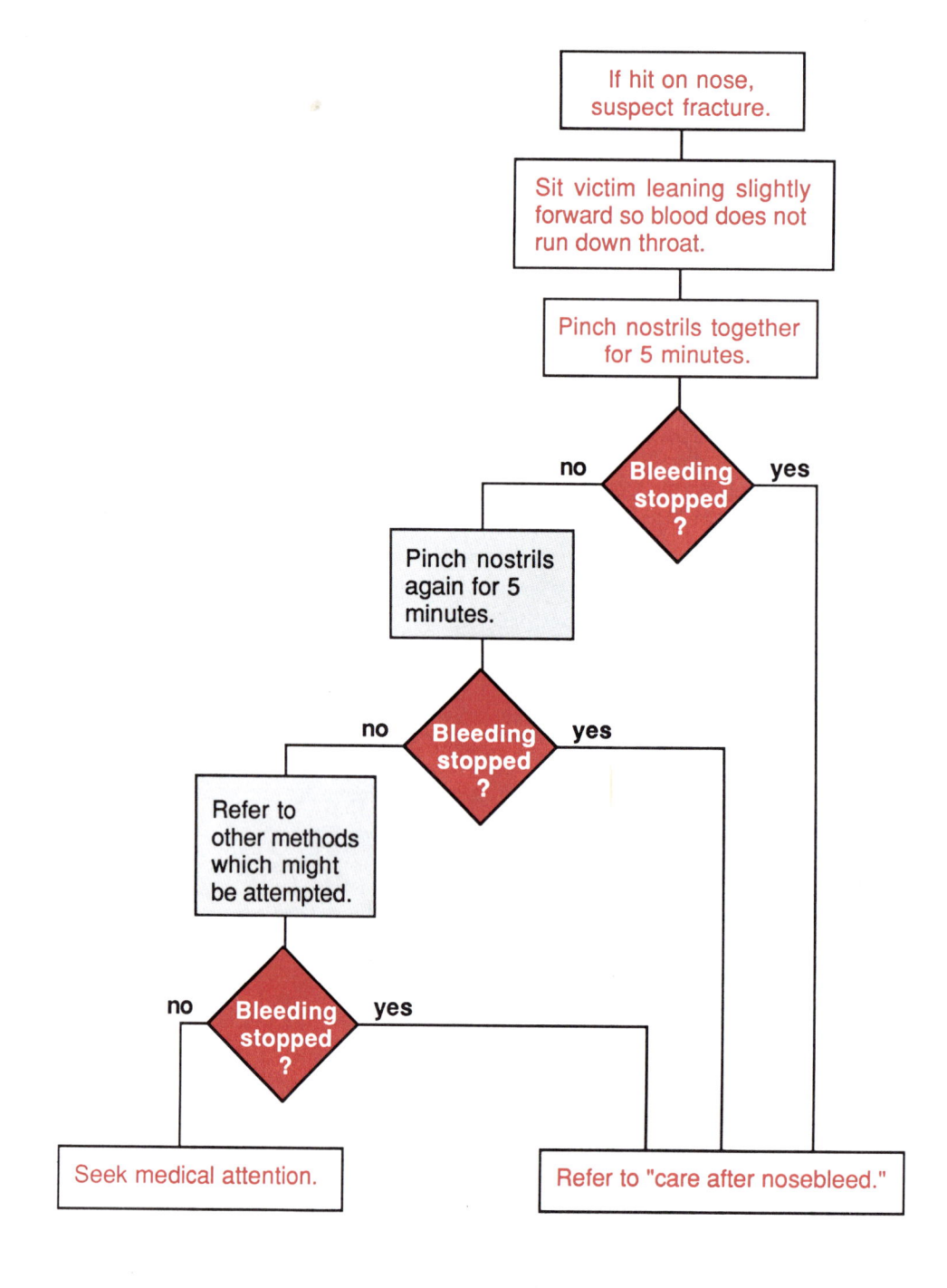

- If hit on nose, suspect fracture.
- Sit victim leaning slightly forward so blood does not run down throat.
- Pinch nostrils together for 5 minutes.
- **Bleeding stopped?**
  - yes → Refer to "care after nosebleed."
  - no → Pinch nostrils again for 5 minutes.
    - **Bleeding stopped?**
      - yes → Refer to "care after nosebleed."
      - no → Refer to other methods which might be attempted.
        - **Bleeding stopped?**
          - yes → Refer to "care after nosebleed."
          - no → Seek medical attention.

Tooth Injury

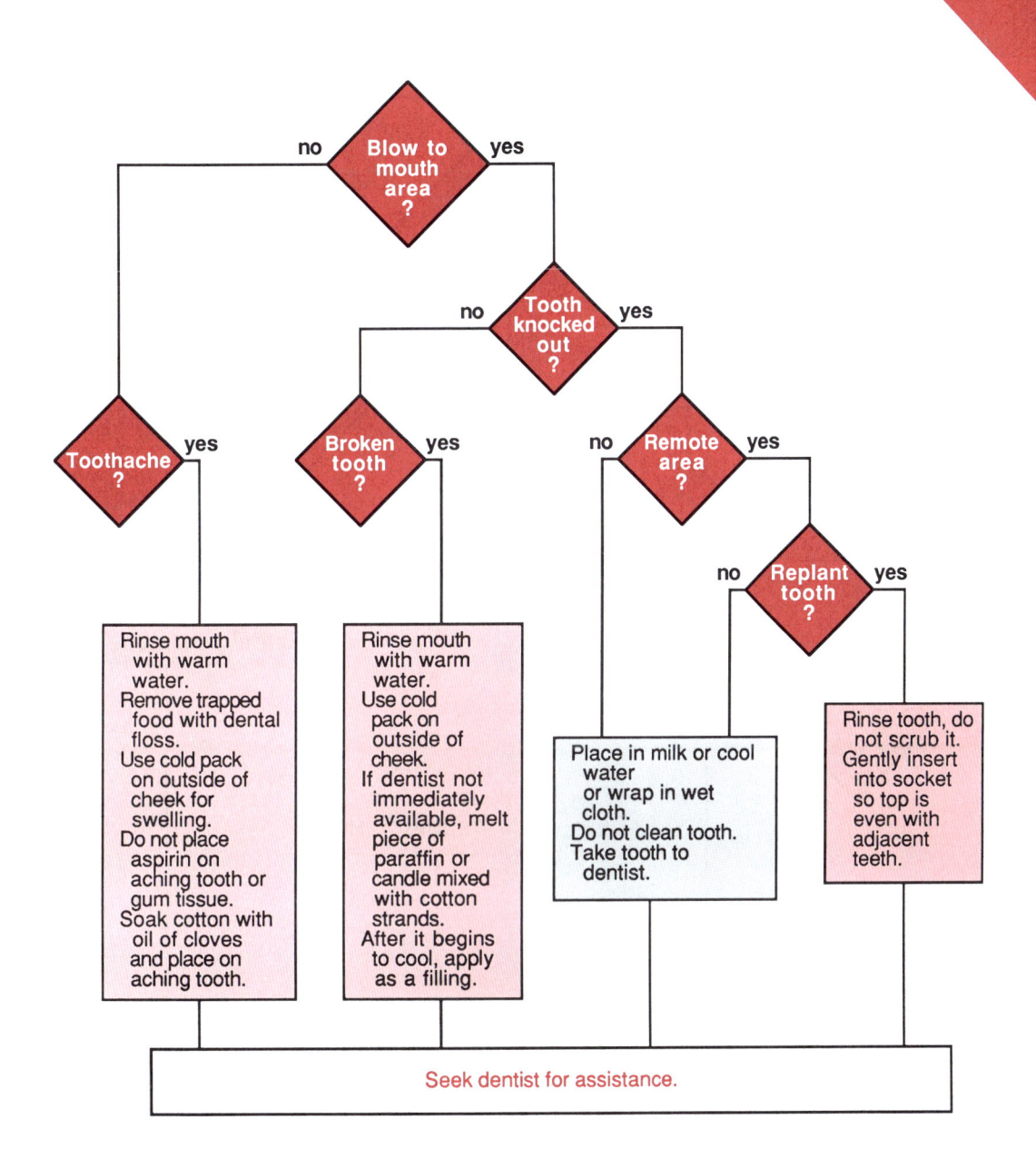

```
                        Blow to
              no        mouth       yes
         ┌──────────────  area  ──────────────┐
         │                  ?                 │
         │                                    │
         │                               Tooth
         │                    no       knocked      yes
         │              ┌───────────────  out  ───────────────┐
         │              │                  ?                  │
         │              │                                     │
      Toothache    Broken                              Remote
         ?   yes    tooth    yes                  no    area     yes
         ◆─────┐     ?  ─────┐                   ┌─────   ?   ─────┐
                                                 │                 │
                                                 │              Replant
                                                 │         no    tooth    yes
                                                 │        ┌───────  ?  ───────┐
```

Toothache path (yes):
Rinse mouth with warm water.
Remove trapped food with dental floss.
Use cold pack on outside of cheek for swelling.
Do not place aspirin on aching tooth or gum tissue.
Soak cotton with oil of cloves and place on aching tooth.

Broken tooth path (yes):
Rinse mouth with warm water.
Use cold pack on outside of cheek.
If dentist not immediately available, melt piece of paraffin or candle mixed with cotton strands. After it begins to cool, apply as a filling.

Remote area – no / Replant tooth – no:
Place in milk or cool water or wrap in wet cloth.
Do not clean tooth.
Take tooth to dentist.

Replant tooth – yes:
Rinse tooth, do not scrub it. Gently insert into socket so top is even with adjacent teeth.

Seek dentist for assistance.

91

Chest Injuries

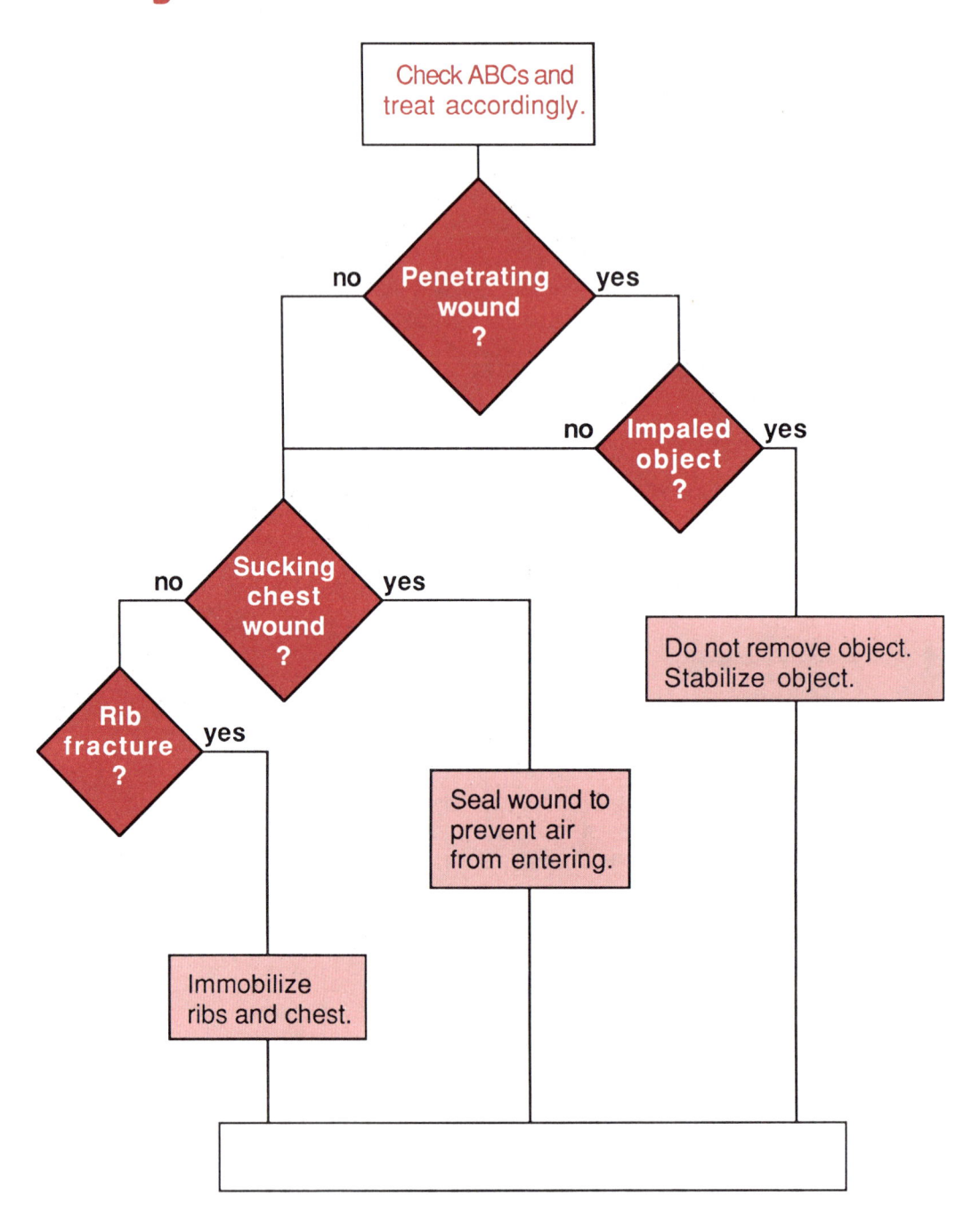

- Check ABCs and treat accordingly.
- Penetrating wound?
  - yes → Impaled object?
    - yes → Do not remove object. Stabilize object.
    - no → Sucking chest wound?
      - yes → Seal wound to prevent air from entering.
      - no → Rib fracture?
        - yes → Immobilize ribs and chest.
  - no → Sucking chest wound? (same as above)

Abdominal Injuries

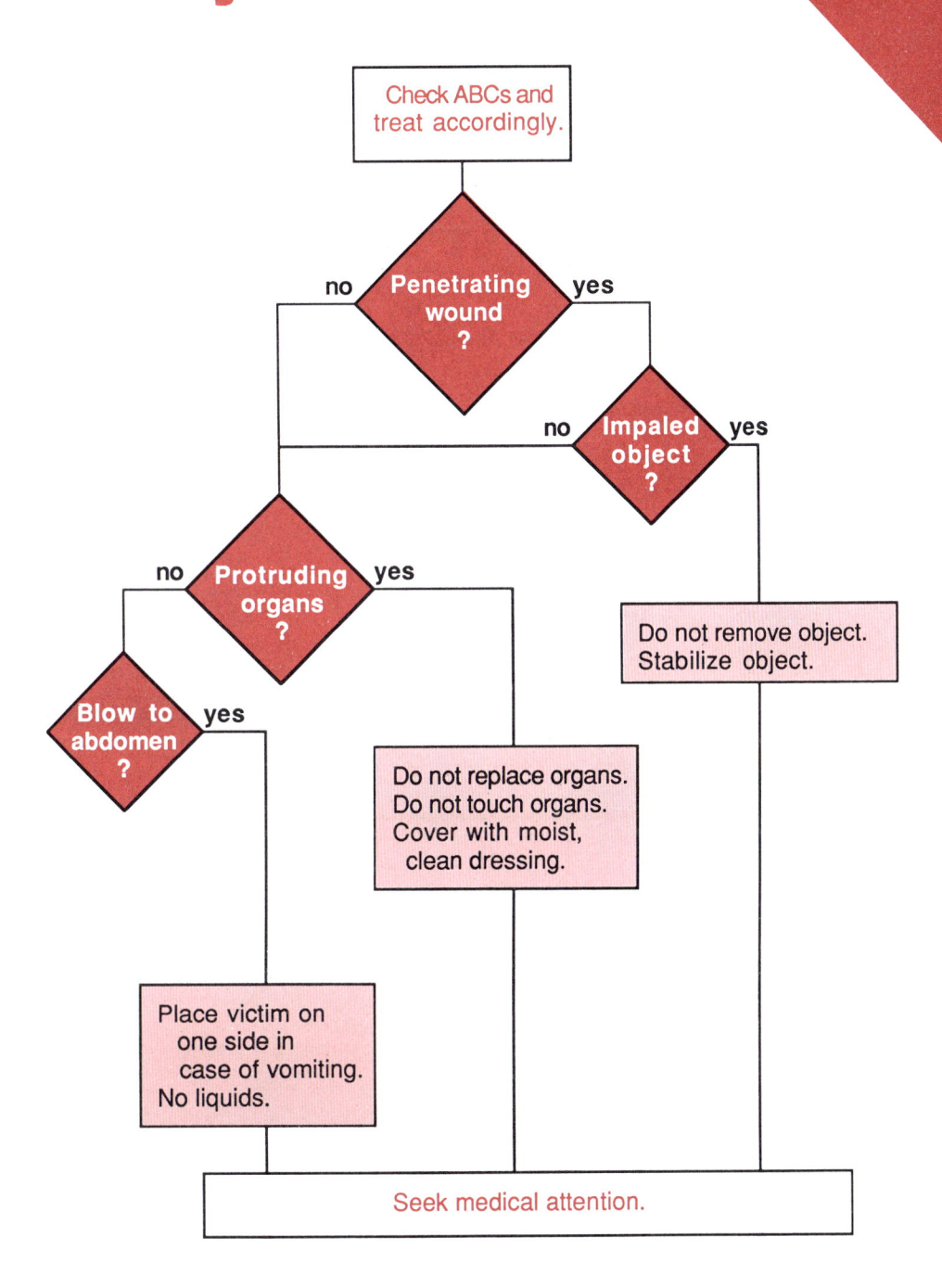

Check ABCs and treat accordingly.

Penetrating wound?
- yes → **Impaled object?**
  - yes → Do not remove object. Stabilize object.
  - no → **Protruding organs?**
    - yes → Do not replace organs. Do not touch organs. Cover with moist, clean dressing.
    - no → (continue)
- no → **Blow to abdomen?**
  - yes → Place victim on one side in case of vomiting. No liquids.

Seek medical attention.

Object In Nose

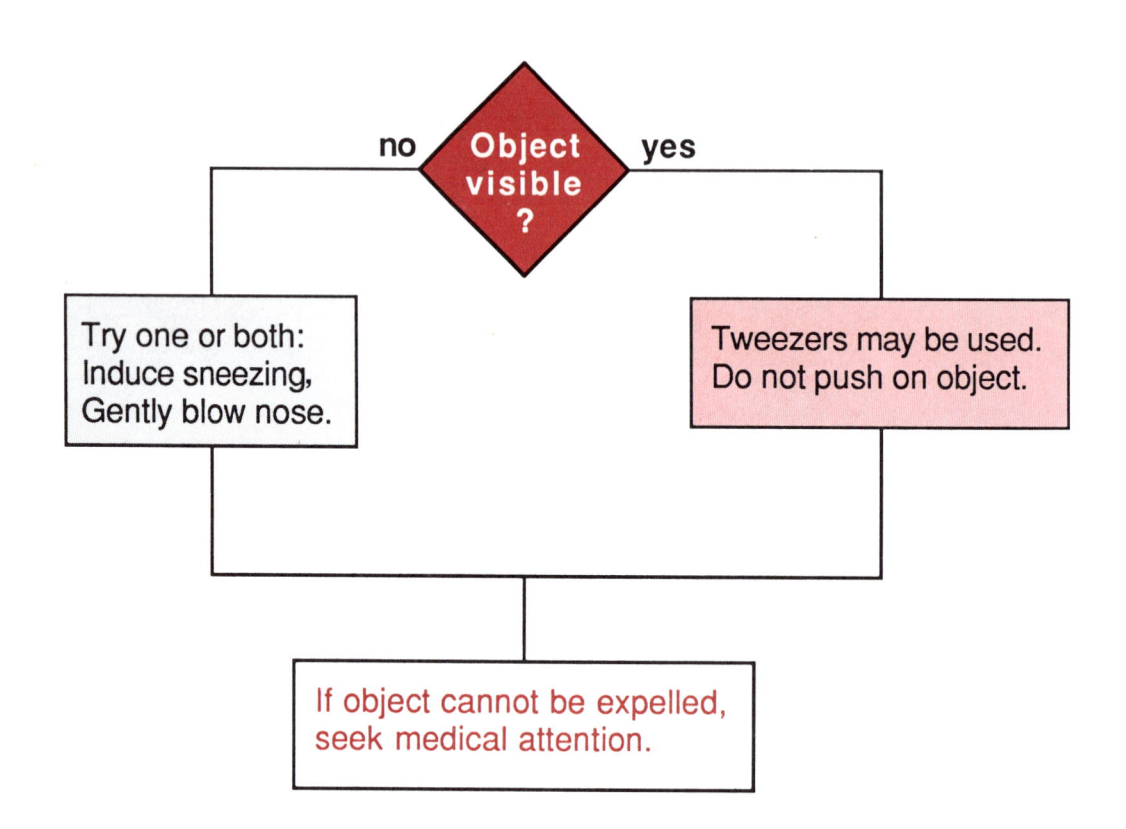

```
         Object
  no     visible    yes
            ?
```

Try one or both:
Induce sneezing,
Gently blow nose.

Tweezers may be used.
Do not push on object.

If object cannot be expelled, seek medical attention.

Object In Ear

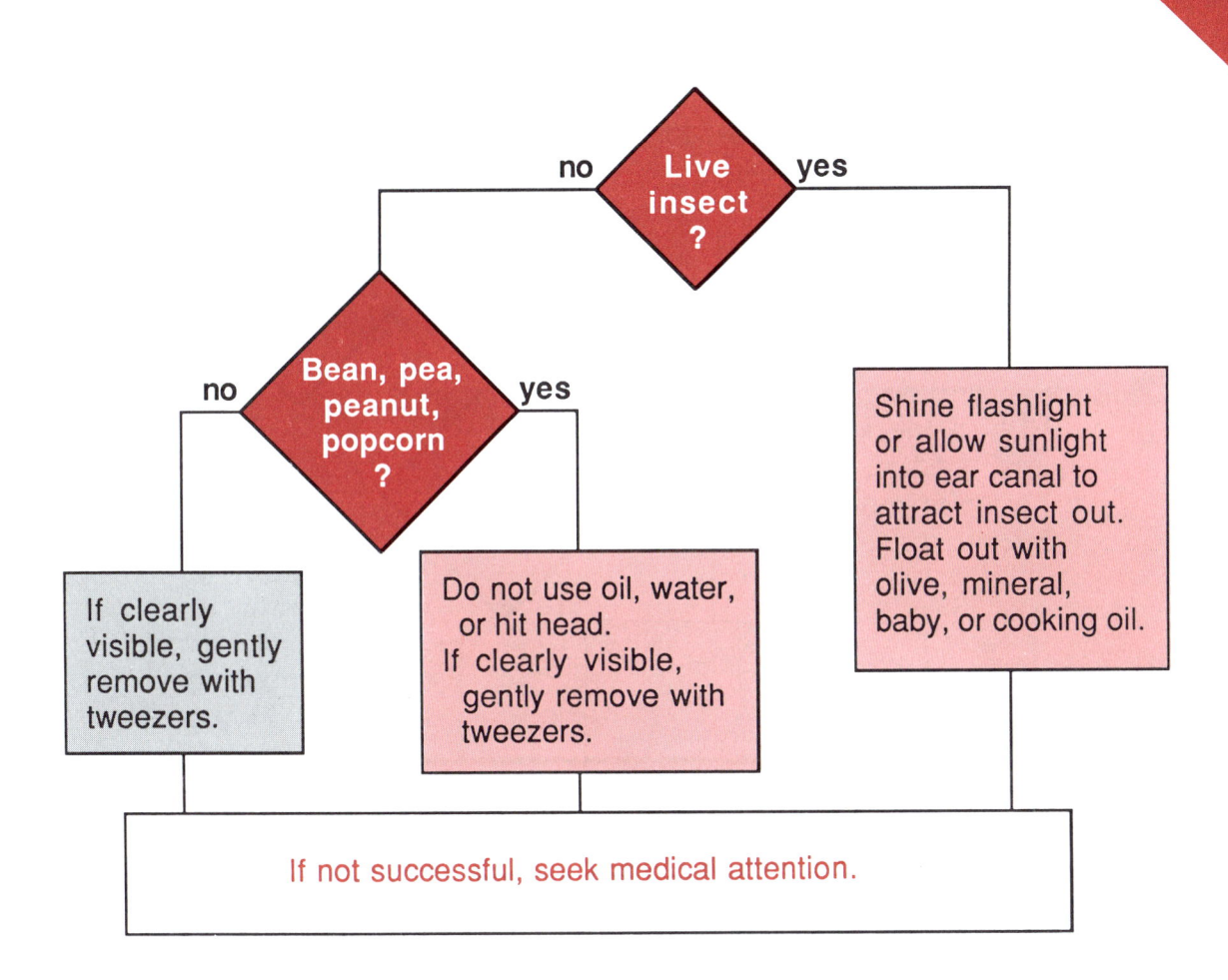

Live insect?
- **yes** → Shine flashlight or allow sunlight into ear canal to attract insect out. Float out with olive, mineral, baby, or cooking oil.
- **no** → **Bean, pea, peanut, popcorn?**
  - **yes** → Do not use oil, water, or hit head. If clearly visible, gently remove with tweezers.
  - **no** → If clearly visible, gently remove with tweezers.

If not successful, seek medical attention.

Fishhook Removal

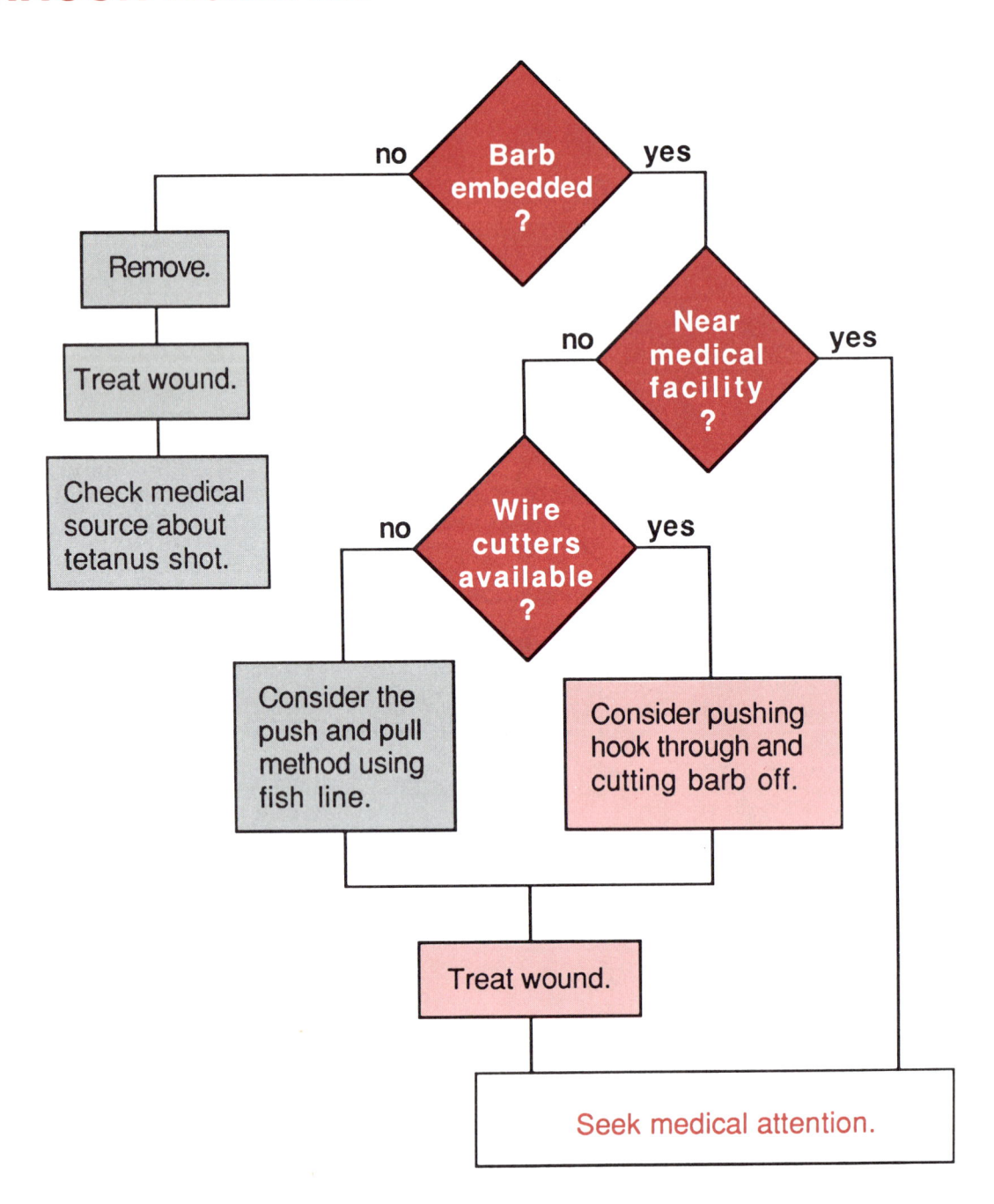

Barb embedded?
- no → Remove. → Treat wound. → Check medical source about tetanus shot.
- yes → **Near medical facility?**
  - yes → Seek medical attention.
  - no → **Wire cutters available?**
    - no → Consider the push and pull method using fish line. → Treat wound. → Seek medical attention.
    - yes → Consider pushing hook through and cutting barb off. → Treat wound. → Seek medical attention.

Blisters

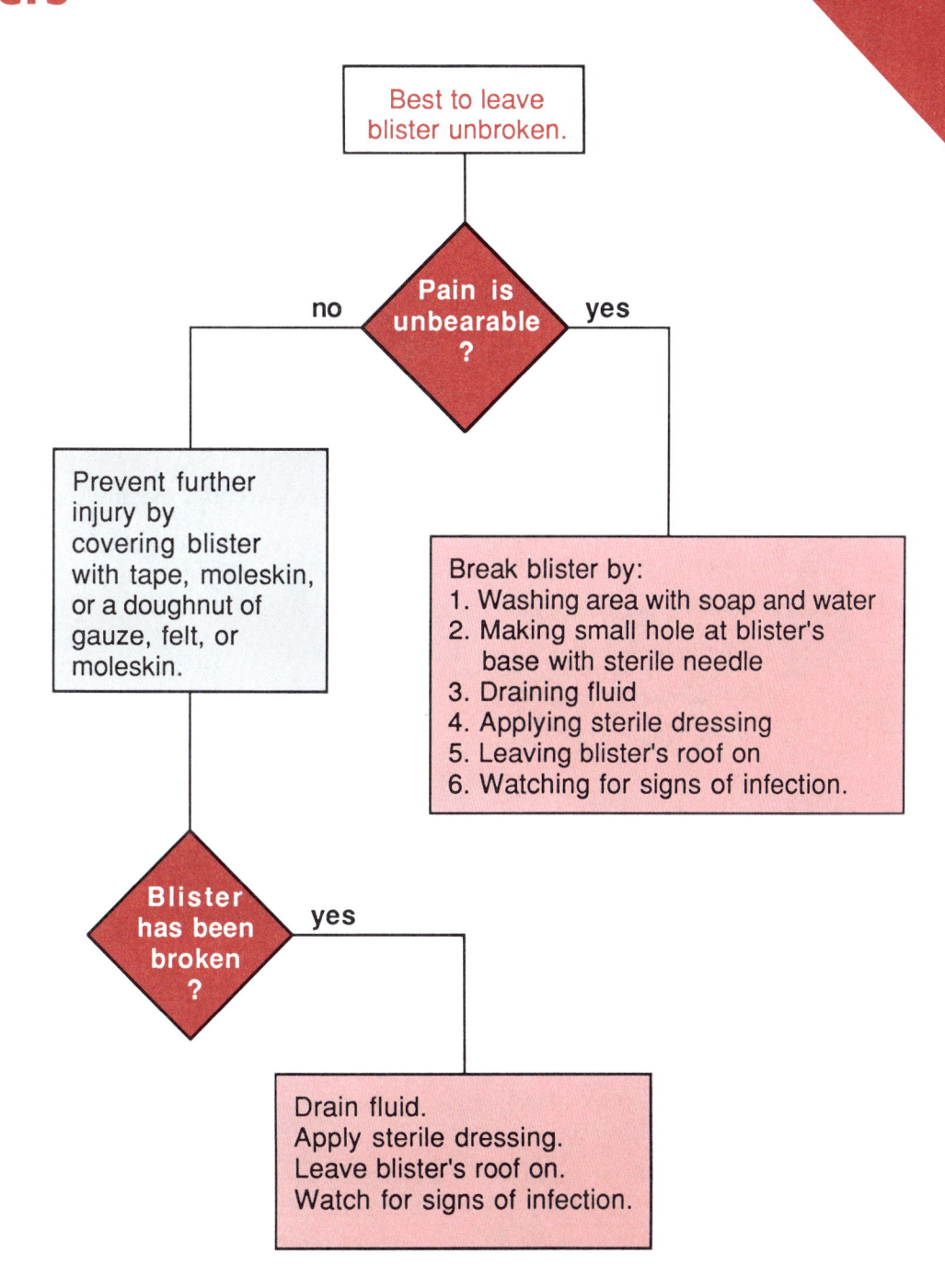

```
                    ┌─────────────────┐
                    │ Best to leave   │
                    │ blister unbroken.│
                    └─────────────────┘
                             │
                         ◇ Pain is
                  no   unbearable?   yes
            ┌────────              ────────┐
            │                              │
┌───────────────────────┐    ┌────────────────────────────────┐
│ Prevent further       │    │ Break blister by:              │
│ injury by             │    │ 1. Washing area with soap and  │
│ covering blister      │    │    water                       │
│ with tape, moleskin,  │    │ 2. Making small hole at blister's│
│ or a doughnut of      │    │    base with sterile needle    │
│ gauze, felt, or       │    │ 3. Draining fluid              │
│ moleskin.             │    │ 4. Applying sterile dressing   │
└───────────────────────┘    │ 5. Leaving blister's roof on   │
            │                │ 6. Watching for signs of infection. │
            │                └────────────────────────────────┘
         ◇ Blister
         has been    yes
         broken? ────────┐
                         │
             ┌──────────────────────────────┐
             │ Drain fluid.                 │
             │ Apply sterile dressing.      │
             │ Leave blister's roof on.     │
             │ Watch for signs of infection.│
             └──────────────────────────────┘
```

SELF-CHECK QUESTIONS

Activity 1: Head Injury

A. Skull Fracture

Choose the signs and symptoms of a skull fracture.

　　Yes　No
1. ☐　☐　Pain at the injury site
2. ☐　☐　Deformed skull
3. ☐　☐　Fluid leaking from ears or nose
4. ☐　☐　Discoloration around eye(s) (black eyes)
5. ☐　☐　Pupil of one eye larger than pupil of the other eye

B. After a head injury, which of the following signs indicate a need for medical attention?

　　Yes　No
1. ☐　☐　Headache lasting more than a day or increased severity
2. ☐　☐　Vomiting beginning hours after the initial injury
3. ☐　☐　One pupil appearing larger than the other
4. ☐　☐　Convulsions or seizures
5. ☐　☐　Seeing "double"

Activity 2: Eye Injury

A. Which represents proper first aid for an embedded object in the eye?

　　Yes　No
1. ☐　☐　Using a damp, sterile or clean cloth to remove an object lying on an eyeball's surface
2. ☐　☐　Using a toothpick, match stick, etc., to remove a foreign object
3. ☐　☐　For an embedded object, using a paper cup or similar item over the eye but not touching the object
4. ☐　☐　Allowing the victim to see by leaving the uninjured eye uncovered

B. Mark each statement true (T) or false (F).
1. ☐ Hitting the eye may cause a black eye.
2. ☐ An ophthalmologist should see blurred vision victims.
3. ☐ For an eyeball knocked out of socket, gently and carefully replace the eyeball in the socket and cover with a dressing.
4. ☐ After a blow to the eye apply a cold compress immediately for about 15 minutes to reduce pain and swelling.

C. A tree limb scraped against an eye results in a cut to the eyeball.

First aid, besides seeking medical help for the victim, includes:

Yes　No
1. ☐　☐ Applying a dressing tightly over the injured eye
2. ☐　☐ Holding the eyelids of the injured eye open
3. ☐　☐ Applying direct pressure to the cut eyeball in order to control the bleeding
4. ☐　☐ Loosely applying dressings over both eyes
5. ☐　☐ Tightly applying a dressing over both eyes

D. Corrosive acid has spilled into a coworker's eyes resulting in severe pain.

☐ Which one of the following actions should you take immediately?
1. Cover both eyes with dressings and immediately obtain medical aid.
2. Hold his eyes open and flood the eye with water for 15 minutes.
3. Allow tears to flush out the chemicals.
4. Pour water into his eyes for about 5 minutes.

☐ Following your initial actions, which one should you do?
1. Place wet dressings over both eyes.
2. Leave both eyes uncovered and seek medical attention.
3. Allow the victim to rest for at least 30 minutes.
4. Apply dressings over both eyes and seek medical attention.

E. A welder suffers ultraviolet light eye burns.

Mark which first aid procedures you should give.
1. ☐ Apply cold, wet dressings.
2. ☐ Have the victim rest with his eyes closed.
3. ☐ Do not cover the eyes.
4. ☐ Seek medical attention.

Activity 3: Nosebleeds

Choose the best techniques for controlling most nosebleeds.

	Choice 1		*Choice 2*
1. ☐	Position victim in a sitting position.	OR ☐	Position victim lying down.
2. ☐	Keep the head tilted or slightly backward.	OR ☐	Keep the head tilted slightly forward.
3. ☐	Pinch both nostrils for 5 minutes.	OR ☐	Pinch only one nostril for 60 seconds.
4. ☐	Always seek medical attention.	OR ☐	Seek medical attention for those taking blood thinners, large doses of aspirin, or those with high blood pressure.

Activity 4: Dental Injuries

Mark each statement true (T) or false (F).

1. ☐ Use dental floss rather than a toothpick to remove an object stuck between teeth.
2. ☐ If a tooth is knocked out, attempt reimplantation (placing tooth back in the socket) if in a remote area with no dentists nearby.
3. ☐ Clean and scrub the tooth before attempting to reimplant.
4. ☐ Put the knocked-out tooth in mouthwash or alcohol to preserve it.

Activity 5: Chest Injuries

A. Which of the following actions serve as effective immediate first aid for a penetrating chest wound?

Yes No
1. ☐ ☐ Remove a penetrating object from the chest.
2. ☐ ☐ Apply a sterile or clean dressing loosely over the wound.
3. ☐ ☐ Leave the wound uncovered.
4. ☐ ☐ Tape a piece of plastic tightly over the wound.

6 / SELF-CHECK QUESTIONS 101

B. You have taped a piece of plastic over a penetrating chest wound.

If difficult breathing occurs, check which action you should take:

1. ☐ Apply a second piece of plastic over the first.
2. ☐ Remove the plastic covering from the wound to allow air to escape from the chest cavity and then reapply.
3. ☐ Leave the plastic in place and check breathing.

C. Choose the correct completions for the following statements.
The aim of first aid for a penetrating chest wound is to:

Choice 1   *Choice 2*

1. ☐ Not cover the wound.   OR   ☐ Cover the chest's hole immediately to prevent air entering into the chest.

The aim of first aid for a flail chest is to:

2. ☐ Stabilize the injured chest wall.   OR   ☐ Not bind the injured chest since it interferes with breathing.

D. Which of the following materials, when taped at the edges, would make an effective covering for a penetrating chest wound?

    Yes   No
1. ☐ ☐ Clear plastic wrap
2. ☐ ☐ A large gauze dressing
3. ☐ ☐ Aluminum foil
4. ☐ ☐ A plastic bag
5. ☐ ☐ A pillow case

E. Flail chest signs and symptoms include:

    Yes   No
1. ☐ ☐ Blood oozing from the injury site
2. ☐ ☐ Victim complaining about pain when breathing
3. ☐ ☐ The victim having a neck injury
4. ☐ ☐ Part of the chest wall moving abnormally during breathing

Activity 6: Abdominal Injuries

A. Which represents proper first aid for a blow to the abdomen? You suspect internal injuries.

Choice 1 | *Choice 2*

1. ☐ Place the victim on his back with a support on his abdomen.   OR   ☐ Place the victim on his side.

2. ☐ Give him ice chips or sips of water to drink.   OR   ☐ Give him nothing to eat or drink.

B. Select the best first aid choice for a victim's abdominal open wound resulting from a penetrating object.

Choice 1 | *Choice 2*

☐ Remove the penetrating object.   OR   ☐ Leave object in place and stabilize it.

C. When protruding organs appear through an abdominal wound, you should

Choice 1 | *Choice 2*

1. ☐ Gently push the organs back into the abdomen   OR   ☐ Not attempt to push them back into the abdomen

2. ☐ Cover the wound with a clean, moist dressing   OR   ☐ Cover the wound with a cotton dressing

Activity 7: Foreign Objects

Which of the following actions are recommended?

Yes   No
1. ☐ ☐ Gently blowing while compressing the opposite nostril can remove a foreign object.
2. ☐ ☐ A foreign object in the nose can be "sneezed" out.
3. ☐ ☐ An insect in the ear may be attracted out by shining a flashlight into the ear.
4. ☐ ☐ Float a bean, pea, or raisin out of an ear with water or oil.
5. ☐ ☐ Remove an impaled object in the cheek.
6. ☐ ☐ A physician should remove an embedded fishhook, if nearby.
7. ☐ ☐ Physicians should remove all embedded fishhooks.

Activity 8: Hand and Finger Injuries

A. Relieve the painful pressure caused by the accumulation of blood under a fingernail or toenail by (check those that apply):

1. ☐ Placing the finger in hot water for several minutes
2. ☐ Drilling a hole through the nail with the point of a knife
3. ☐ Melting a hole through the nail to the site of the blood with a red-hot paper clip

B. Which techniques can be useful in removing a stuck ring?

    Yes No
1. ☐ ☐ Lubricate finger with oil, butter, or other slippery substance.
2. ☐ ☐ Place finger in hot water for several minutes.
3. ☐ ☐ Use string wrapped tightly around finger.
4. ☐ ☐ Cut ring with a fine-toothed hacksaw.
5. ☐ ☐ Cut the skin along the ring to relieve pressure.

C. Positioning for an injured hand (check one):

1. ☐ Fingers kept straight
2. ☐ Fingers closed tightly in a fist
3. ☐ Fingers flexed and supported on a wad of cloth with a board held on the palm side by a roller bandage
4. ☐ Stretched out, with the palm lying on a flat, hard board

Activity 9: Blisters

A. After a blister forms, what should be tried first?

1. ☐ Drain the blister by making a small hole at the blister's edge.
2. ☐ Use scissors to remove the blister's top.
3. ☐ Cover with gauze or tape cut into the shape of a donut.

B. When can a blister be broken?

1. ☐ When very painful
2. ☐ At least three days after its appearance
3. ☐ Never by a first aider

C. Which represents the proper procedure for breaking a blister?
1. ☐ Cut entire roof of blister off.
2. ☐ Drain the fluid by making a small hole at the blister's edge.
3. ☐ Use a red-hot paper clip to puncture the skin.
4. ☐ Pinch or squeeze the blister off.
5. ☐ Soak the blister off in hot water.
6. ☐ None of these since blisters should never be broken.

7
Poisoning

- Poisoning by Ingestion • Insect Stings • Snakebites
- Spider Bites • Scorpion Stings • Tick Removal
- Poison Ivy, Oak, and Sumac • Carbon Monoxide • Alcohol
- Drugs

POISONING BY INGESTION

Of the one million poisonings reported in the United States each year, about 75% occur in children under five, and most are caused by household products. Suicidal and homicidal attempts account for most adult poisonings.

It is beyond the scope of this book to provide an encyclopedia of poisons. Detailed information can be obtained from all local poison control centers, which are staffed by experienced people with access to information on the thousands of poisonous substances.

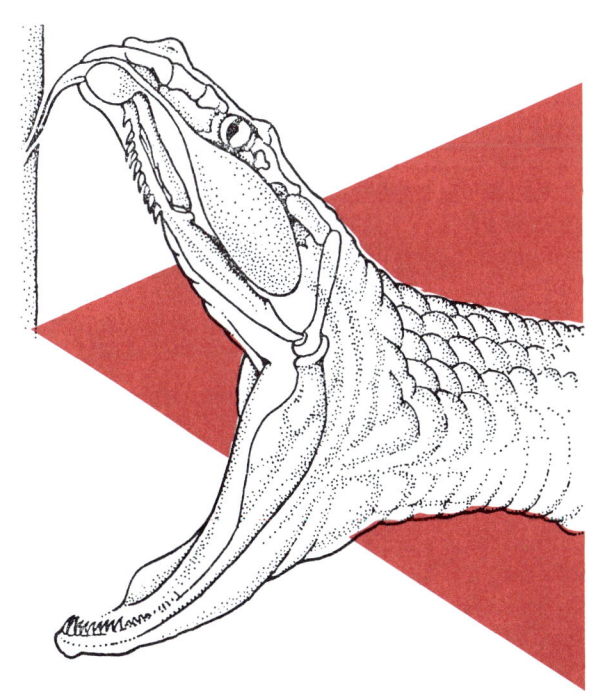

This section provides guidelines for the first aid and emergency care of poisoning in general. For each case, however, the first aider should seek advice from the local poison control center.

Poisons can enter the body through ingestion, inhalation, skin absorption, or injection. Ingested poisons usually remain in the stomach only a short time, and the stomach absorbs only small amounts. Most absorption takes place after the poison passes into the small intestine. Suspect poisoning in any person who suddenly has an onset of unexplained illness, especially an illness characterized by abdominal pain, nausea, and vomiting. Thus first aid is aimed at trying to rid the body of the poison before it reaches the intestines.

To manage a poisoned person, the first aider should obtain answers to the following questions:

1. What was ingested? The poison container and all its remaining contents, the plant, or a sample of what was ingested should be brought to the emergency department. If the person has vomited, save a sample of the vomitus in a clean, closed container and take it to the hospital with the victim.
2. When was the substance taken?
3. How much of the substance was taken?

105

The first aider should keep three basic principles in mind when managing the victim who has ingested a poison:

1. Maintain an open airway.
2. If possible, identify the poison and answer the questions of when was the poison taken and how much was ingested. Then call the local poison control center (refer to Table 7-1 or telephone directory) for advice on proper procedures.
3. If inducing vomiting is advised by a medical authority, do so.

As a general rule, if the victim has ingested a poison within the past three to four hours, the stomach should be emptied, but there are important exceptions. Never induce vomiting in:

- The unresponsive, unconscious, or potentially unconscious victim
- The victim with seizures
- The pregnant woman
- The person with possible heart attack or a history of heart disease
- The victim who has ingested corrosives (strong acids or alkalies)
- The victim who has ingested petroleum products (e.g., kerosene, gasoline, lighter fluid, furniture polish)

For practically all other ingested poisons, the first aider should promptly empty the victim's stomach, if advised by a poison control center. Studies have shown that vomiting is the most effective way to empty the stomach of ingested poisons. To empty the victim's stomach in this way, you should:

1. Give syrup of ipecac—one tablespoonful (use the type used for cooking because household tablespoons hold less) with one to two glasses of water for a child over one year old, and two tablespoonfuls with two to three glasses of water to an adult. Other methods (e.g., salt water or gagging) are not reliable and may be dangerous.
2. Place the victim face down, with the head lower than the hips, to reduce the possibility of the victim's breathing in the vomitus.
3. If vomiting does not occur within twenty minutes, repeat the dose of ipecac and water once.
4. If vomiting stops, give activated charcoal.

The dose of charcoal should be eight to ten times the amount of poison ingested. When the exact quantity of poison is unknown, a general guideline is to give about one-half of a lightly packed 8 ounce glass in about two cups of water for children. Double the amounts for an adult victim. The consistency should be similar to a thin milk shake so the victim can drink it. Mix the charcoal and water by shaking it well in a jar. Children may require some persuasion to drink the mixture because of its uninviting appearance. A firm, positive approach generally works. Do not give activated charcoal with syrup of ipecac because the charcoal will inactivate the syrup of ipecac.

A shortcoming of ipecac is that it only removes 30%–40% of the poison, leaving the remaining 60%–70% to be absorbed and produce possible toxic effects. Therefore, the procedure for handling the remaining poison is the use of activated charcoal, which has a huge capability to bind chemicals. Ordinary charcoal is "activated" by heating it in carbon dioxide. This causes each grain of charcoal powder to expand like a sponge. Substances such as burnt toast, fireplace ashes, and charcoal briquettes are all ineffective in treating poisoning. Even though activated charcoal is effective and should be used more frequently, most pharmacies do not stock it because of a lack of demand.

Diluting poison with water or milk is often recommended. For many chemicals, especially those with corrosive effects (e.g., acids and alkalies), giving water or milk is appropriate. Water or milk dilutes the corrosive agent and decreases its potential for damaging tissues. However, dilution may actually increase the rate of absorption of tablets, capsules and other "dry poisons" by causing them to dissolve more rapidly in the stomach. Also, large amounts of fluid can distend the stomach, which allows the contents to move into the small intestines faster, increasing the rate of absorption.

TABLE 7-1. American Association of Poison Control Centers: 1988 Certified Regional Poison Centers

Alabama Poison Center
809 University Boulevard East
Tuscaloosa, AL 35401

Arizona Poison Control System
College of Pharmacy
University of Arizona
Tucson, AZ 85721
Component Centers
- Arizona Poison and Drug Information Center
  Health Sciences Center, Room 3204K
  Tucson, AZ 85724
- Samaritan Regional Poison Center
  Good Samaritan Medical Center
  1130 East McDowell Road
  Phoenix, AZ 85006

Blodgett Regional Poison Center
1840 Wealthy S.E.
Grand Rapids, MI 49506

Cardinal Glennon Children's Hospital
Regional Poison Center
1465 South Grand Boulevard
St. Louis, MO 63104

Central Ohio Poison Center
700 Children's Drive
Columbus, OH 43205

Children's Hospital of Alabama Poison Control Center
1600 – 7th Avenue South
Birmingham, AL 35233

Delaware Valley Regional Poison Control Program
One Children's Center
Philadelphia, PA 19104

Duke Regional Poison Control Center
Box 3007
Durham, NC 27710

Florida Poison Information Center
The Tampa General Hospital
Davis Islands
Tampa, FL 33606

Georgia Poison Control Center
80 Butler Street, SE
Post Office Box 26066
Atlanta, GA 30335

Hennepin Regional Poison Center
Hennepin County Medical Center
710 Park Avenue South
Minneapolis, MN 55415

Intermountain Regional Poison Control Center
50 North Medical Drive
Salt Lake City, UT 84132

Kentucky Regional Poison Center of Kosair Children's Hospital
Post Office Box 35070
Louisville, KY 40232-5070

Los Angeles County Medical Association
Regional Poison Center
1925 Wilshire Boulevard
Los Angeles, CA 90057

Louisiana Regional Poison Center
LSU Medical Center
Post Office Box 33932
Shreveport, LA 71130

Maryland Poison Center
20 North Pine Street
Baltimore, MD 21201

Massachusetts Poison Control System
300 Longwood Avenue
Boston, MA 02115

Mid-Plains Poison Center
8301 Dodge Street
Omaha, NE 68114

Minnesota Regional Poison Center
St. Paul-Ramsey Medical Center
St. Paul, MN 55101

Nassau County Medical Center's Long Island Regional Poison Control Center
2201 Hempstead Turnpike
East Meadow, NY 11554

National Capital Poison Center
Georgetown University Hospital
3800 Reservoir Road, N.W.
Washington, DC 20007

New Jersey Poison Information and Education System
201 Lyons Avenue
Newark, NJ 07112

New Mexico Poison and Drug Information Center
University of New Mexico
Albuquerque, NM 87131

New York City Poison Center
455 First Avenue
Room 123
New York, NY 10016

North Texas Poison Center
Post Office Box 35926
Dallas, TX 75235

Oregon Poison Center
The Oregon Health Sciences University
3181 SW Sam Jackson Park Road
Portland, OR 97201

Pittsburgh Poison Center
One Children's Place
3705 5th Avenue at DeSoto
Pittsburgh, PA 15213

Poison Control Center
Children's Hospital of Michigan
3901 Beaubien Boulevard
Detroit, MI 48201

Rhode Island Poison Center
593 Eddy Street
Providence, RI 02902

Rocky Mountain Poison and Drug Center
645 Bannock Street
Denver, CO 80204-4507

San Diego Regional Poison Center
UCSD Medical Center
225 Dickinson Street
H925
San Diego, CA 92103

San Francisco Bay Area Regional Poison Center
San Francisco General Hospital
1001 Potrero Avenue
San Francisco, CA 94110

Regional Poison Control System and Cincinnati Drug and Poison Information Center
231 Bethesda Avenue
ML 144
Cincinnati, OH 45267

Texas State Poison Center
University of Texas Medical Branch
Galveston, TX 77550-2780

UC Davis Regional Poison Control Center
2315 Stockton Boulevard
Sacramento, CA 95817

West Virginia Poison Center
3110 MacCorkle Avenue, S.E.
Charleston, WV 25304

Therefore, dilution with water or milk should *not* be an automatic first aid procedure unless the poison control center advises, a corrosive is swallowed, or vomiting is to be induced immediately after dilution through the use of syrup of ipecac, which requires water to be effective.

Do not rely on the antidote printed on the label of the poison. These labels are frequently incorrect.

INSECT STINGS

The number of deaths definitely known to have resulted from insect stings averages about forty a year; however, many deaths identified as natural causes or heart attack may actually have been from insect stings.

For a severely allergic person, a single sting may be fatal within 15 minutes. Although there are accounts of individuals who have survived some 2,000 stings, generally 500 or more will bring about the death of those not allergic to stinging insects.

First aiders need to know more about this important problem. Refer to Table 7-3 for more information. First aiders need to know if a reaction is dangerous and when a victim should be seen by a physician. A knowledge of emergency care procedures, as well as preventive measures, is also important.

Fatalities from insect stings most frequently occur during the summer months when exposure is maximum. Most stings are on the head, neck, or feet. About two-thirds of those who die from insect stings die within one hour, which stresses the importance and the need for immediate medical treatment.

Types of Reactions

- Usual reactions—momentary pain, redness around sting site, itching, heat.
- Worrisome reactions—skin flush, hives, localized swelling of lips or tongue, "tickle" in throat, wheezing, abdominal cramps, diarrhea.
- Life-threatening reactions—cyanosis (bluish or grayish skin color), inability to breathe due to swelling of vocal cords, seizures, unconsciousness.

First Aid

Carefully examine the sting site to determine whether a stinger is still embedded in the skin. If it is embedded, remove it to prevent further injection of toxin into the skin. If the stinger is left in the skin (only honeybees leave a stinger), it will continue to inject venom through spasmodic muscle contractions for two or three minutes unless immediately removed. Scrape off the stinger with your fingernail or a knife (*see* Figure 7-1). Removal with the fingers or tweezers exerts pressure on the venom sac, and the victim will get the full amount of venom.

After examining the sting site and removing any stinger, place an ice pack over the affected area to slow absorption of the toxin into the bloodstream. An ice pack relieves some of the pain associated with the sting. Wash the site with soap and water to cleanse the area of bacteria.

Full strength household ammonia or sodium bicarbonate (baking soda) paste usually helps control the pain. Some suggest smearing a paste of water and meat tenderizer on the sting site to reduce discomfort. An antihistamine may prevent some local symptoms if administered early, and an analgesic may be needed for pain relief. The victim should be observed for at least thirty minutes for signs of an allergic reaction.

The only effective treatment for insect sting anaphylaxis is the injection of epinephrine. Epinephrine should not be used to treat a sting unless anaphylaxis ensues, and on many occasions untrained persons might use the drug inappropriately. Finally, epinephrine has a limited shelf life of one to three years or when it has turned brown; therefore, over-the-counter kits would become outdated and ineffective. Such kits are, however, available through a prescription from a medical doctor.

These emergency insect sting kits contain a preloaded syringe of aqueous epinephrine and fast-acting antihistamine capsules or tablets. Antihistamines are of little value in treating the immediate and life-threatening reaction. The epinephrine (0.3 ml) is given subcutaneously at

TABLE 7-4. Facts About Troublesome Insects

Description	Habitat	Problem	Severity	Treatment	Protection
Chigger Oval with red velvety covering. Sometimes almost colorless. Larva has six legs. Harmless adult has eight and resembles a small spider. Very tiny—about 1/20-inch long.	Found in low damp places covered with vegetation: shaded woods, high grass or weeds, fruit orchards. Also lawns and golf courses. From Canada to Argentina.	Attaches itself to the skin by inserting mouthparts into a hair follicle. Injects a digestive fluid that causes cells to disintegrate. Then feeds on cell parts. It does not suck blood.	Itching from secreted enzymes results several hours after contact. Small red welts appear. Secondary infection often follows. Degree of irritation varies with individuals.	Lather with soap and rinse several times to remove chiggers. If welts have formed, dab antiseptic on area. Severe lesions may require antihistamine ointment.	Apply proper repellent to clothing, particularly near uncovered areas such as wrists and ankles. Apply to skin. Spray or dust infested areas (lawns, plants) with suitable chemicals.
Bedbug Flat oval body with short broad head and six legs. Adult is reddish brown. Young are yellowish white. Unpleasant pungent odor. From 1/8- to 1/4-inch in length.	Hides in crevices, mattresses, under loose wallpaper during day. At night travels considerable distance to find victims. Widely distributed throughout the world.	Punctures the skin with piercing organs and sucks blood. Local inflammation and welts result from anticoagulant enzyme that bug secretes from salivary glands while feeding.	Affects people differently. Some have marked swelling and considerable irritation, others aren't bothered. Sometimes transmits serious diseases.	Apply antiseptic to prevent possible infection. Bug usually bites sleeping victim, gorges itself completely in 3 to 5 minutes and departs. It's rarely necessary to remove one.	Spray beds, mattresses, bed springs, and baseboards with insecticide. Bugs live in large groups. They migrate to new homes on water pipes and clothing.
Brown Recluse Spider Oval body with eight legs. Light yellow to medium dark brown. Has distinctive mark shaped like a fiddle on its back. Body from 3/8- to 1/2-inch long, 1/4-inch wide, 3/4-inch from toe-to-toe.	Prefers dark places where it's seldom disturbed. Outdoors: old trash piles, debris, and rough ground. Indoors: attics, storerooms, closets. Found in Southern and Midwestern United States.	Bites producing an almost painless sting that may not be noticed at first. Shy, it bites only when annoyed or surprised. Left alone, it won't bite. Victim rarely sees the spider.	In 2 to 8 hours pain may be noticed followed by blisters, swelling, hemorrhage, or ulceration. Some people experience rash, nausea, jaundice, chills, fever, cramps, or joint pain.	Summon doctor. Bite may require hospitalization for a few days. Full healing may take from 6 to 8 weeks. Weak adults and children have been known to die.	Use caution when cleaning secluded areas in the home or using machinery usually left idle. Check firewood, inside shoes, packed clothing and bedrolls—frequent hideaways.
Black Widow Spider Color varies from dark brown to glossy black. Densely covered with short microscopic hairs. Red or yellow hourglass marking on the underside of the female's abdomen. Male does not have this mark and is not poisonous. Overall length with legs extended is 1½ inch. Body is ¼-inch wide.	Found with eggs and web. Outside: in vacant rodent holes, under stones, logs, in long grass, hollow stumps, and brush piles. Inside: in dark corners of barns, garages, piles of stone, wood. Most bites occur in outhouses. Found in Southern Canada, throughout United States, except Alaska.	Bites causing local redness. Two tiny red spots may appear. Pain follows almost immediately. Larger muscles become rigid. Body temperature rises slightly. Profuse perspiration and tendency toward nausea follow. It's usually difficult to breathe or talk. May cause constipation, urine retention.	Venom is more dangerous than a rattlesnake's but is given in much smaller amounts. About 5% of bite cases result in death. Death is from asphyxiation due to respiratory paralysis. More dangerous for children; to adults its worst feature is pain. Convulsions result in some cases.	Use an antiseptic such as alcohol or hydrogen peroxide on the bitten area to prevent secondary infection. Keep victim quiet and call a doctor. Do not treat as you would a snakebite since this will only increase the pain and chance of infection; bleeding will not remove the venom.	Wear gloves when working in areas where there might be spiders. Destroy any egg sacs you find. Spray insecticide in any area where spiders are usually found, especially under privy seats. Check them out regularly. General cleanliness, paint, and light discourage spiders.
Scorpion Crablike appearance with claw-like pincers. Fleshy post-abdomen or "tail" has five segments, ending in a bulbous sac. and stinger. Two poisonous types: solid straw yellow or yellow with irregular black stripes on back. From 2½ to 4 inches long.	Spends days under loose stones, bark, boards, floors of outhouses. Burrows in the sand. Roams freely at night. Crawls under doors into homes. Lethal types are found only in the warm desert-like climate of Arizona and adjacent areas.	Stings by thrusting its tail forward over its head. Swelling or discoloration of the area indicates a nondangerous, though painful, sting. A dangerously toxic sting doesn't change the appearance of the area, which does become hypersensitive.	Excessive salivation and facial contortions may follow. Temperature rises to over 104°F. Tongue becomes sluggish. Convulsions, in waves of increasing intensity, may lead to death from nervous exhaustion. First 3 hours most critical.	Apply constriction. Keep victim quiet and call a doctor immediately. Do not cut the skin or give pain killers. They increase the killing power of the venom. Antitoxin, readily available to doctors, has proved to be very effective.	Apply a petroleum distillate to any dwelling places that cannot be destroyed. Cats are considered effective predators, as are ducks and chickens, though the latter are more likely to be stung and killed. Don't go barefoot at night.

7 / POISONING 111

Bee Winged body with yellow and black stripes. Covered with branched or feathery hairs. Makes a buzzing sound. Different species vary from ½ to 1 inch in length.	Lives in aerial or underground nests or hives. Widely distributed throughout the world wherever there are flowering plants—from the polar regions to the equator.	Stings with tail when annoyed. Burning and itching with localized swelling occur. Usually leaves venom sac in victim. It takes between 2 and 3 minutes to inject all the venom.	If a person is allergic, more serious reactions occur—nausea, shock, unconsciousness. Swelling may occur in another part of the body. Death may result.	Gently scrape (don't pluck) the stinger so venom sac won't be squeezed. Wash with soap and antiseptic. If swelling occurs, contact doctor. Keep victim warm while resting.	Have exterminator destroy nests and hives. Avoid wearing sweet fragrances and bright clothing. Keep food covered. Move slowly or stand still in the vicinity of bees.
Mosquito Small dark fragile body with transparent wings and elongated mouthparts. From ⅛- to ¼-inch long.	Found in temperate climates throughout the world where the water necessary for breeding is available.	Bites and sucks blood. Itching and localized swelling result. Bite may turn red. Only the female is equipped to bite.	Sometimes transmits yellow fever, malaria, encephalitis, and other diseases. Scratching can cause secondary infections.	Don't scratch. Lather with soap and rinse to avoid infection. Apply antiseptic to relieve itching.	Destroy available breeding water to check multiplication. Place nets on windows and beds. Use proper repellent.
Tarantula Large dark "spider" with a furry covering. From 6 to 7 inches in toe-to-toe diameter.	Found in Southwestern United States and the tropical varieties are poisonous.	Bites produce pin-prick sensation with negligible effect. It will not bite unless teased.	Usually no more dangerous than a pin prick. Has only local effects.	Wash and apply antiseptic to prevent the possibility of secondary infection.	Harmless to man, the tarantula is beneficial since it destroys harmful insects.
Tick Oval with small head; the body is not divided into definite segments. Grey or brown. Measures from ¼ to ⅜ inch when mature.	Found in all United States areas and in parts of Southern Canada, on low shrubs, grass, and trees. Carried around by both wild and domestic animals.	Attaches itself to the skin and sucks blood. After removal there is danger of infection, especially if the mouthparts are left in the wound.	Sometimes carries and spreads Rocky Mountain spotted fever, tularemia and Colorado tick fever. In a few rare cases, causes paralysis until removed.	Gently remove with tweezers so none of the mouthparts are left in skin. Wash with soap and water; apply antiseptic.	Cover exposed parts of body when in tick-infested areas. Use proper repellent. Remove ticks attached to clothes, body. Check neck and hair. Bathe.

Source: National Safety Council, *Family Safety*, Spring 1980, pp. 20–21.

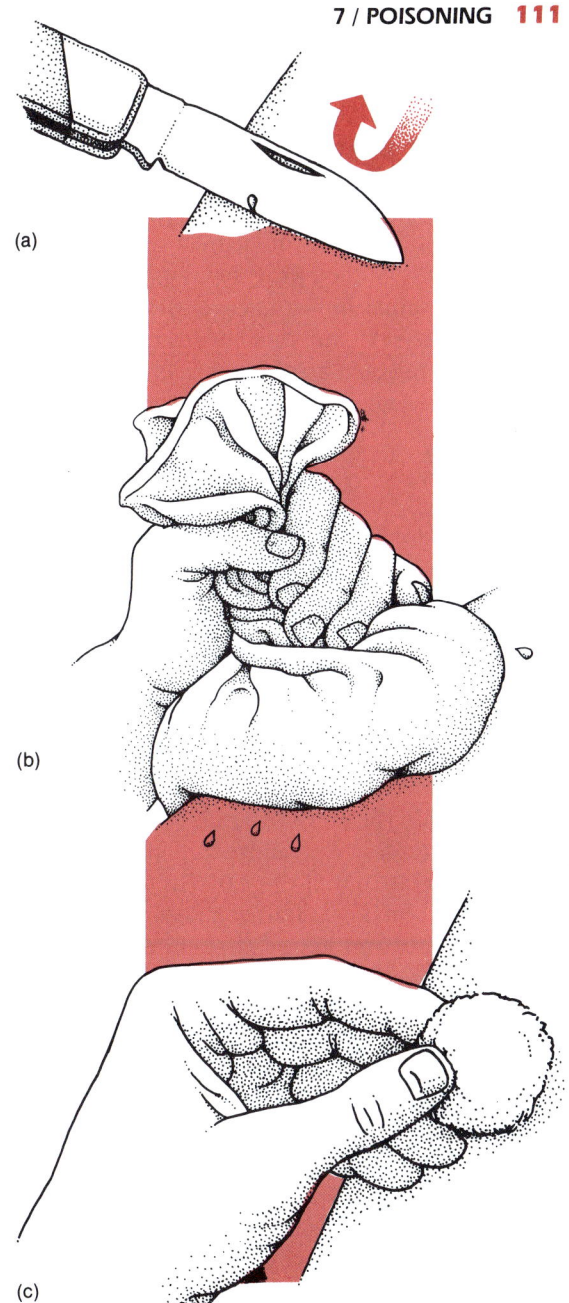

(a)

(b)

(c)

7-1. Bee stings
(a) If stinger is visible, carefully remove it with the edge of a knife or fingernail. Do not squeeze the stinger.
(b) Wash bee sting site with soap and water and put ice or a cold compress on the sting.
(c) Relieve the pain with a baking soda paste or full strength household ammonia.

the sting site. Many kits also contain a constriction band. The kits contain simple instructions that almost any layman could follow.

Victims having had moderate to severe reactions with insect stings in the past should always be told to go to the nearest medical facility after a sting. Since epinephrine is short acting, the victim must be watched closely for signs of returning shock, and small doses of epinephrine should be injected as often as every fifteen minutes as needed.

SNAKEBITES

"Cut; don't cut." "Use a tourniquet; don't use a tourniquet."

"Capture the snake; don't capture the snake." "Use ice; don't use ice." "Use antivenin; don't use antivenin." "Apply mouth suction; don't apply mouth suction."

All these are offered in first aid and medical literature as proper first aid procedures for snakebite. With the maze of confusion about what to do in the event of a poisonous snakebite, it is amazing that only a dozen people die yearly from snakebite out of the 8,000 annual bitten by poisonous snakes. Rattlesnakes account for about 60% of venomous snakebites and for almost all the deaths.

Since opinions vary as to the correct first aid procedures, some of these opinions are misleading and occasionally dangerous.

Do not cool the bite site with ice: Some medical experts believe that cooling the bite with ice water or ice packs will slow the spread of venom. The cold treatment of snakebite has fallen into disrepute. When it was thought that the only harmful substances in venom were enzymes, use of cold seemed reasonable. However, the more toxic effect of peptides in venom were overlooked, and it was found that they are not affected by cold temperatures.

A second problem with using ice is the freezing of tissue, thus the snakebite victim may receive frostbite as well. A third reason for not using a cold treatment is that the enzymes produced in any animal body generally are active at that animal's average body temperature. Snakes are cold-blooded animals. Thus, enzymes produced by cold-blooded animals are active at low temperatures.

Do not cut through the bite wound: Do not perform cuts unless the victim is several hours from a medical facility—just quietly transport the victim. Since most bites occur at home, not in the wild, cutting should seldom be done. If thirty minutes has elapsed since the bite occurred, no cutting should be performed.

In situations other than the preceding ones, cutting over the fang marks should be done. The cut should be carefully done along the fang's path. Do *not* make cross cuts. Cuts should not be deeper ($1/8$ inch) than the skin because of the closeness of nerves and muscles. Cuts should be no more than $1/4$ inch long. Cuts should not be made elsewhere. (*See* Figure 7-2.)

Apply suction over the cut: Suction cups found in a snakebite kit are usually adequate. However, you could use mouth suction, but the danger of introducing infection to the wound is much greater. If you have sores or unfilled tooth caries, you could contract venom from the bite. Rinsing the mouth between suctions is suggested. Suction is only effective for about the first thirty minutes. Suction without cuts is ineffective.

First aiders should not give antivenin: Only qualified medical personnel should administer antivenin because many people are allergic to it. Antivenin can be helpful if given within four hours, but it is of doubtful value if administered later than that.

Do not apply a tourniquet: A tourniquet is tight enough to stop arterial and venous blood flow which may result in the loss of the limb. Rather, you should apply a constriction band which allows a finger to be wedged under it in order to allow some arterial blood flow. Loosen the constriction band slightly as swelling appears, but do not release.

Do not capture the snake: The type of snake should be identified, but do not waste time if it is elusive. A pit viper bite can usually be identified by two large puncture wounds, blood oozing, and progressive swelling and discoloration.

Other considerations in snakebite treatement are: immobilize the arm or leg below the heart; wash the wound thoroughly with soap and water; and carry the victim if possible, or have him move slowly if he must walk.

Summary

- Get the victim away from the snake. Snakes have been known to bite more than once. Transport the victim to a physician or emergency department as rapidly and carefully as possible.
- Apply a constriction band above the bite area. Be sure that a finger can pass under the band, showing that it is not too tight. Do not periodically release it, but loosen it if swelling increases.
- If feasible, do not allow the victim to walk, thus lessening the spread of the venom.
- If you are more than one and one-half hours from an emergency medical facility, or if a large snake is the offender, immediately use incision and suction. You can remove 20% to 50% of the venom with this method, if it is done within three minutes; a lesser quantity can be removed up to thirty minutes. A ¼-inch incision going lengthwise through each fang mark, no more than ⅛ inch deep, is all that is necessary. Crosscut incisions are not recommended. Use mouth suction if no other method is available.
- Transport the victim as rapidly as possible. If feasible, call ahead to report an extreme emergency.
- Perform CPR if the victim stops breathing or has no pulse.
- Use absolutely no form of cooling.
- Antivenin should not be used in the field due to a possible allergic reaction to horse serum.

7-2. Snakebite
(a) Pit vipers inject their fangs in a slanting, shallow penetration.
(b) Do *not* use cross cuts when cutting and sucking are needed in snakebite cases.
(c) If incisions are to be used, make two parallel cuts starting at the punctures and extending along the presumed path of the fangs. Cuts are ⅛ inch deep and about ¼ inch long.

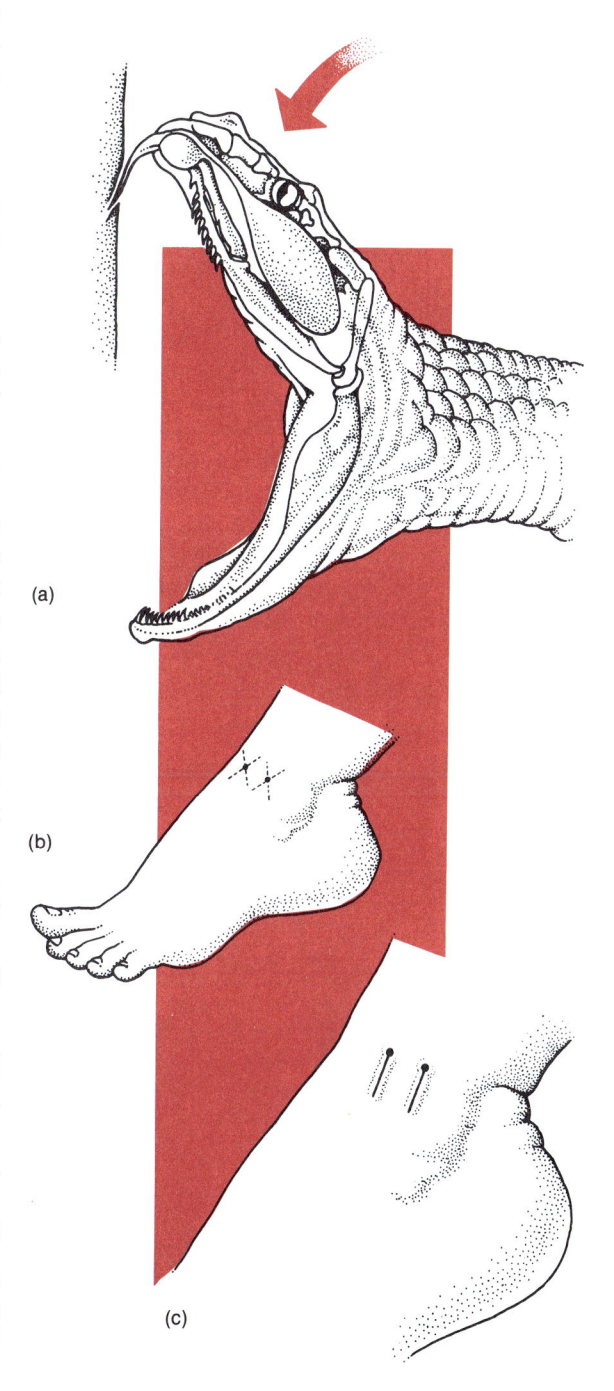

Coral Snakebite

The coral snake is America's most venomous snake. This snake has short fangs and "chews" its venom into the victim. First aid includes washing the bitten area, transporting the victim to a hospital quickly, and not using a constriction band nor incision or suction.

SPIDER BITES

Just about all spiders are venomous—that is how they paralyze and kill their prey. Very few spiders, however, have fangs long enough to endanger the health of man.

The few fatal spider bites seen in this country are attributable to the black widow or to the brown recluse spider. (Refer to Table 7-3.) For a long time the black widow was thought to be the only highly poisonous spider in North America. In the late 1950s, reports began to appear about the bite of the brown recluse.

Black Widow Spider

Black widow spiders live in all states but Alaska. The female can be identified by a red spot on the abdomen—she is the one that bites. (Males do not have fangs large enough to puncture the site.) She has a coal black body. (*See* Figure 7-3.)

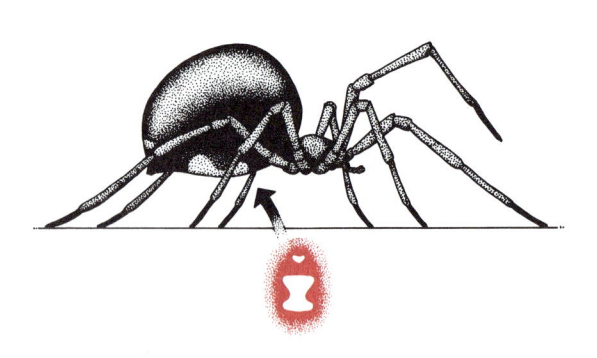

7-3. Female black widow spider with typical hourglass on the abdomen

They hide in the wood and brush piles, long grass, and under stones and logs. Most bites occur on the hands and forearms between April and October when humans are outside rooting around in seldom-used places.

Determining whether a person has been bitten by a black widow spider is difficult. After a sharp pinprick of the spider's bite is felt, it usually takes no more than fifteen minutes for a dull, numbing pain to develop in the bitten extremity. Muscle cramps occur next, usually affecting the abdomen when the bite is in the lower extremities and the shoulders, back, or chest when it is on the upper. Headache, heavy sweating, dizziness, nausea, and vomiting also can occur.

Even without treatment, most healthy adults will survive. However, black widow bites threaten the lives of children and the elderly.

By volume, black widow spider venom is more deadly than the rattlesnake's, but it is injected in much smaller amounts.

If possible, the spider should be caught to confirm its identity. Even if the body is crushed, save it for identification.

Victims of black widow spider bites should get medical help immediately. At the hospital, the wound is cleaned, muscle relaxants are given, and calcium gluconate is administered to relieve cramping. There is an antivenin for black widow bites. The antivenin brings relief of symptoms within one to three hours, especially if given as soon as possible after the victim was bitten.

The bitten area can be cleaned with alcohol. Do not apply a constricting band because the black widow venom's action is swift, and there is little to be gained by trying to slow absorption with a constriction band. In fact, it will hasten tissue death. An ice pack may be placed over the bite to relieve pain. Keep the victim quiet, and be alert for any respiratory difficulty.

Brown Recluse Spider

The brown recluse spider has a brown, possibly purplish, violin-shape figure on its back. (*See* Figure 7-4.) Brown recluse bites are rarely fatal, except

7 / POISONING

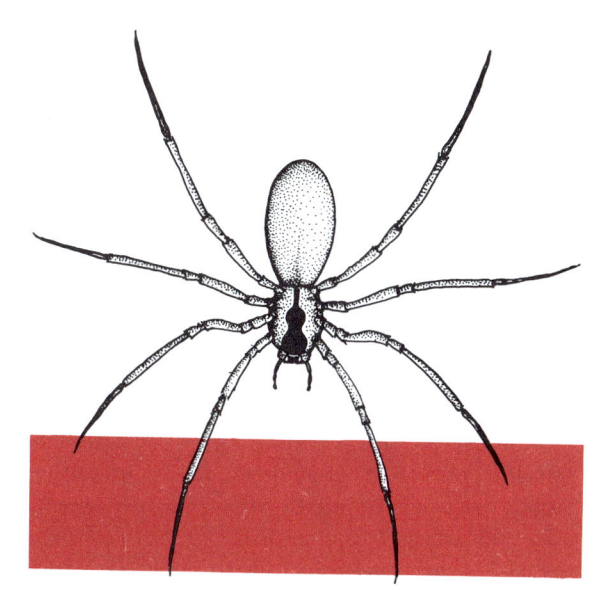

7-4. Brown recluse spider with typical violin-shaped marking on top

for hypersensitive people, or for children, the elderly, or those with chronic health problems.

The initial pain felt from a brown recluse spider may be slight enough to be overlooked at first. The first signs are usually a blister at the bite site, along with redness and swelling. Pain, which may remain mild but can become severe, develops within two to eight hours. Days later the bite site hardens, and within a week the flesh forms an ulcer. Gangrene may develop in some cases.

First aid consists of cold packs and disinfecting the bite site. The victim should be transported to a medical facility as quickly as possible. If possible, the biting spider should be captured and taken with the victim for accurate physician diagnosis and treatment.

Tarantula Spider

The tarantula is far more ominous looking than the other two poisonous spiders, but its bite rarely produces symptoms other than mild to moderate pain. Clean the bite wound to prevent infection. (Refer to Table 7-3.)

SCORPION STINGS

Scorpions are nocturnal and live under buildings, logs, and debris in hot dry areas of California, Arizona, New Mexico, and Mexico. (*See* Figure 7-5.) Death from the sting of the scorpion is rare in the United States. Apply an ice pack over the wound and take the victim to a medical facility. (Refer to Table 7-3.)

Its sting causes immediate pain around the sting site, followed by numbness or tingling. Severe cases may entail paralysis, spasms, or respiratory difficulties. Children are at greatest risk.

TICK REMOVAL

Four popular folk methods of tick removal—ways of inducing the tick to back out of the skin of its host—failed to work in a study carried out by Glen R. Needham.[*] Even if they worked, Dr. Needham says, the safest way to remove a tick is still to pull it off because that method lessens the

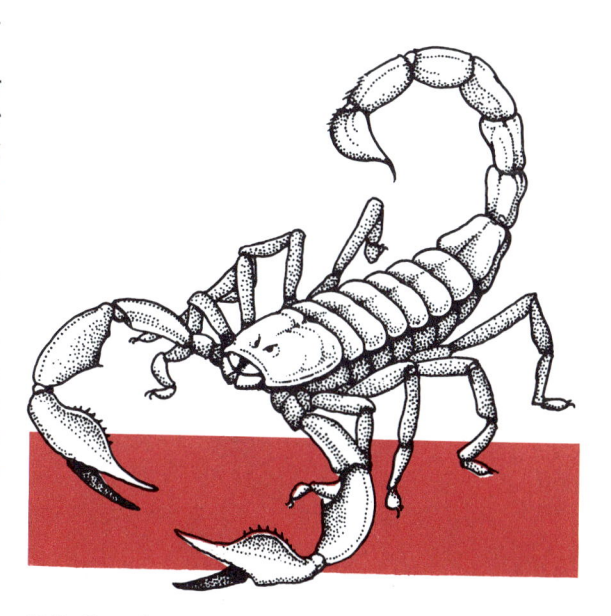

7-5. Scorpion

---

[*]Glen R. Needham, "Evaluation of Five Popular Methods of Tick Removal," *Pediatrics*, Vol. 75, 1985, pp. 997–1002.

likelihood of leaving behind tick secretions that later could lead to infection.

Dr. Needham tested the application of petroleum jelly, fingernail polish, 70% isopropyl alcohol, and a hot kitchen match as well as removal with tweezers or a protected hand as ways to remove ticks from a sheep.

After allowing a group of ticks to remain attached to the host for 72 to 96 hours, Dr. Needham attempted to remove them using the previously named methods. None of the ticks detached in a two-hour period.

To see whether any of these methods would work with ticks less firmly anchored, Dr. Needham applied them to a second group of sixteen that had been attached to the host for 12 to 15 hours. None of the ticks detached itself within 24 hours after application. Dr. Needham subsequently removed all of them intact by pulling with tweezers or protected fingers.

The strategy behind the use of petroleum jelly and perhaps behind the use of fingernail polish is presumably to deprive the tick of respiratory gas exchange, Dr. Needham says, but he points out that the tick breathes only a few times per hour when at rest and that a tick covered with fingernail polish probably cannot move on its own. The notion about getting ticks to back out persist, "probably because most people prefer not to touch them," he says.

Dr. Needham suggests the following removal method which you might want to use:

- Use tweezers or, if you have to use your fingers, protect your skin by using a paper towel or disposable tissue. Although few people ever encounter ticks infected with Rocky Mountain spotted fever or other disease, the person removing the tick may become infected by pathogens entering through breaks in the skin or through mucous membranes. For this reason, children should not be allowed to remove ticks from family pets.

- Grasp the tick as close to the skin surface as possible and pull away from the skin with a steady pressure or lift the tick slightly upward and pull parallel to the skin until the tick detaches. Do not twist or jerk the tick since this may result in incomplete removal. (*See* Figure 7-6.)

- Dispose of the tick by flushing it down a drain or wadding it in adhesive tape before placing it in the trash.

- Wash the bite site and your hands well with soap and water. Apply alcohol to further disinfect the area. Then apply a cold pack to reduce pain. Calamine lotion might aid in relieving any itching. Keep the area clean.

Dr. Needham says that in most instances you need not be overly concerned if the tick's cement

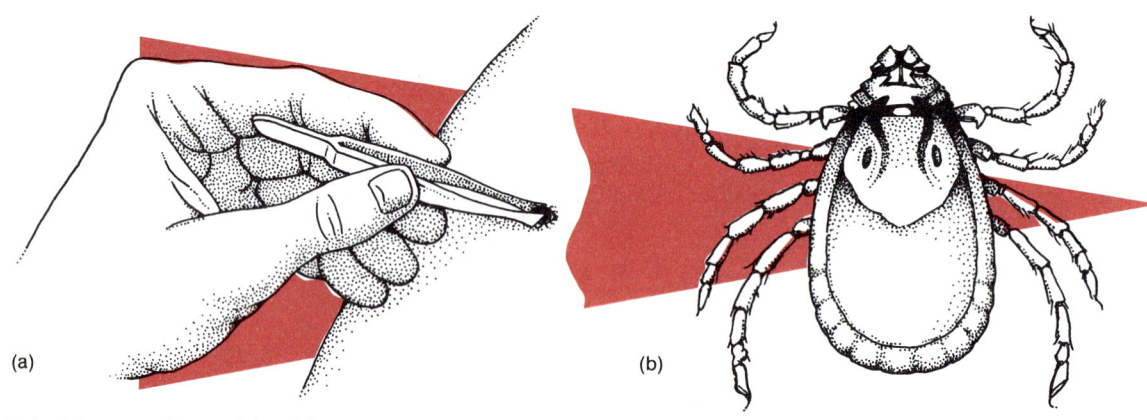

(a)

(b)

7-6. (a) Removing a tick with tweezers (b) A Tick

is not removed or if the mouthpiece breaks off and remains in the skin.

Watch for signs of infection or unexplained symptoms, such as severe headaches, fever, or rash, which may develop three to ten days later. If these symptoms appear, seek medical care immediately.

POISON IVY, OAK, AND SUMAC

Two million Americans will suffer allergic contact dermatitis from poison ivy, poison oak, or poison sumac this year. (*See* Figure 7-7.)

Resistance, or immunity, varies greatly from one person to another and even in the same person at different times, but probably no one is completely immune. Most people thought to be immune have just not been exposed under the right conditions.

Signs and Symptoms

Although the limbs, face, and neck are common sites of the dermatitis, all areas of the skin that come in contact with the sensitizing substance can be affected. However, different parts of the body may not have the same sensitivity; thus, the dermatitis may appear first in one area and later in another. The phenomenon is often called "spreading," but this description is inaccurate. Often, parts of the body that may sustain a heavy concentration of the allergen and exhibit more severe reactions will remain "hypersensitive" for years.

The characteristic burning, itching, rash, and swelling resulting from poison ivy, oak, or sumac contact may not follow for as long as ten days after exposure. A day or two is the usual interval between exposure and onset of signs and symptoms.

The rash first consists of streaks or patches of red discoloration of the skin associated with itching. Later, blisters develop which break down, resulting in oozing and crusting from the surface. Usually swelling of the tissue, burning, and itching are present. Avoid scratching because it can introduce infection or cause scarring. Scratching does not spread the rash. The blisters are filled with serum, not with urushiol, which causes the dermatitis.

First Aid

It has been demonstrated that washing delayed only five minutes after exposure does very little good.

Generally, the local treatment should be adapted to the stage or severity of the lesions.

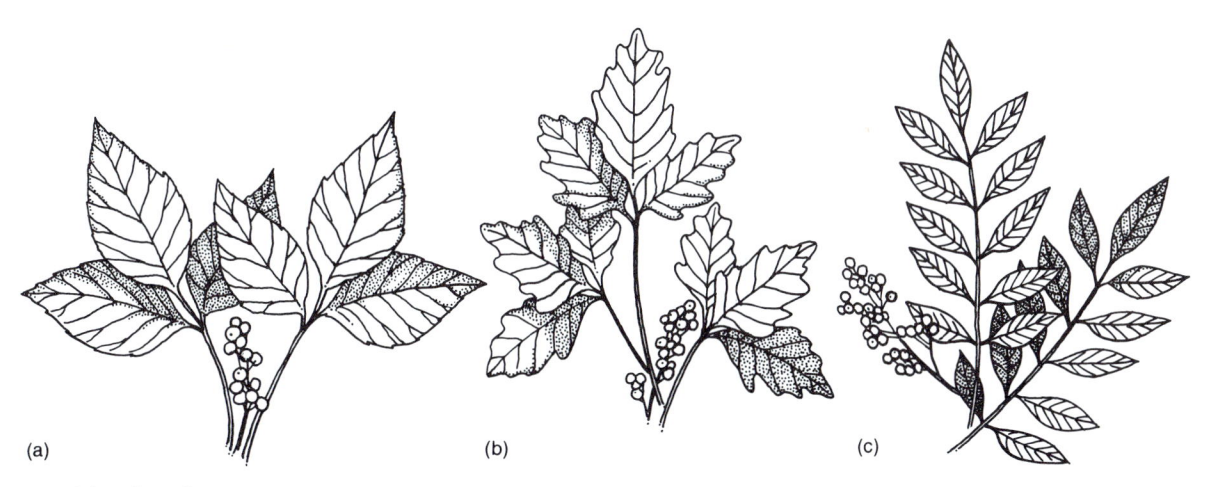

7-7. (a) Poison ivy
(b) Poison oak
(c) Poison sumac

During the acute weeping and oozing stage, sodium bicarbonate (baking soda) solution should be used either as a soak, bath, or wet dressing for thirty minutes, three or four times a day. "Shake" lotions (calamine, zinc oxide) are used at night or when wet dressings are not desirable. Greasy ointments should not be used during active oozing. Unfortunately, there is no convincing evidence that any of the numerous over-the-counter preparations are more effective than these few simple procedures.

Reassure the victim that the fluid from the blisters will not lead to spreading of the dermatitis, nor will touching someone with the dermatitis produce irritation. During the healing phase, application of a neutral soothing cream (such as cold cream) helps prevent crusting and scaling.

Studies indicate that not one medication tested was more effective than tap water compresses and "shake" lotions containing a soothing ingredient, such as zinc oxide or calamine. Antihistamines appeared to have no value taken by mouth or in ointments and lotions. In fact, ointments and lotions could even cause their own allergic reactions on top of the poison plant eruption.

When the dermatitis eruption affects a large part of the body, corticosteroids taken under the care of a physician may benefit most severely affected victims.

For severe itching, hot water—hot enough to redden the skin temporarily—may relieve discomfort. Heat releases histamine, the substance in the cells of the skin that causes the intense itching. Therefore, a hot shower or bath causes intense itching as the histamine is released. This depletes the cells of histamine and the victim will obtain up to eight hours of relief from itching. Using this method does not require frequent applications of ointment.

CARBON MONOXIDE

Carbon monoxide (CO) is produced by the incomplete combustion (burning) of any organic (carbon-containing) material. Incomplete combustion may occur with the burning of any fuel containing carbon, including coal, gas, kerosene, oil, wood, paper, and charcoal. Carbon monoxide is a nonirritating, colorless, tasteless, and odorless gas.

When you inhale air into your lungs, oxygen is transferred from the air to your blood. Oxygen attaches to a component of blood called hemoglobin; the hemoglobin carries the oxygen to the body's tissues. Carbon monoxide is also capable of attaching to the hemoglobin in the blood. The affinity of red blood cells (hemoglobin) for CO is more than two hundred times that for oxygen. When CO is attached to red blood cells instead of oxygen, the body is deprived. Therefore, a lethal concentration could be produced in as short a time as ten minutes.

The symptoms of carbon monoxide exposure include dizziness, headache, nausea, and vomiting followed or accompanied by loss of consciousness. In cases of massive exposures, consciousness may be lost with few or no other symptoms. Those who survive near lethal exposure will, if conscious, look and act intoxicated.

The traditionally cited sign of CO poisoning has been cherry-red color of the skin and lips. However, several studies indicate that the cherry-red color occurs at death and is, therefore, a poor initial indicator as to whether or not a person has been CO poisoned.

Children are affected worse than adults with CO poisoning. It is not unusual for a youngster, especially an infant, to have severe symptoms including unconsciousness, while adults subjected to exactly the same exposure may show little effect.

Women, because they are usually comparatively anemic, tend to fare less well than men. A person at complete rest is likely to be less affected than someone who was fairly active at the time of exposure.

Carbon monoxide poisoning can be fatal; all have probably heard of accidental deaths from carbon monoxide exposure. In such cases, the carbon monoxide level in the blood became so high that the person could not get enough oxygen to stay alive.

Sometimes people are exposed to carbon monoxide in amounts that do not threaten their lives but do make them feel dizzy or sick. Since the symptoms are indistinguishable from those of a viral infection such as the flu (headache, nausea, chills, dizziness, and tiredness), the person may not even realize what is causing the discomfort.

If you suspect carbon monoxide poisoning, remove the person from the source of the carbon monoxide and ventilate the area. Then, base your actions on the victim's condition:

- If the person is conscious, take him to a doctor who will perform a blood test to determine the level of carbon monoxide.
- If the person is unconscious, place him on his side with his head resting on his arm. Loosen tight clothing and maintain body heat with a blanket.
- If the person has stopped breathing, administer mouth-to-mouth respiration and CPR if you have been trained in cardiopulmonary resuscitation.

The *victim needs 100% oxygen as quickly as possible.* This will improve oxygenation and it also will disassociate the linkage between the carbon monoxide and the red blood cell. Therefore, either transport the victim to a hospital or call for an ambulance that carries oxygen.

Even when there are only mild symptoms, such as headache or nausea, it may be a good idea to check with a doctor if you suspect carbon monoxide poisoning.

ALCOHOL

Alcohol is a depressant, not a stimulant. Many people think alcohol is a stimulant because its first effect is to reduce tension and give a mild feeling of euphoria or exhilaration.

Alcohol affects a person's judgment, vision, reaction time, and coordination. In very large quantities, it can cause death by paralyzing the respiratory center of the brain.

The signs of alcohol intoxication are familiar to all. Some of them are:

1. Odor of alcohol on breath
2. Swaying and unsteadiness
3. Slurred speech
4. Nausea and vomiting
5. Flushed face

These signs can mean illnesses or injuries other than alcohol abuse (e.g., epilepsy, diabetes, or head injury). It is, therefore, especially important that you not immediately dismiss the person with apparent alcohol on his or her breath (which can smell like the fruity breath of a diabetic) as a drunk. Check the person carefully for other illnesses and injuries, and give the intoxicated victim the same attention you would give to those with other illnesses and/or injuries. The intoxicated victim needs constant watching to be sure that he or she does not aspirate vomitus and that respiration is maintained.

DRUGS

Vomiting should be induced if the overdose was taken in the preceding thirty minutes and if advised by a medical authority. Hyperactive victims should be protected from hurting themselves and others. They should be reassured and treated calmly. Respirations should be monitored because overdoses of depressants can cause respiratory depression and death. The first aider should instill confidence. The victim should be assured that he or she will be all right. The first aider should be alert for possible allergic reactions and shock. Evidence should be preserved for the legal authorities. Prompt transportation is required to a medical facility.

Poisoning (Ingestion)

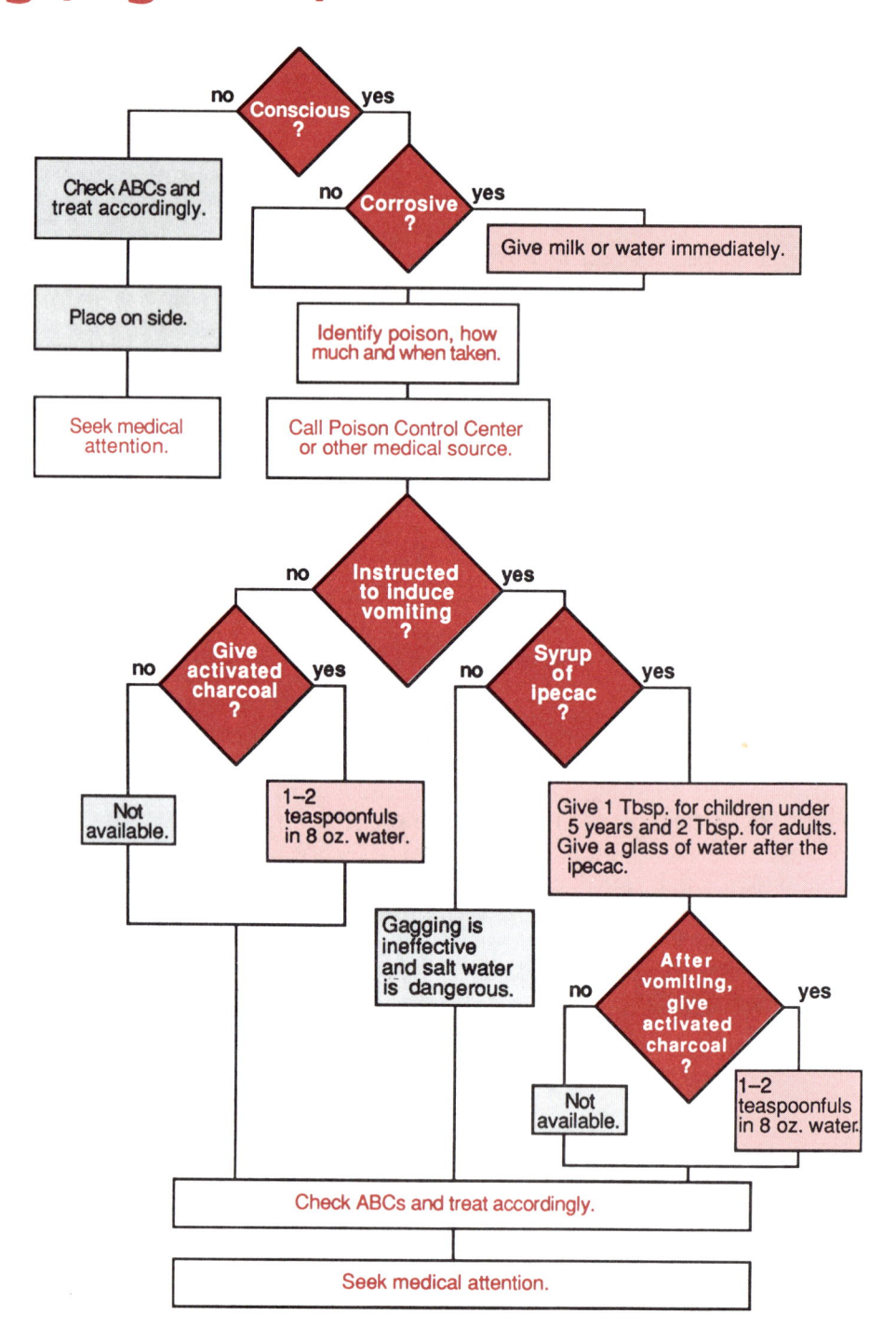

- **Conscious?**
  - **no** → Check ABCs and treat accordingly. → Place on side. → Seek medical attention.
  - **yes** → **Corrosive?**
    - **yes** → Give milk or water immediately.
    - **no** → Identify poison, how much and when taken. → Call Poison Control Center or other medical source. → **Instructed to induce vomiting?**
      - **no** → **Give activated charcoal?**
        - **no** → Not available.
        - **yes** → 1–2 teaspoonfuls in 8 oz. water.
      - **yes** → **Syrup of ipecac?**
        - **no** → Gagging is ineffective and salt water is dangerous.
        - **yes** → Give 1 Tbsp. for children under 5 years and 2 Tbsp. for adults. Give a glass of water after the ipecac. → **After vomiting, give activated charcoal?**
          - **no** → Not available.
          - **yes** → 1–2 teaspoonfuls in 8 oz. water.

Check ABCs and treat accordingly.

Seek medical attention.

Poisoning (Inhaled)

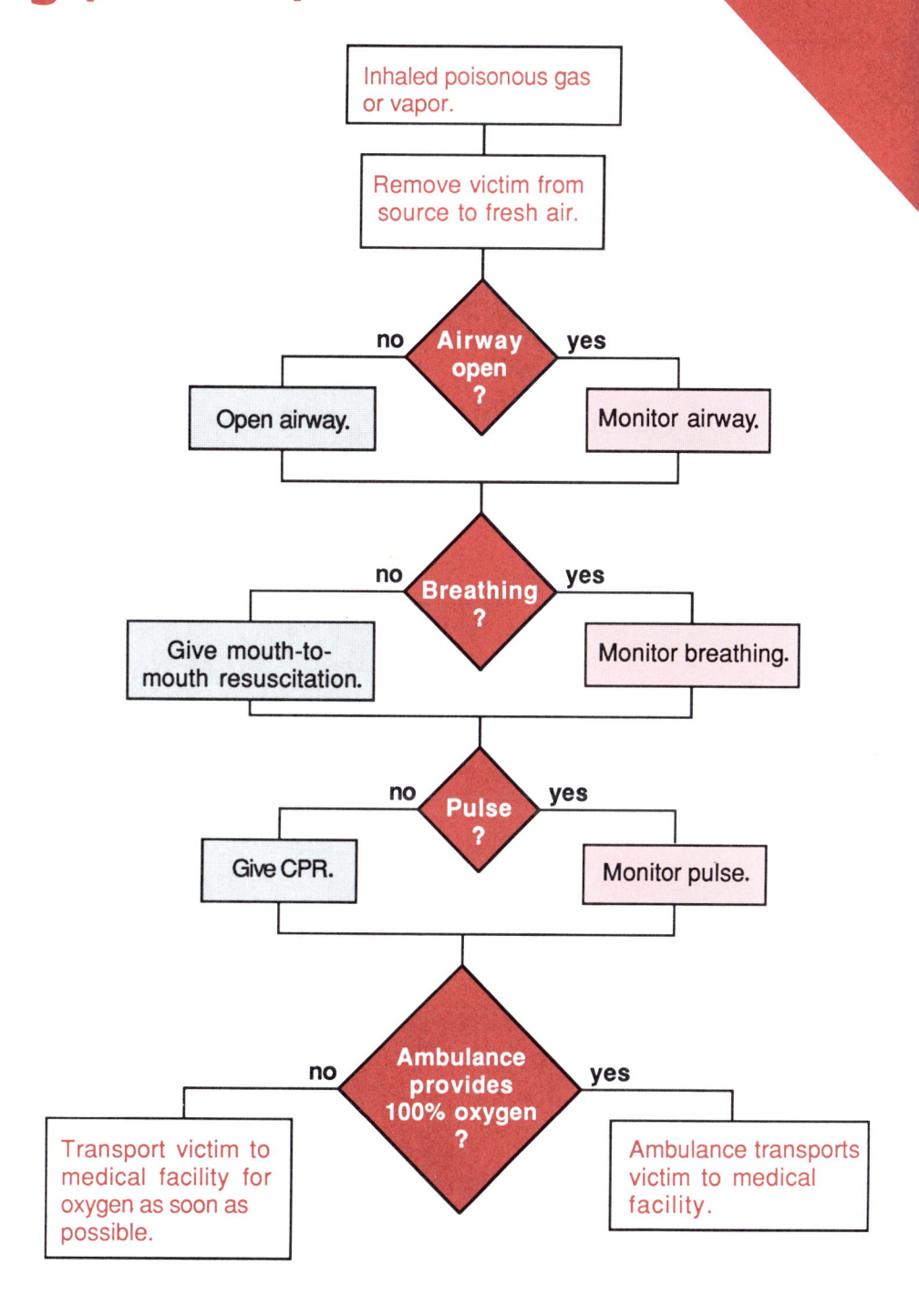

```
Inhaled poisonous gas or vapor.
            │
            ▼
Remove victim from source to fresh air.
            │
            ▼
        Airway open?
   no ──┤         ├── yes
Open airway.        Monitor airway.
            │
            ▼
        Breathing?
   no ──┤         ├── yes
Give mouth-to-mouth    Monitor breathing.
resuscitation.
            │
            ▼
         Pulse?
   no ──┤         ├── yes
Give CPR.           Monitor pulse.
            │
            ▼
   Ambulance provides 100% oxygen?
   no ──┤         ├── yes
Transport victim to     Ambulance transports
medical facility for    victim to medical
oxygen as soon as       facility.
possible.
```

121

Insect Stings (Flying Insects)

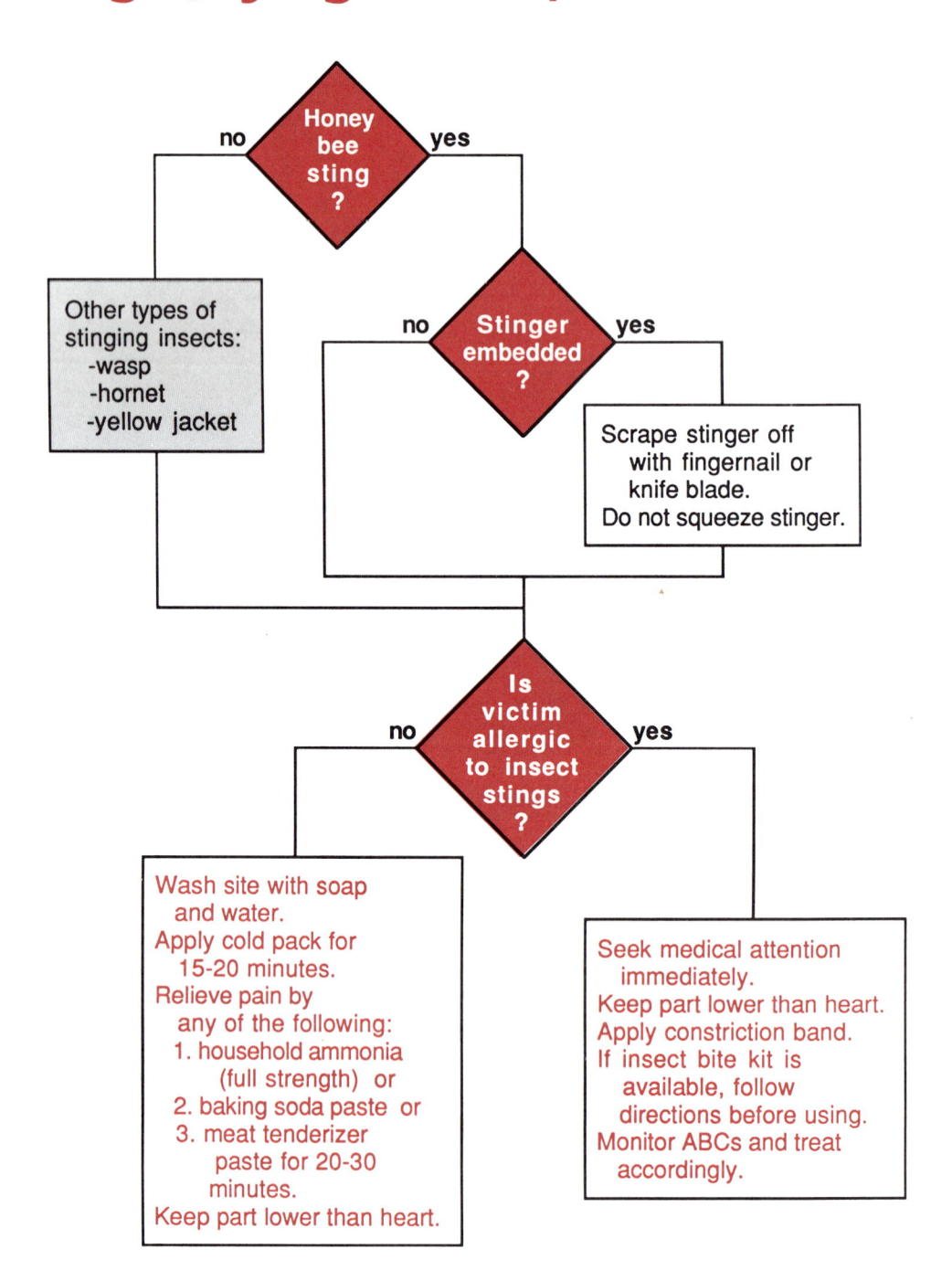

Honey bee sting?
- **no** → Other types of stinging insects:
  - wasp
  - hornet
  - yellow jacket
- **yes** → **Stinger embedded?**
  - **no**
  - **yes** → Scrape stinger off with fingernail or knife blade. Do not squeeze stinger.

Is victim allergic to insect stings?

- **no** →
  Wash site with soap and water.
  Apply cold pack for 15-20 minutes.
  Relieve pain by any of the following:
  1. household ammonia (full strength) or
  2. baking soda paste or
  3. meat tenderizer paste for 20-30 minutes.
  Keep part lower than heart.

- **yes** →
  Seek medical attention immediately.
  Keep part lower than heart.
  Apply constriction band.
  If insect bite kit is available, follow directions before using.
  Monitor ABCs and treat accordingly.

Snakebite

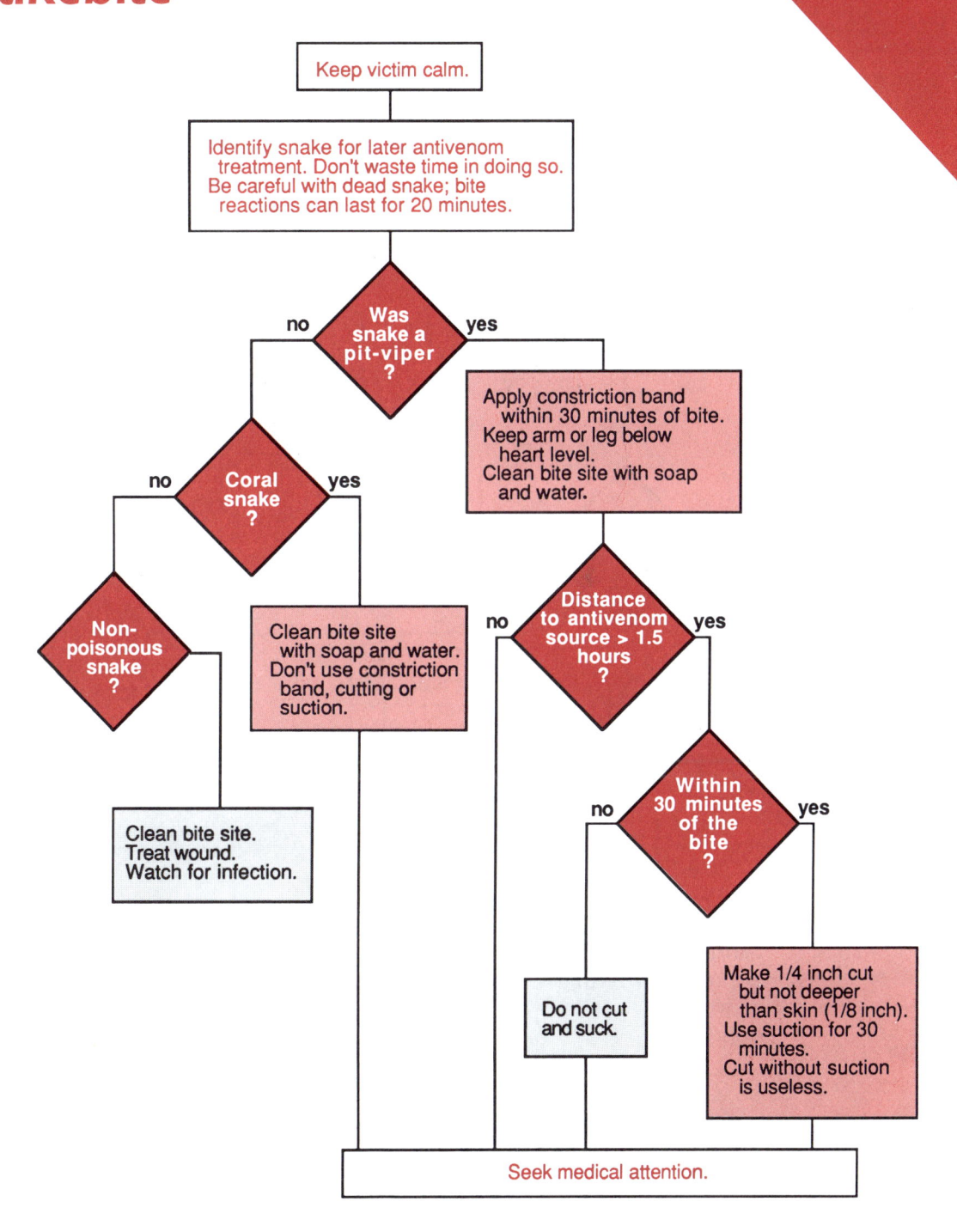

Keep victim calm.

Identify snake for later antivenom treatment. Don't waste time in doing so. Be careful with dead snake; bite reactions can last for 20 minutes.

Was snake a pit-viper?

- **yes** → Apply constriction band within 30 minutes of bite. Keep arm or leg below heart level. Clean bite site with soap and water.
- **no** → **Coral snake?**
  - **yes** → Clean bite site with soap and water. Don't use constriction band, cutting or suction.
  - **no** → **Non-poisonous snake?**
    - Clean bite site. Treat wound. Watch for infection.

From pit-viper path: **Distance to antivenom source > 1.5 hours?**
- **no** → Seek medical attention.
- **yes** → **Within 30 minutes of the bite?**
  - **no** → Do not cut and suck.
  - **yes** → Make 1/4 inch cut but not deeper than skin (1/8 inch). Use suction for 30 minutes. Cut without suction is useless.

Seek medical attention.

Spider Bites and Scorpion Stings

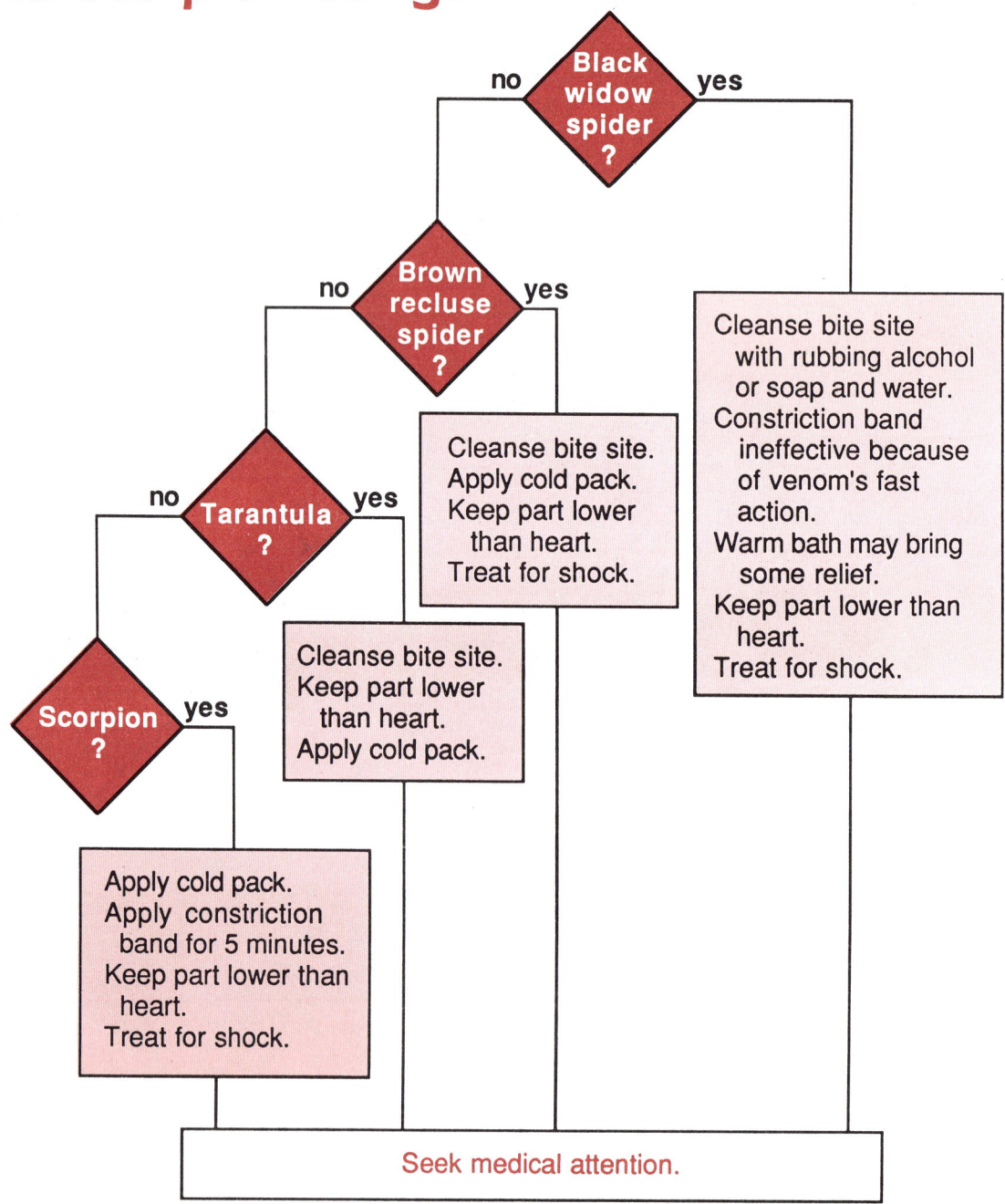

Black widow spider?
- yes → Cleanse bite site with rubbing alcohol or soap and water. Constriction band ineffective because of venom's fast action. Warm bath may bring some relief. Keep part lower than heart. Treat for shock.
- no → **Brown recluse spider?**
  - yes → Cleanse bite site. Apply cold pack. Keep part lower than heart. Treat for shock.
  - no → **Tarantula?**
    - yes → Cleanse bite site. Keep part lower than heart. Apply cold pack.
    - no → **Scorpion?**
      - yes → Apply cold pack. Apply constriction band for 5 minutes. Keep part lower than heart. Treat for shock.

Seek medical attention.

Tick Removal

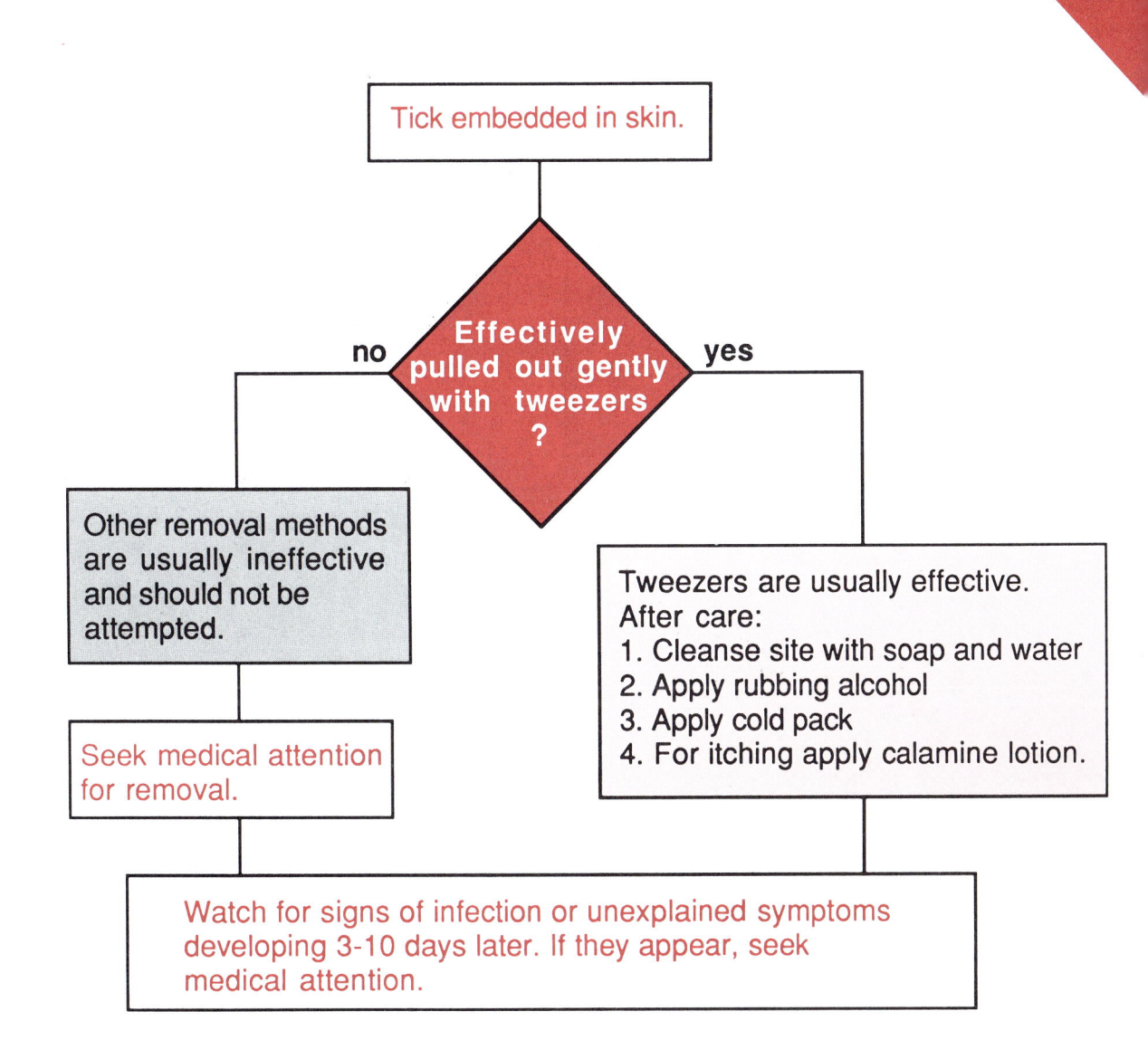

```
Tick embedded in skin.
        │
        ▼
   ◇ Effectively pulled out gently with tweezers? ◇
   no ←              → yes
```

no → Other removal methods are usually ineffective and should not be attempted.

Seek medical attention for removal.

yes → Tweezers are usually effective. After care:
1. Cleanse site with soap and water
2. Apply rubbing alcohol
3. Apply cold pack
4. For itching apply calamine lotion.

Watch for signs of infection or unexplained symptoms developing 3-10 days later. If they appear, seek medical attention.

125

Poison Ivy, Poison Oak, and Poison Sumac

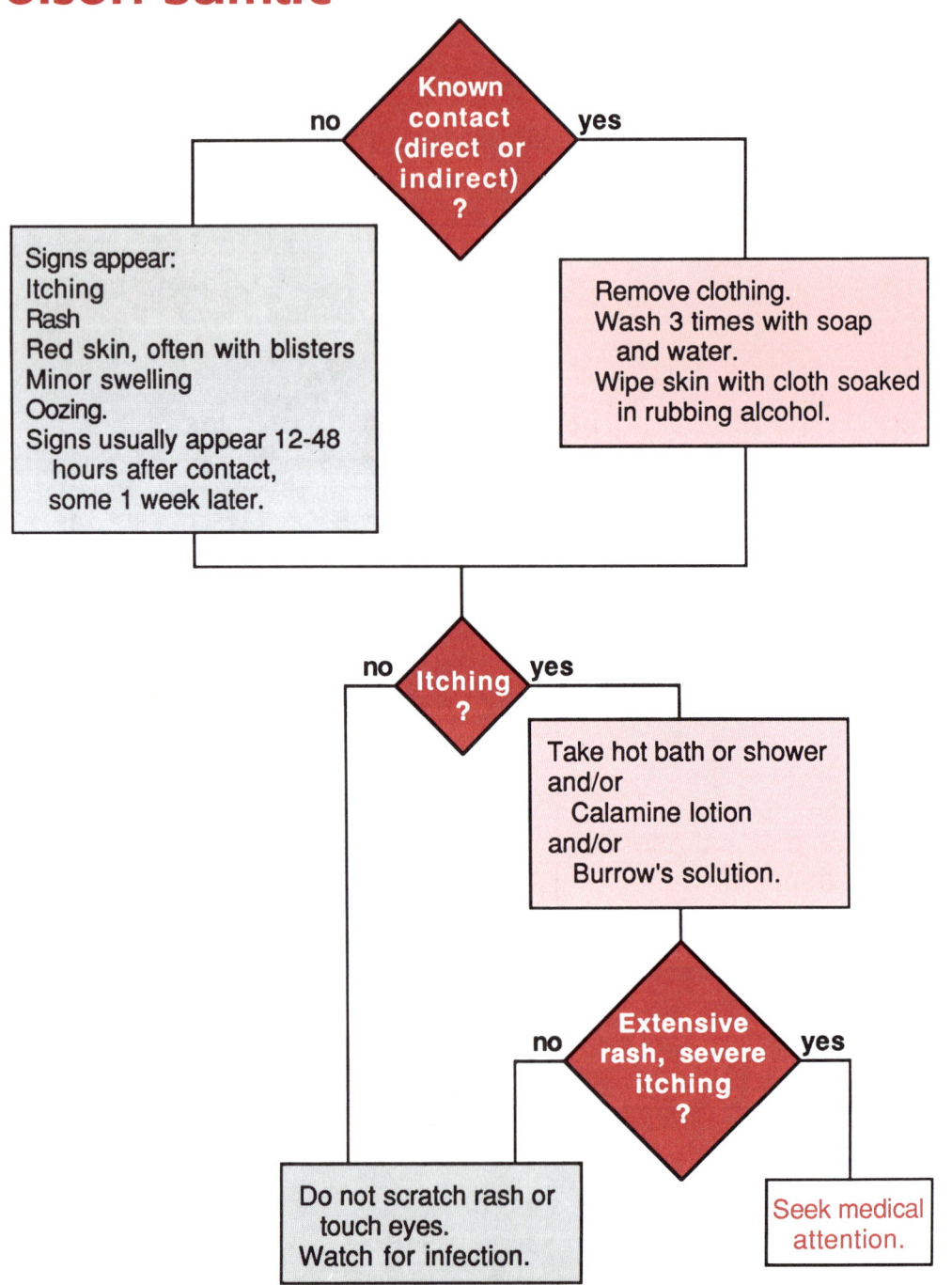

Known contact (direct or indirect)?
- no →
  - Signs appear:
    Itching
    Rash
    Red skin, often with blisters
    Minor swelling
    Oozing.
    Signs usually appear 12-48 hours after contact, some 1 week later.
- yes → Remove clothing. Wash 3 times with soap and water. Wipe skin with cloth soaked in rubbing alcohol.

Itching?
- yes → Take hot bath or shower and/or Calamine lotion and/or Burrow's solution.
- no → Do not scratch rash or touch eyes. Watch for infection.

Extensive rash, severe itching?
- no → Do not scratch rash or touch eyes. Watch for infection.
- yes → Seek medical attention.

SELF-CHECK QUESTIONS

Activity 1: Ingested Poison

A. You suspect a 3-year-old boy has swallowed aspirin from an opened bottle.

   What information should you immediately attempt to find out?

   1. ☐ Did he eat any aspirin?
   2. ☐ How many tablets, if any, did he eat?
   3. ☐ If he ate any aspirin, how long has it been?

B. An elderly man reports he swallowed a substance you know is poisonous.

   You should . . .
      Yes No
   1. ☐ ☐ Ask him how much he took, and when.
   2. ☐ ☐ Give him a glass of milk to drink.
   3. ☐ ☐ Telephone the Poison Control Center and tell them what you know about the poisoning.
   4. ☐ ☐ Empty the victim's stomach before attempting to contact a medical authority.

C. Mark the following statements true (T) or false (F).

   1. ☐ Induce vomiting for swallowed gasoline victims.
   2. ☐ Induce vomiting immediately for those who have swallowed a strong acid.
   3. ☐ A Poison Control Center's instructions include inducing vomiting for an unconscious person who has swallowed a poison.
   4. ☐ Throat damage can result if vomiting occurs after swallowing a poison.
   5. ☐ Immediately dilute with milk or water any swallowed corrosive.

D. Mark the following statements true (T) or false (F).

   1. ☐ Induce vomiting with syrup of ipecac in a conscious person who has swallowed a poison.
   2. ☐ Give syrup of ipecac for poisoning only after receiving medical advice or when told to do so by a Poison Control Center.
   3. ☐ Syrup of ipecac alone causes vomiting.
   4. ☐ Gagging or drinking warm salt water are as effective and safe as syrup of ipecac for inducing vomiting.

E. Mark each statement true (T) or false (F).
1. ☐ Syrup of ipecac removes only 30%–40% of the poison.
2. ☐ Activated charcoal binds chemicals.
3. ☐ Burnt toast, fireplace ashes, and charcoal briquettes represent activated charcoal.
4. ☐ The victim drinks the activated charcoal and water mixed
5. ☐ Give activated charcoal before inducing vomiting.

Activity 2: Insect Stings

Which are appropriate first aid measures for insect stings?

　　　Yes　No
1. ☐ ☐ Remove a stinger with tweezers or fingers.
2. ☐ ☐ Wash the stung areas with soap and water.
3. ☐ ☐ Place a warm pack over the stung area.
4. ☐ ☐ Immediately seek medical attention for the victim.
5. ☐ ☐ For allergic reactions, use epinephrine from an "emergency insect sting kit."

Activity 3: Snakebites

Which should you do for a venomous snakebite?

Choice 1　　　　　　　　　　　　　　　　　　　　*Choice 2*

1. ☐ Cool the bite site with ice.　　　OR　☐ Avoid using cold on the bite site.
2. ☐ Cut through the bite wound if several hours from a medical facility.　　　OR　☐ Avoid cutting through any snakebite wound.
3. ☐ First aiders can give antivenin.　　　OR　☐ Only qualified medical personnel should give antivenin.
4. ☐ Apply a tourniquet.　　　OR　☐ Apply a constriction band.
5. ☐ If possible, identify the snake and its size.　　　OR　☐ Information about the snake isn't usually needed.

Activity 4: Spider Bites and Scorpion Stings

Which of the following first aid procedures are appropriate for spider bites and scorpion stings?

Yes No
1. ☐ ☐ Apply a cold or ice pack over the bite site.
2. ☐ ☐ Seek medical attention immediately.
3. ☐ ☐ Apply a constriction band 2–4 inches above the bite.
4. ☐ ☐ Capture the spider or have a definite identification.
5. ☐ ☐ Apply calamine lotion to relieve pain.
6. ☐ ☐ Wash area with soap and water or rubbing alcohol.

Activity 5: Tick Removal

Choose which of the following methods are most likely to be successful in removing an embedded tick.

1. ☐ Apply a substance (i.e., oil, grease, etc.) to smother the tick causing it to disengage its head.
2. ☐ Apply fingernail polish and allow it to harden. Peel the polish off and the tick will come with it.
3. ☐ Apply heat by holding a heated needle or a blown out, glowing match head to the tick.
4. ☐ Pull the embedded tick out with tweezers.
5. ☐ Pry a tick out with a needle.
6. ☐ Put some gasoline or rubbing alcohol on a cotton ball and tape it loosely over the tick for 15 minutes.
7. ☐ Apply an ice cube over the tick.

Activity 6: Poison Ivy, Oak, and Sumac

Check which of the following may be useful in alleviating the itching from poison ivy.
1. ☐ Apply rubbing alcohol to the rash and all affected areas.
2. ☐ Apply calamine lotion to the rash.
3. ☐ Apply petroleum jelly to the affected area.
4. ☐ Apply buttermilk or cream to the affected area.
5. ☐ Apply hot water (don't burn victim) even though intense itching will initially be felt.
6. ☐ Only a physician's prescription for cortisone works.
7. ☐ Wash the affected area with soap and water.

Activity 7: Carbon Monoxide Poisoning

Mark the statement true (T) or false (F).
1. ☐ Carbon monoxide (CO) from automobiles is easily detected by its odor.
2. ☐ Headache characterizes carbon monoxide poisoning.
3. ☐ Carbon monoxide victims need pure oxygen as quickly as possible.
4. ☐ Check with a physician whenever carbon monoxide poisoning is suspected.
5. ☐ Carbon monoxide poisoning symptoms can be confused with those of viral infections (flu).

8

Burns

- Thermal Burns • Chemical Burns • Electrical Burns

THERMAL BURN

Burn injury often generates extraordinary anxiety, not only in the victim and bystanders but in the first aider as well. Inexperience may explain some of the apprehension felt by most first aiders. With two million people burned each year, most first aiders will eventually be called upon to treat this type of injury.

Initially, most burns are minor problems. But without aggressive emergency care, these injuries can progress to serious conditions. Early assessment and emergency care of the burn victim is critical in minimizing pain, long-term disability, and disfigurement.

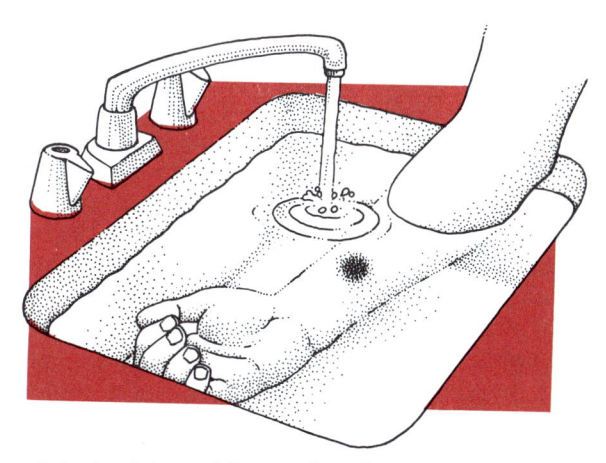

8-1. Applying cold water for a burn

First Aid

When a first aider encounters a burned victim, establish that the victim is not in any life threatening danger by quickly assessing the airway, pulse, and external bleeding and by treating any life threatening problems. The flames should be extinguished. During assessment, remove rings, bracelets, or other jewelry before edema (swelling) makes removal difficult. Take off burned clothing, cutting around and leaving fabric that adheres to wounds. Avoid unnecessary contamination, but since burn wounds are not life threatening at this point, cleansing is not recommended. If possible, elevate burned areas such as hands or feet to minimize swelling.

Quickly and carefully remove any of the victim's clothing. Do not pull stuck fabric; cut around where it adheres to the skin. Later removal could be difficult and painful if swelling develops. Do not apply petroleum jelly, butter, or any burn medication. Ointments seal in the heat; may have to be scrubbed off in the hospital, causing unnecessary pain if the burn is serious; and offer little real pain relief.

For most minor burns, a continuous flow of cool tap water stops pain. (*See* Figure 8-1.) Prompt cooling may lessen local tissue destruction and the severity of the burn. In fact, if the burned skin has cold applied to it within thirty seconds of being burned, skin temperature drops to normal within three seconds. Cool water can help even when applied up to forty-five minutes after the burn. Have the victim immerse the burned area in cool water while keeping the tap on to maintain a cool temperature. If the site of the injury (e.g., the face) renders this awkward, cool compresses refreshed frequently under cool water will suffice.

The victim with a major burn—one involving more than 10% of the body surface or roughly the equivalent of the surface of one arm—should be transported immediately to the nearest emergency facility. Once a burn has been cooled, covering the area with a dressing will help control pain.

There is a controversy over whether to keep extensively burned areas wet or dry. One school of thought maintains that you should wrap the burned area with a moist dressing. The other school of thought prefers to keep the area dry because a wet victim easily becomes hypothermic. It seems reasonable that moist dressings can be used on small burned areas (<10%) and avoid such dressings on larger burned areas. Do not break any blisters because infection can be introduced.

When transporting the victim to an emergency facility, apply ice wrapped in several layers of towels. It takes from thirty minutes to three hours to stop the pain, depending on the depth and extent of the wound. Cooling is no longer necessary if pain does not recur when the compresses are removed from the burn for a five minute period.

Assessing the Burn

One of the first things for a first aider to do when confronted with a burned victim is to assess the severity of the burn. It should be stressed, however, that you should have already checked and taken care of breathing problems and severe bleeding.

In assessing a burn, you should appraise the following (remember, even experienced physicians have difficulty in assessing burns):

- *How large is the burn?* The extent of the burn is expressed as a percentage of the total body surface. The familiar "Rule of Nines" defines each hand and arm as 9% of the body surface. Each leg counts as 18% of the body surface. The front and back torso are each valued at 18% with the genital area at 1%. The victim's hand size is about 1% and this surface area can be used for calculating most burns. (*See* Figure 8-2.)

The Rule of Nines is accurate for adults, but it does not make allowances for the different proportions of a child. In small children the head accounts for 18% and each leg 14%. You will have to allow for that.

- *How deep is the burn?*

First-Degree Burns. These burns affect only the outer layer of skin (epidermis). Characteristics include redness, mild swelling, tenderness, and pain. These burns often result from sunburn, hot water scalding, and flash burns. Healing occurs without scarring within a week.

Second-Degree Burns. These burns extend through the entire outer skin layer (epidermis) and into the inner skin layer (dermis). Blister formation, swelling, weeping of fluids, and severe pain characterize second-degree burns. Healing with little scarring takes about three weeks.

Third-Degree Burns. These severe burns extend through the epidermis, dermis, and into the underlying fat, muscle, and bone. Discoloration (charred, white, or cherry red), leathery, and dryness indicate this degree of burn. Absence of pain occurs because of the destruction of nerve endings. Any pain found with this burn results from accompanying lesser degrees of burns (first- and/or second-degree). These burns result from ignited clothing, electricity, explosions, and petroleum fires. Proper healing requires skin grafting.

- *What parts of the body are burned?* Areas of most importance are the face (especially the eyelids), the hands, the feet, and the genitals. Burns of the respiratory tract are particular serious if associated with the inhalation of fumes or blast effects.

- *How old is the burned victim?* A burn is considered more serious in a young infant and in an

8-2. The "Rule of Nines"

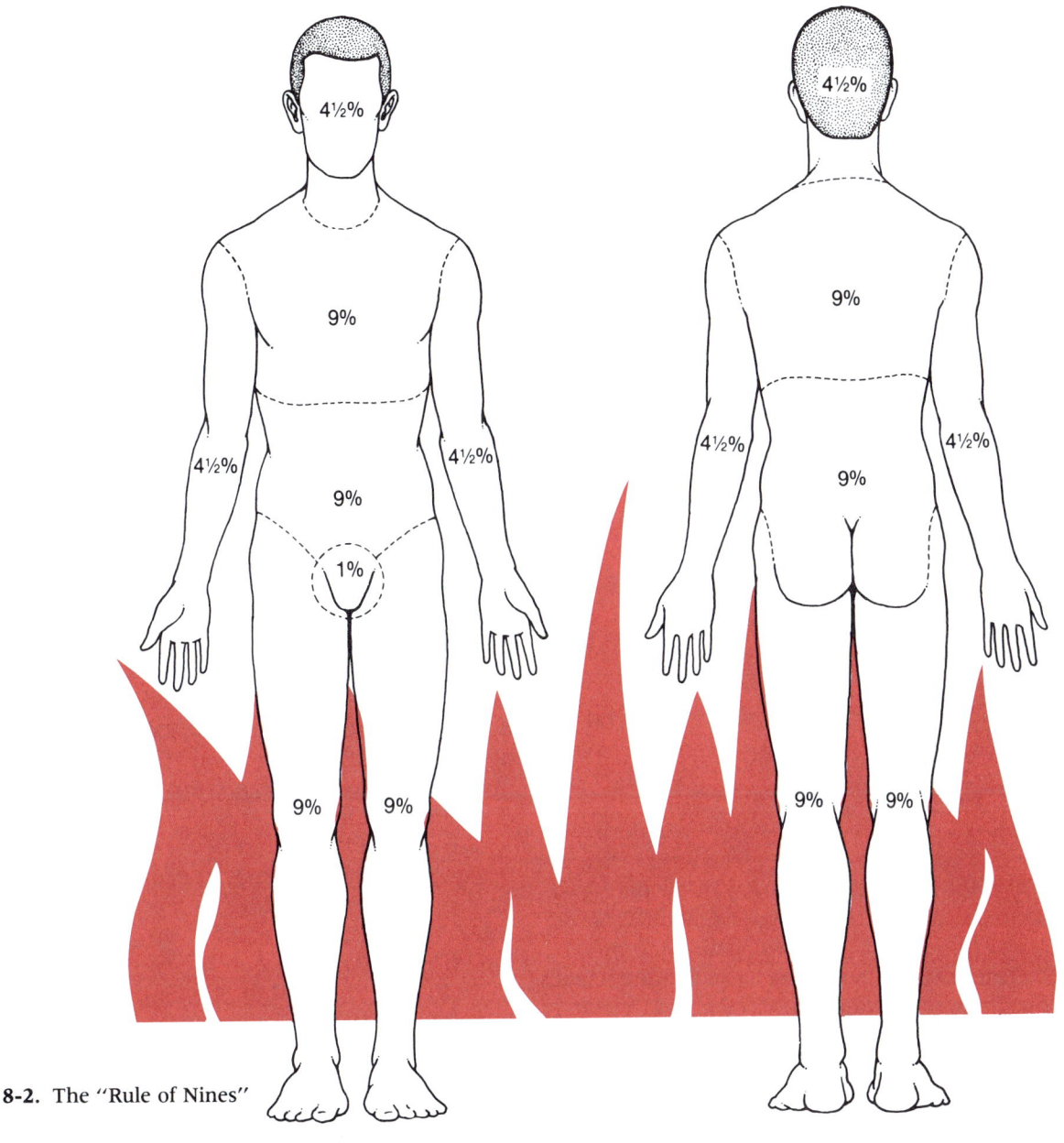

elderly person (over 65) than in other victims. Younger victims have poor antibody response to infection. In older victims, serious burns aggravate other health problems (e.g., heart disease).

• *Does the victim have any injuries or medical problems?* Burns can aggravate diabetes, rheumatic heart disease, chronic obstructive pulmonary disease, as well as other medical problems. Injuries received (other than the burn) such as extensive lacerations can complicate the victim's recovery. With this information and reference to Table 8-1, you can determine the severity of a burn on a victim.

TABLE 8-1. Burn Severity

Burn classification	Characteristics
Minor burn	1° burns
	2° burns <15% BSA adults
	2° burns <5% BSA in children/elderly persons
	3° burn <2% BSA
Moderate burn	2° burn 15%–25% BSA in adults
	2° burn 10%–20% BSA in children/elderly persons
	3° burn <10% BSA
Major burn	2° burn >25% BSA in adults
	2° burn >20% BSA in children/elderly persons
	3° burn >10% BSA
	Burns of hands, face, eyes, feet, or perineum
	Most victims with inhalation injury, electrical injury, major trauma, or significant preexisting diseases

BSA = Body surface area
Adapted from the American Burn Association categorization.

Most burn information centers upon the immediate care of the damaged tissue rather than instructions about caring for that tissue during the subsequent days. Use of information in Table 8-2 serves as a guide to proper first aid for burns.

The quality of burn care has a definite impact on the eventual outcome. One should certainly follow a physician's recommendations about caring for the burn, but many burns are never seen by a doctor. That is why the following suggestions are so relevant:

1. Wash hands thoroughly before changing any dressing.

2. Attempt to leave unbroken blisters intact.

3. Change dressings two times a day unless otherwise specified by a physician.

4. Change a dressing by:

   a. Removing old dressings. If it adheres, soak it off with cool, clean water.

   b. Cleanse area gently with mild soap (e.g., Ivory™) and water.

   c. Pat dry with clean, dry cloth.

   d. Apply a thin layer of antibacterial cream to the burn.

   e. Apply clean dressings.

5. Watch for signs of infection. Call a physician if any of these appear:

   a. Increased redness, pain, tenderness, swelling, or red streaks near burn

   b. Pus

   c. Elevated temperature (fever)

6. Keep the area and dressing as clean and dry as possible.

7. Elevate the burned area, if possible, for the first twenty-four hours.

8. Administer a pain medication, if necessary.

Proper burn care will decrease the chance of infection and speed the healing process.

The time needed for the wound to heal varies according to the wound. A relatively minor partial-thickness burn may close in five to seven days; a deep partial-thickness burn may take up to thirty days to heal. When the wound is closed, apply moisturizing cream as needed to prevent excessive drying and itching.

Damaged skin cannot tolerate daily wear and tear even though it appears healed. An injury on an exposed area of the body is especially vulnerable. Total healing requires up to eighteen months, and the burned area must be hypersensitive to heat and cold for a long time after the injury occurred.

Vitamin E ointment has been promoted by some as useful for treating superficial burns; yet there are no known controlled studies to support the claim.

Extracts of the Aloe vera plant are widely believed by the public to be useful in the treatment of first-degree burns (e.g., sunburn). This is supported by a long history of use in Mexico. Even though scientific documentation of its effectiveness is extremely limited, researchers are

TABLE 8-2. First Aid for Burns

Burn	Do	Don't
First Degree (redness, mild swelling, and pain)	Apply cold water and/or dry sterile dressing.	Apply butter, oleomargarine, etc.
Second Degree (deeper; blisters develop)	Immerse in cold water, blot dry with sterile cloth for protection. Treat for shock. Obtain medical attention if severe.	Break blisters. Remove shreds of tissue. Use antiseptic preparation, ointment spray, or home remedy on severe burn.
Third Degree (deeper destruction, skin layers destroyed)	Cover with sterile cloth to protect. Treat for shock. Watch for breathing difficulty. Obtain medical attention quickly.	Remove charred clothing that is stuck to burn. Apply ice. Use home medication.
Chemical Burn	Remove by flushing with large quantities of water for at least 5 minutes. Remove surrounding clothing. Obtain medical attention.	

Source: U.S. Coast Guard.

finding support for its use in the treatment of minor burns after the burned part has been first cooled.

CHEMICAL BURNS

You need not have training in toxicology to treat all of the common chemical burns, because emergency care is the same for all except a few special burns for which something has to be added to neutralize the chemical.

All acids, alkalies, and caustic agents are best treated by washing with large quantities of water. In acid and alkali burns, damage is practically set within three minutes after the victim comes in contact with the chemical, so if you get the victim in the water in the first minute or two after the injury, the damage will be substantially reduced. Removal of contaminated clothing takes any absorbed chemicals away from the skin. This can be done during washing.

Nevertheless, prolonged washing may do a great deal of good, even when it is started late. Prolonged washing means washing for no less than twenty minutes. That is a long time and it is difficult to do, even in the best of circumstances.

Try to avoid applying water under any type of pressure because it drives the chemical deeper into the tissue. Use a faucet or hose under low pressure and simply wash with a gently flow for long periods of time.

The washing technique must be modified for dry lime and white phosphorus burns. Before washing, the lime should be brushed away gently. Water mixed with lime reacts chemically to produce heat, which may further burn the skin. White phosphorus continues to burn as long as it is exposed to oxygen. The only way to stop the burning is to close off the air supply to the affected area. This can be done by submerging it in water or covering with an airtight wet dressing.

Do not attempt to neutralize a chemical because the neutralizatiion process may produce heat, which can cause further damage. Some product label directions for neutralizing may be wrong. Call a Poison Control Center to find out other steps you can take. Additional treatments would be the same as for any thermal burn of the same extent and depth.

ELECTRICAL BURNS

When electrical current passes through tissue, it creates heat, causing internal burns. These burns are actually worse than they look from the outside. Third-degree burns will be seen where the current entered and exited the body. The current can travel along blood vessels and nerves as well as muscles. Electricity does its major damage inside the body.

If a person grabs hold of a "hot" wire, the electrical current causes the muscles in the hand to contract (fingers close around the cord), making it impossible for the person to remove his or her hand. The only safe way to "free" such a person is to stop the current. In addition, the current may paralyze the nerves and muscles that control breathing and heartbeat. Unconsciousness and death can occur even from house current.

When someone is in contact with electrical current, it is not safe to touch him or her until the current has stopped. You may unplug the appliance if the plug is not damaged, or turn off the power at the switch box if you are afraid to touch the cord. *Do not touch the appliance or the victim until the current is off.*

Current crossing the heart by taking a hand-to-hand pathway is more dangerous than current taking a hand-to-foot or foot-to-foot pathway. Electricity takes the path of least resistance, which is going to involve the nerves and blood vessels. Hands are most likely to be one of the entrance or exit points of the electricity since they tend to be uncovered, wet, and used to touch things.

The first priority at the scene of an electrical injury is prevention of injury to rescuers and bystanders. If there is a fallen wire at the scene, treat it as live. Do not approach the victim until the power is disconnected, the wire removed from the victim, or the wire is dead. Do not attempt to remove the wire with ropes or wooden poles or to cut the wire. Wait until the electric company or qualified rescue unit arrives to handle the situation.

If the victim is involved in a motor vehicle accident and the downed wire is making contact with the car, do not let the victim get out of the car or let bystanders try to help the victim out of the car. The only exception to this rule is when there is a potential of the car igniting. In this case, instruct the victim to jump out of the car carefully without making contact with the car or wire.

Once the danger of causing injury to the rescuers has passed, treatment can begin. The first priority is to check the ABCs—airway, breathing and circulation. Give mouth-to-mouth resuscitation and/or cardiopulmonary resuscitation, whichever is needed. The two most common causes of death from electrical injury are asphyxiation and cardiac arrest.

Asphyxiation results from the muscular contractions produced by alternating current. The spasms not only affect the victim's ability to let go of the energized object, but also they impair the victim's ability to breathe.

Electrical current may result in loss of consciousness lasting from several minutes to hours. If the current passes directly through the brain, it may cause a seizure.

When vital signs are stable, you can check for burns. You may relieve the pain of first- and second-degree burns by applying cold water, but most electrical burns are third-degree burns. If the skin is charred or white, cover with sterile material, elevate the part, and treat for shock by elevating the legs about twelve inches and keeping the victim warm. Seek medical aid for the victim.

The victim should be transported to the nearest hospital capable of handling such an injury.

The severity of electrical burns often is difficult to determine because the deeper layers of the skin, muscles, and internal organs may be involved.

Thermal Burns

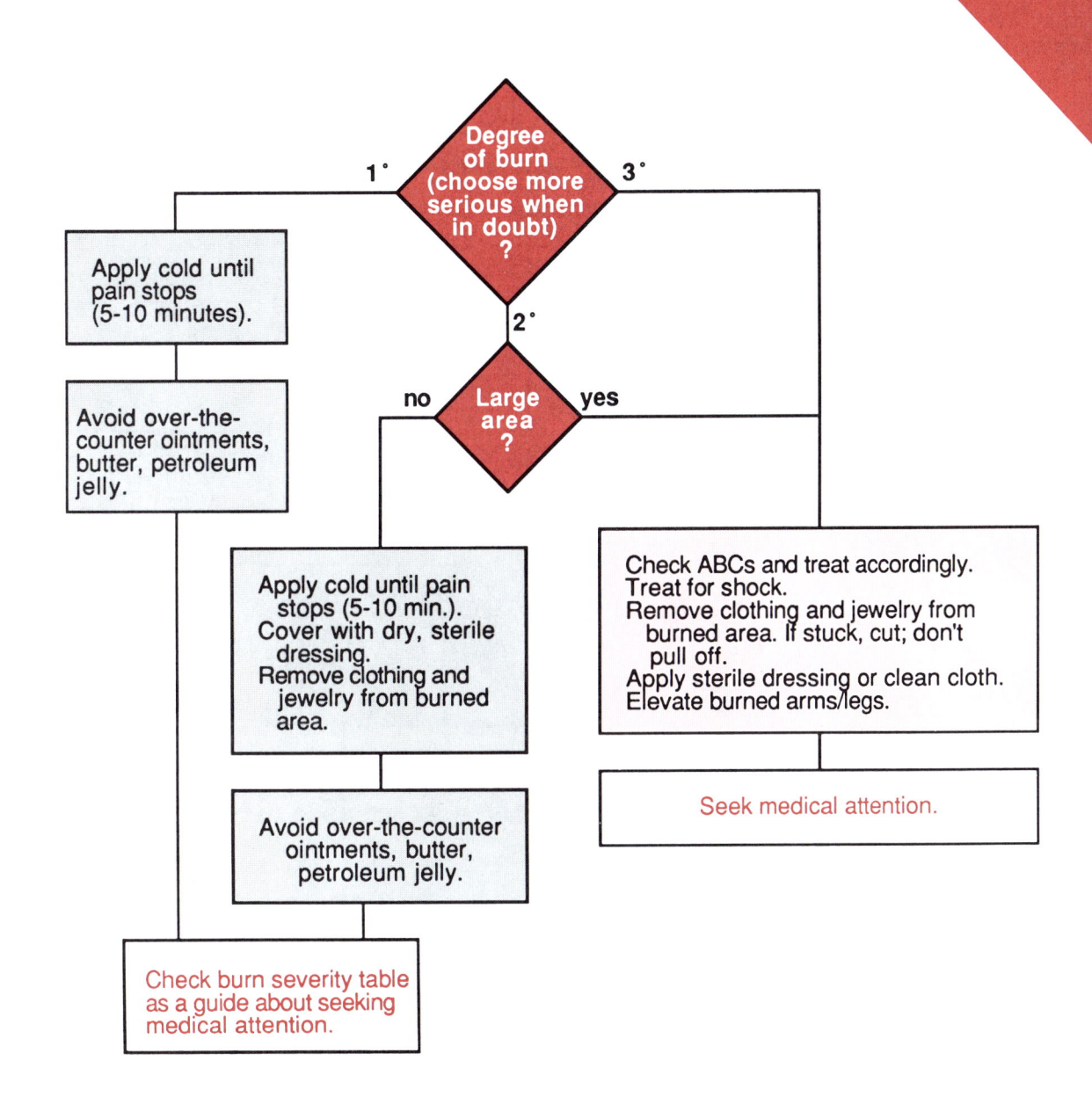

Degree of burn (choose more serious when in doubt)?

- **1°**:
  - Apply cold until pain stops (5-10 minutes).
  - Avoid over-the-counter ointments, butter, petroleum jelly.

- **2°** — **Large area?**
  - **no**:
    - Apply cold until pain stops (5-10 min.). Cover with dry, sterile dressing. Remove clothing and jewelry from burned area.
    - Avoid over-the-counter ointments, butter, petroleum jelly.
    - Check burn severity table as a guide about seeking medical attention.
  - **yes**:
    - Check ABCs and treat accordingly. Treat for shock. Remove clothing and jewelry from burned area. If stuck, cut; don't pull off. Apply sterile dressing or clean cloth. Elevate burned arms/legs.
    - Seek medical attention.

- **3°**:
  - Check ABCs and treat accordingly. Treat for shock. Remove clothing and jewelry from burned area. If stuck, cut; don't pull off. Apply sterile dressing or clean cloth. Elevate burned arms/legs.
  - Seek medical attention.

Chemical Burns

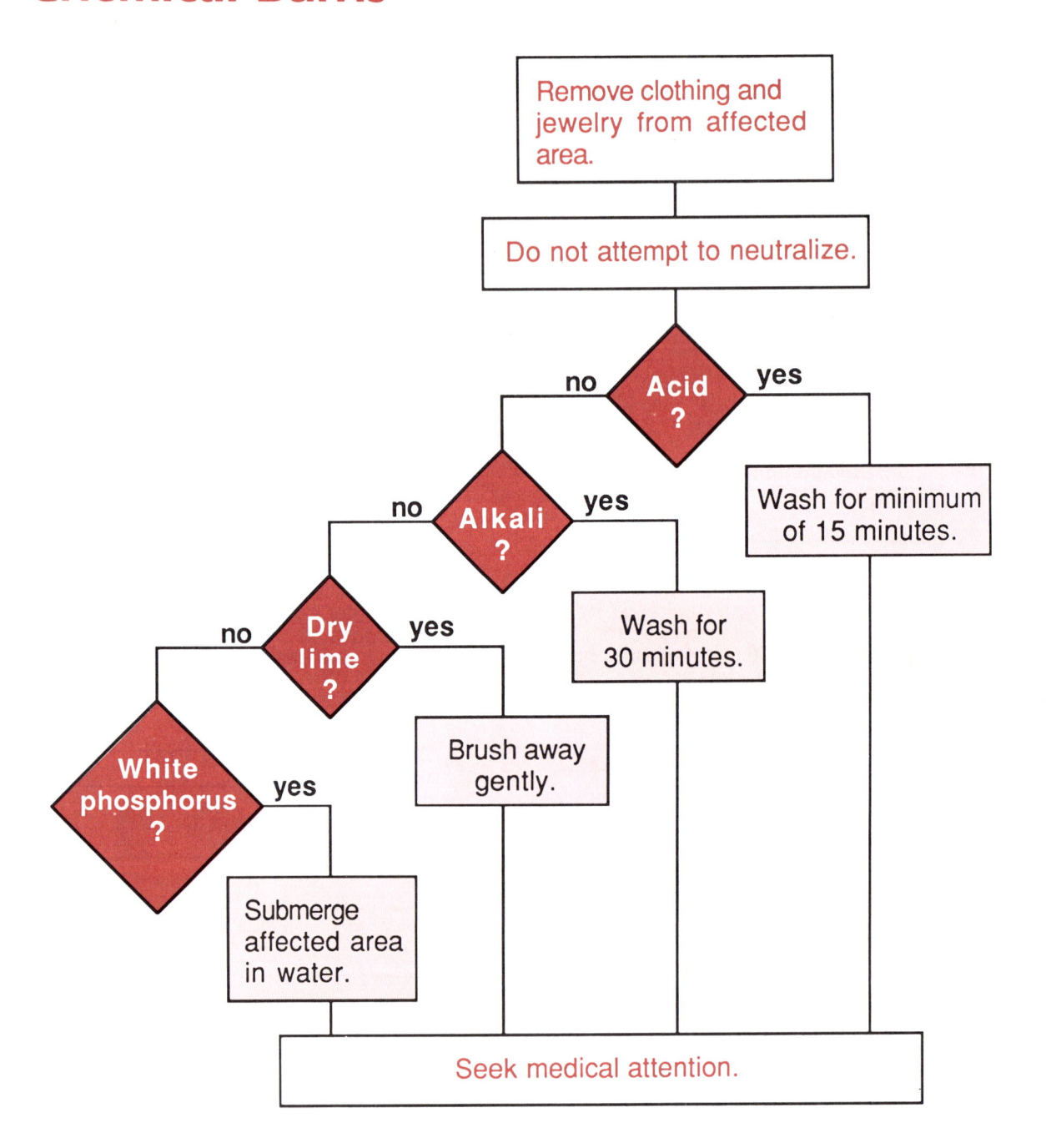

```
Remove clothing and jewelry from affected area.
        │
Do not attempt to neutralize.
        │
      Acid?
      ├── yes → Wash for minimum of 15 minutes.
      └── no
           │
         Alkali?
         ├── yes → Wash for 30 minutes.
         └── no
              │
            Dry lime?
            ├── yes → Brush away gently.
            └── no
                 │
               White phosphorus?
               └── yes → Submerge affected area in water.
```

Seek medical attention.

Electrical Burns

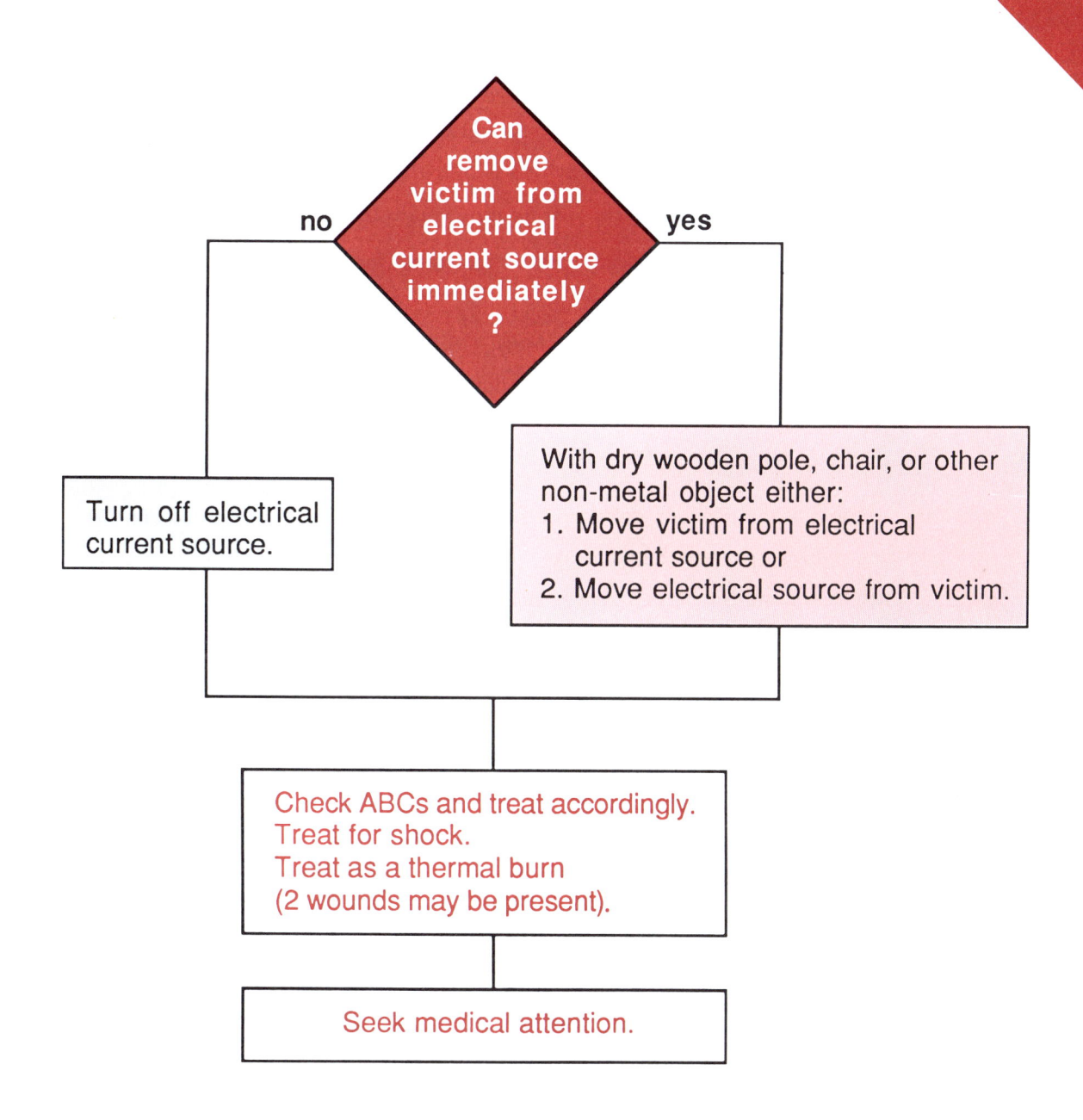

```
                    Can
                  remove
                 victim from
      no         electrical        yes
                current source
                 immediately
                      ?
```

Turn off electrical current source.

With dry wooden pole, chair, or other non-metal object either:
1. Move victim from electrical current source or
2. Move electrical source from victim.

**Check ABCs and treat accordingly.
Treat for shock.
Treat as a thermal burn
(2 wounds may be present).**

Seek medical attention.

The above procedures apply only for low voltage situations (i.e., households). Otherwise, never attempt to move a downed wire. Wait for the power company or specially trained personnel with the necessary equipment to handle the electrical hazard.

139

SELF-CHECK QUESTIONS

Activity 1: Thermal Burns

A. You just burned your hand by falling onto a hot cooking grill. What should you do first to ease the pain?
   1. ☐ Hold the hand in a sink filled with lukewarm water.
   2. ☐ Cover the burned area with a clean dressing.
   3. ☐ Cover the burn with petroleum jelly or any over-the-counter burn ointment.
   4. ☐ Place your hand in a sink filled with running cold water.

B. How could you lessen pain while seeking medical assistance for a burned victim?
   1. ☐ Soak burned area in warm water.
   2. ☐ Cover small burned areas with wet cloths.
   3. ☐ Cover large burned areas with wet dressings.
   4. ☐ Pinch the area.
   5. ☐ Immerse in cold salt water.

C. Which one of the following actions should you perform while soaking your burned hand?
   1. ☐ Remove any rings from the hand.
   2. ☐ Pinch or squeeze the burned area to relieve pain.
   3. ☐ Add salt to lower the water temperature.

D. Classify each of the following actions as *Do* or *Do Not* when giving first aid for a burn.

	Do	Do Not	
1.	☐	☐	Apply petroleum jelly to the burn.
2.	☐	☐	Pull a piece of clothing stuck to a burn.
3.	☐	☐	Apply a clean dressing and secure it in place.
4.	☐	☐	Blow on a burned area to cool it.
5.	☐	☐	Use your fingers to remove pieces of burned skin.
6.	☐	☐	Open blisters before apply a dressing.
7.	☐	☐	Apply cool water to the burn.

Activity 2: Chemical Burns

Which of the following procedures apply to proper chemical burn care?

1. ☐ Put on butter, an over-the-counter ointment, or spray to relieve pain.
2. ☐ Neutralize an acid with an alkali or vice versa.
3. ☐ Flood area immediately with cool water for at least 10 minutes.
4. ☐ Remove contaminated clothing as flooding takes place.
5. ☐ A strong spray of water effectively removes chemicals.
6. ☐ Do nothing except seek medical attention immediately.

Activity 3: Electrical Burns

Mark each of the following statements true (T) or false (F).

1. ☐ Most electrical burns cause third-degree burns.
2. ☐ Electrical burns produce both entrance and exit wounds.
3. ☐ Jump from a vehicle if it is likely to ignite.
4. ☐ Heart stoppage may result from an electrocution.

9

Exposure to Cold and Heat

• Frostbite • Hypothermia • Heat-Related Emergencies

FROSTBITE

As the body tries to conserve heat for vital internal organs in bitter cold, the flow of warming blood to the extremities is reduced. Eventually, if the temperature in the tissue drops low enough, tiny ice crystals begin to form in the watery spaces between the cells. Expanding outward in all directions, the ice ruptures cell membranes and kills the tissue, which turns white, stiff, and insensitive to the touch. Furthermore, the reduced blood flow (due to sludging and clotting of blood inside small blood vessels) raises the possibility of gangrene occurring.

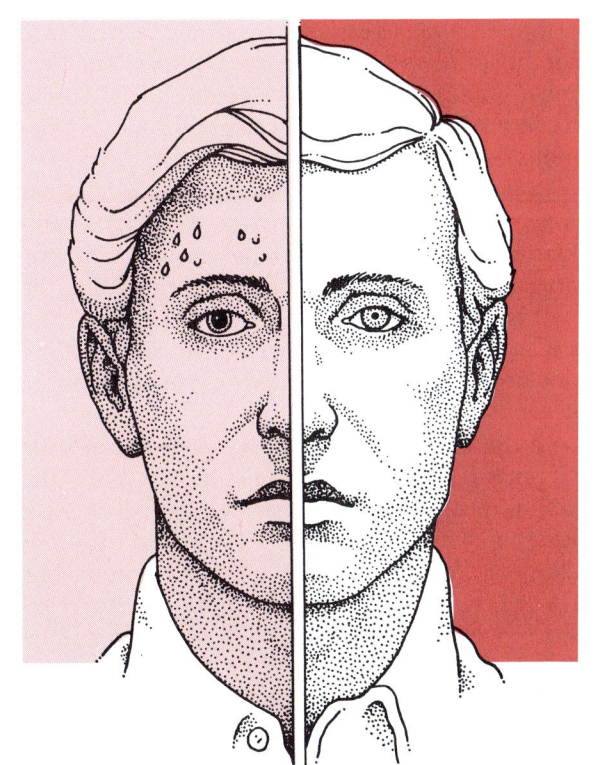

The extent of the injury depends on such factors as temperature, duration of exposure, wind velocity, humidity, lack of protective clothing, and the presence of wet clothing. Use Tables 9-1 and 9-2 as aids in determining actual temperatures. Also, the harmful effects of exposure to cold are intensified by fatigue, individual susceptibility, existing injuries, emotional stress, smoking, and drinking alcoholic beverages.

Types of Frostbite

The extent of injury is not usually known at first glance. At one time, some effort was made to describe frostbite injury in terms of degrees, as is presently done with burns (e.g., first, second, third degree). Frostbite injuries are now classified as either superficial or deep. Even these designations are somewhat limited because it is difficult initially to tell the extent of injury. Classifying may not matter, however, because the treatment for both types is basically the same.

Superficial: Fingers, cheeks, ears, and nose are the most commonly affected body parts. If the

143

TABLE 9-1. Wind-Chill Factor

Estimated Wind Speed (in MPH)	Actual Thermometer Reading (°F.)										
	50	40	30	20	10	0	−10	−20	−30	−40	−50	−60
	Equivalent Temperature (°F.)										
calm	50	40	30	20	10	0	−10	−20	−30	−40	−50	−60
5	40	37	27	16	6	−5	−15	−26	−36	−47	−57	−68
10	40	28	16	4	−9	−24	−33	−46	−58	−70	−83	−95
15	36	22	9	−5	−18	−32	−45	−58	−72	−85	−99	−112
20	32	18	4	−10	−25	−39	−53	−67	−82	−96	−110	−124
25	30	16	0	−15	−29	−44	−59	−74	−88	−104	−118	−133
30	25	13	−2	−18	−33	−48	−63	−79	−94	−109	−125	−140
35	27	11	−4	−20	−35	−51	−67	−82	−98	−113	−129	−145
40	26	10	−6	−21	−37	−53	−69	−85	−100	−116	−132	−148

(Wind speeds greater than 40 mph have little additonal effect.) | Little danger (for properly clothed person). Maximum danger of false sense of security. | Increasing danger. (Flesh may freeze within 1 minute.) | Great danger. (Flesh may freeze within 30 seconds.)

exposure is prolonged, the freezing may extend up the arms and legs. Ice crystals in the skin and other tissues cause the area to appear a white or grayish-yellow color. Pain may occur early and subside. Often, the part will feel only very cold and numb; and there may be a tingling, stinging, or aching sensation. The victim may not be aware of frostbite until someone mentions it. When the damage is superficial, the surface will feel hard and underlying tissue soft when depressed gently and firmly. After thawing, the part becomes flushed and sometimes deep purple in color. It later sheds by flaking.

Deep: In deep, unthawed frostbite, the area (mainly the hands and feet) will feel hard, solid, and cannot be depressed. It will be cold, pale, and numb. Blisters will appear on the surface and in the underlying tissues in twelve to thirty-six hours. After thawing, it may be blue, purple, or black in color. The area will become swollen when it thaws, and later gangrene may occur. There will be a loss of tissue. Time alone will reveal the kind of frostbite that has been present.

First Aid

All frostbite injuries follow the same sequence in treatment: initial care, rapid rewarming, and post care. You should also assess the victim for hypothermia because it is a life-threatening condition for which priority treatment should be given.

Initial Care: The principles of emergency care for frostbite injury are relatively few. The two most important aspects are getting the victim to a place of permanent treatment as soon as possible, and then rewarming.

If the victim is out in the field—but not too far away from a medical facility—and the part is still frozen, transport the victim as he is and make no attempt to thaw the injured part. Be sure that the part is kept frozen. If partial thawing and refreezing occurs, ice crystals formed the second time are larger, and therefore, tissue damage is more severe.

If the injury occurs in a remote area and the victim's feet are frostbitten, you can allow the victim to walk on frostbitten feet only if the feet have not started to thaw. Otherwise, do not allow the victim to walk. Once rewarming has started, warming must be maintained. Refreezing or walking on a partially thawed part can be very harmful.

During transportation and initial treatment, do not permit the use of alcoholic beverages because they dilate capillaries and cause a loss of body heat. Do not let the victim smoke because

9 / EXPOSURE TO COLD AND HEAT

TABLE 9-2. Estimating Wind Velocity from Simple Observations

If you see ...	The wind is probably blowing
Flags or pennants hanging limp from their staffs; smoke rising vertically from chimneys and open fires	0–1 mph
Flags and pennants barely moving; leaves moving slightly on trees; smoke drifting lazily with the wind	0–3 mph
Flags and pennants moving slightly out from their staffs; leaves rustling in trees; if you feel wind on your face	4–7 mph
Flags and pennants standing out from their staffs at an angle of 30° to 40°; or leaves and twigs in constant motion	8–12 mph
Small branches moving in trees; dust and paper being blown about	13–18 mph
Flags and pennants flying at 90° angle; small trees swaying	19–24 mph
Flags and pennants standing straight out from their staffs and fluttering vigorously; large tree branches in motion; or if you hear whistling in power lines	25–31 mph
Flags and pennants whipping about widely on the staffs; whole trees in motion; loose objects being picked up and blown about; or if you find it somewhat difficult to walk when facing the wind	32–38 mph
Twigs being broken from trees; drivers having a problem in controlling their vehicles; or if you hear power lines whining loudly	39–46 mph
Trees bending sharply; structural damage occurring in buildings; the progress of vehicles and pedestrians alike being seriously impeded.	47–54 mph
Trees being uprooted; considerable structural damage occurring	55–63 mph
Buildings suffering severe damage	63–72 mph
Widespread destruction; or if walking is virtually impossible	more than 72 mph

smoking constricts capillaries and thus provides poor circulation.

Do not rub the affected part to restore circulation, and especially do not rub it with snow. Rubbing or massage increases the injury to frozen tissue; rubbing it with snow just intensifies the damage.

Rapid Rewarming: There are two techniques of rapid rewarming: wet and dry.

1. *The wet rapid rewarming technique* is preferred because it preserves the greatest amount of tissue. It is accomplished by completely immersing the part in an adequate amount of water at a temperature between 102°F and 106°F. Different authorities have suggested temperatures as low as 90°F to as high as 108°F. The water bath should be tested frequently with a thermometer. If a thermometer is not available, pour some of the water over the inner portion of your wrist or arm to make sure the water is not too hot. Discontinue warming when the part becomes flushed, usually within twenty minutes with the wet method. Further rapid wet rewarming is not necessary. For injuries involving the face or ears, you can apply warm moist cloths (frequently changed to maintain heat).

The thawing process is quick but usually quite painful. As thawing proceeds, a pink flushing progresses down the extremity; continue thawing until the tip of the thawed part flushes, is warm to the touch, and remains flushed when removed from the warm bath.

2. *The dry rapid rewarming technique* takes three to four times as long as the wet technique and is best accomplished by the use of natural body warmth as exemplified by putting the victim's hands in another person's axilla (armpit) or sharing warm clothing. Also, the victim can be exposed to warm room air.

The first aider should remember certain procedures *not* to take:

146 FIRST AID ESSENTIALS

1. Do *not* allow the victim to walk nor massage a body part.

2. Do *not* use water hotter than 110°F (may cause massive tissue destruction).

3. Do *not* expose the extremity near an open flame or fire.

Post-Care: After rewarming frostbite of a lower extremity, treat the victim as a stretcher case. Remove any of the victim's constricting clothing, maintain total body warmth, and encourage sleep. Protect the injured part(s) from direct contact with clothing, bedding, and so on.

After rewarming, take care to leave any blisters intact. Place dry, sterile gauze between toes and fingers to keep them separated. Elevate the affected part(s), and protect them from being bumped or rubbed.

Depending on circumstances, anyone exposed to temperatures below 32°F is a candidate for frostbite. This means that a large portion of the population are potential victims of frostbite injury.

HYPOTHERMIA

The *Guinness Book of World Records* reports two cases of victims surviving body temperatures as low as 60.8°F. One example is Dorothy Mae Stevens who was found alive in an alley in Chicago on February 1, 1951. In 1956, Vickie Mary Davis of Milwaukee, Wisconsin, at age two years and one month, was found unconscious on the floor of an unheated house and the air temperature had dropped to 24°F. Her temperature returned to normal after twelve hours, but it may have been as low as 59°F when she was first found.

Hypothermia (low body temperature) occurs when the body loses more heat than it produces. Subfreezing temperatures are not needed for hypothermia to occur. If body temperature falls to 80°F, most people die.

Types of Hypothermia

Mild hypothermia in the range of 90° to 95°F, may have few or no symptoms, abnormal drowsiness, slurred speech, memory lapses, incoherence, and fumbling hands. Persons suffering from mild hypothermia can walk but will frequently stumble and stagger. They are usually conscious and can talk. In healthy persons, there is almost no mortality. Though many people have cold extremities in winter, a hypothermic person has a cold abdomen and back. The hands and feet are the first body parts to get cold and the last to warm up.

Persons suffering from *severe* hypothermia with a temperature below 90°F must be considered at serious risk of dying. The following may be present: coldness to touch; pulselessness; cyanotic appearance; unresponsiveness to pain; and fixed, dilated pupils. Shivering usually stops. Muscles may become stiff and rigid, similar to rigor mortis.

Such findings make it difficult to distinguish a dead person from the hypothermic person who has a chance for complete recovery. The victim should not be considered dead unless he fails to respond to cardiopulmonary resuscitation after being rewarmed.

The victim's temperature should be taken rectally because oral and axillary temperatures reflect shell rather than core temperature. The standard clinical thermometer is calibrated from 94° to 108°F. A rectal thermometer reading from 84° to 108°F is available, though not commonly found.

Types of Exposure

The different types of exposure are based on heat loss rate.

Acute exposure occurs when the individual loses body heat very rapidly, usually in water immersion. Acute exposure is considered to be six hours or less in duration. An individual who plunges into cold water that causes his body core temperature to drop swiftly is an example.

Subacute exposure is defined as longer than six hours, but less than twenty-four hours, and it involves a land based experience or immersion in water warmer than 70°F. For example, a person who is lost in a sparsely populated area, or incapacitated for some reason elsewhere, who lies exposed much of the night to snow, rain, or cold, with insufficient clothing or shelter to maintain body core temperature.

Chronic hypothermia implies long-term cooling, generally occurring on land and lasting more than twenty-four hours. For example, a person could suffer from this as a result of drugs, disease, or failure of the body's temperature-regulating mechanism, perhaps combined with age. The person experiences a slow cooling over a period of days. This might occur without ever leaving a house where room temperatures are lower than the person can safely tolerate.

What You Need To Know About Hypothermia

Remember that subfreezing temperatures are not required for a person to succumb to hypothermia. It may develop within a few minutes by immersion in cold water, in a matter of hours by exposure to cold weather, or in a matter of days by continuous exposure to milder cold temperatures.

In the United States, hypothermia is most frequently seen among alcoholics, victims of drug abuse, and the elderly. One of the most common problems in the emergency care of hypothermia is the failure to recognize it. This is due, in part, to the inadequacy of standard thermometers. Oral thermometers (those found in most homes) register only as low as 94°F. Lower reading thermometers are used by emergency response teams and hospital emergency departments.

First Aid

The emergency care of hypothermia is aimed at rewarming the victim as well as treating complications that may arise. The hypothermic victim's heart is very susceptible to ventricular fibrillation which, therefore, is usually the ultimate cause of death in hypothermia. Keep this in mind while handling the hypothermic victim.

Guidelines (refer to Table 9-3) have been established and published for use by rescuers dealing with cold problems. They evolved from a conference conducted by the State of Alaska Emergency Medical Services Section.

TABLE 9-3. Treatment for Hypothermia by First Aiders and the General Public

1. Treat the victim very gently.
2. Remove wet clothing. Replace with dry clothing or dry coverings of some kind.
3. Insulate from the cold.
4. Add heat to the head, neck, chest, and groin externally (hot water bottles, warm bodies, warm packs—taking care not to burn the victim) or internally, if a system for breathing warm moist air is available. Avoid attempts to warm the extremities.
5. Do not rub or manipulate extremities.
6. Do not give coffee or alcohol.
7. Do not put victim in a shower or bath.
8. Warm fluids can be given only after uncontrollable shivering stops and the victim has a clear level of consciousness, the ability to swallow, and evidence of rewarming already.
9. If *severe hypothermia* is present, treat as above and transport to a medical facility.
10. If there is no way to get to a better medical facility, rewarm the victim slowly, cautiously, and gradually.

Treatment for Severe Hypothermia with No Life Signs (CPR Required)

1. Provide basic treatment as indicated above.
2. Carefully assess the presence or absence of pulse or respiration for one to two minutes.
3. If no pulse or respiration, start CPR.
4. Use mouth-to-mouth breathing.
5. Obtain a rectal temperature, if possible.
6. If you are less than fifteen minutes from a medical facility, do not bother trying to add heat.
7. If you are more than fifteen minutes from a medical facility, add heat gradually and gently.
8. Reassess the physical status (pulse and respiration) periodically.
9. Transfer to a medical facility in all cases.

Treatment for Severe Hypothermia with Signs of Life Pulse and Respirations Present (CPR Not Required)

1. Provide treatment as indicated in the first section.
2. If you are more than fifteen minutes from a medical facility, add heat gradually and gently.
3. Transfer to a medical facility.

Source: "State of Alaska Hypothermia and Cold Water Near Drowning Guidelines." Emergency Medical Services Section, Alaska Department of Health and Social Services. Reprinted with permission.

HEAT-RELATED EMERGENCIES

Heat afflicts people of all ages. However, the severity of the reaction tends to increase with age—heat cramps in a 17-year-old may be heat exhaustion in a 40-year-old and heat stroke in a person over 60.

The body tries to adapt to varying temperatures by adjusting the amount of salt in its perspiration. In hot weather, the idea is to lose enough water to keep the body cool, but to create the least possible chemical disturbances. Salt helps body tissues retain water, and if the body loses too much salt through perspiration, the person may be subject to dehydration and the further overheating that follows.

You should know the signs and symptoms of heat-related injuries and be able to administer first aid to others. Refer to Table 9-4 and see Figure 9-1. You must deal with heat exhaustion and heat stroke quickly or the victim can be in real trouble.

Heat Cramps

Heat cramps—muscle spasms occuring in the arms or legs after exertion—are the most painful, but least dangerous heat-related injury. They may occur when an excessive amount of body fluid is lost through sweating. The sodium and potassium lost from excessive sweating creates low amounts of these important minerals in the fluid surrounding the muscle cells. This changes the electrical sensitivity of the muscle, sometimes causing it to contract without warning and stay contracted, which can be very painful.

Cramping may recur because the mineral imbalance that caused the problem cannot be corrected immediately. A diet of fresh fruit and vegetables can help prevent potassium and sodium shortage. Dehydration must be prevented by drinking enough water to keep the body weight constant. Commercial exercise drinks contain the necessary minerals and fluids, but they should be used after exercising, rather than before or during it, when water is best.

Massage rarely provides relief and sometimes actually worsens pain; gentle stretching occasionally may be helpful. A salt water solution (one teaspon per quart of water) provides the proper balance. About one-half glassful should be given every 15 minutes for an hour. Discontinue if the victim vomits. A soft drink mix (e.g., Kool-Aid) can help the drink's taste. For the next few days, the victim should avoid the activity that brought on the cramps.

Heat Exhaustion

Heat exhaustion implies the inability of the circulatory and thermoregulatory systems to keep pace with the demands of work in the heat. It is less critical than heat stroke, but it requires prompt attention because it can progress to heat stroke if left untreated.

TABLE 9-4. Heat Exposure Emergencies

Indicators	Heat Cramps (Least Serious)	Heat Exhaustion (Serious)	Heat Stroke (Most Serious)
Cause	Salt and water loss	Salt and water loss	Failure of heat-regulating mechanisms
Cramping	Present	May be present	Absent
Skin	Cool, moist	Cool, pale, moist	Hot, flushed, dry
Temperature	Normal	Normal or low	Very high
Pulse	Rapid	Rapid, weak	Rapid, bounding
First aid	Salt water solution, unless on medical restriction. Commercial exercise drinks may be used.	Cooling Reclining position, elevate legs If conscious, cold liquids may be used.	Rapid cooling Semireclining position Obtain medical care immediately.

9 / EXPOSURE TO COLD AND HEAT

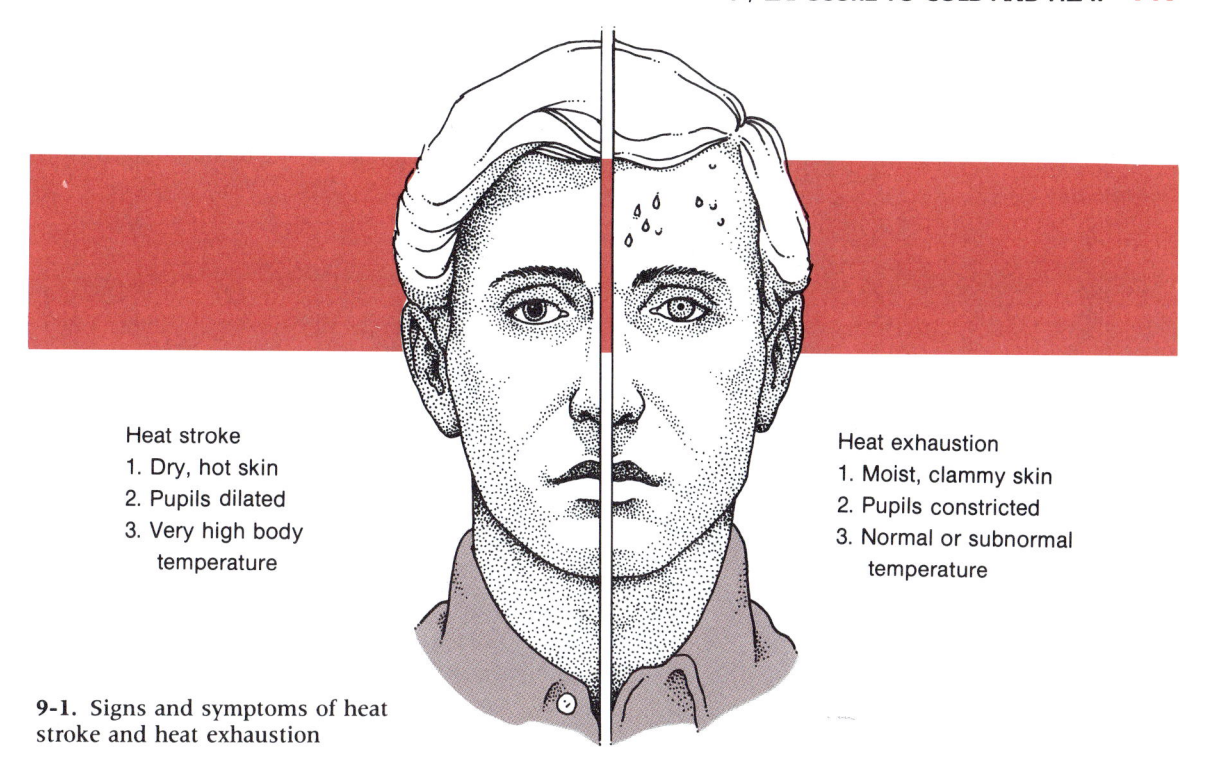

Heat stroke
1. Dry, hot skin
2. Pupils dilated
3. Very high body temperature

Heat exhaustion
1. Moist, clammy skin
2. Pupils constricted
3. Normal or subnormal temperature

9-1. Signs and symptoms of heat stroke and heat exhaustion

The skin is pale, cool, and wet. Heat exhaustion is especially serious and may be fatal in older people and people with heart problems. The victim must discontinue physical activity and be cooled immediately by applying cold to the skin, giving cold liquids by mouth, and exposing the skin to air (especially fans or air conditioners). The need for hospitalization is rare.

Heat Stroke

Heat stroke is the most dangerous heat emergency. The death rate from this condition approaches 50%, even with appropriate therapy.

Most victims are unconcious. The best sign of heat stroke is the victim's hot, dry skin and high body temperature. Heat stroke victims do not sweat because of severe electrolyte imbalance and impaired hypothalamus function. In addition, some experts believe that sweat glands actually become "fatigued" following periods of excessive perspiration. The victim may also reveal fixed, unreactive pupils of the eyes, blotchy redness of the face and skin.

Simply moving the person with heat stroke to a cooler environment is not usually enough to reverse the internal overheating. Quick action must be taken to lower the core body temperature. Immersion in tubs of ice water used to be the standard treatment for heat stroke victims. Many experts now recommend a simpler and more effective treatment. It can be started quickly and applied while transporting the victim to a medical facility.

Undress the heat stroke victim to allow air to circulate around the body (keep modesty in mind), and wrap him in wet towels. Then place ice packs at areas with abundant blood supply (e.g., neck, armpits, and groin). If driving to the hospital, leave the car windows open and have someone fan the victim, if possible. These maneuvers facilitate evaporation and begin the cooling process.

TABLE 9-5. Apparent Temperature

| Relative Humidity | Air Temperature |||||||||||
	70	75	80	85	90	95	100	105	110	115	120
	Apparent Temperature*										
0%	64	69	73	78	83	87	91	95	99	103	107
10%	65	70	75	80	85	90	95	100	105	111	116
20%	66	72	77	82	87	93	99	105	112	120	130
30%	67	73	78	84	90	96	104	113	123	135	148
40%	68	74	79	86	93	101	110	123	137	151	
50%	69	75	81	88	96	107	120	135	150		
60%	70	76	82	90	100	114	132	149			
70%	70	77	85	93	106	124	144				
80%	71	78	86	97	113	136					
90%	71	79	88	102	122						
100%	72	80	91	108							

*Degrees Fahrenheit.
Source: National Weather Service.

In addition to cooling the victim, check and treat accordingly any breathing stoppage and protect the victim during seizures, if they occur. Continue cooling the victim until his temperature drops to 102°F. Stop at this point in order to prevent seizures from occuring. All heat stroke victims should be hospitalized.

It is important to prevent heat-related injuries through adequate water and mineral intake to prevent the dehydration and chemical imbalances. If a heat-related injury occurs, prompt and adequate treatment are even more important to keep the condition from becoming a life-threatening one.

Table 9-5 shows the apparent temperature (how hot the weather feels) at various combinations of temperature and humidity. When the apparent temperature rises above 130°F, heat stroke may be imminent. Between 105° and 130°F, heat cramps or heat exhaustion are likely. With prolonged exposure and physical activity, heat stroke is also possible. Between 90° and 105°F, heat cramps and heat exhaustion are possible with lengthy exposure and activity. Between 80° and 90°F fatigue occurs during prolonged activity and/or exposure. Heat stress varies with age, health, and body characteristics.

Frostbite

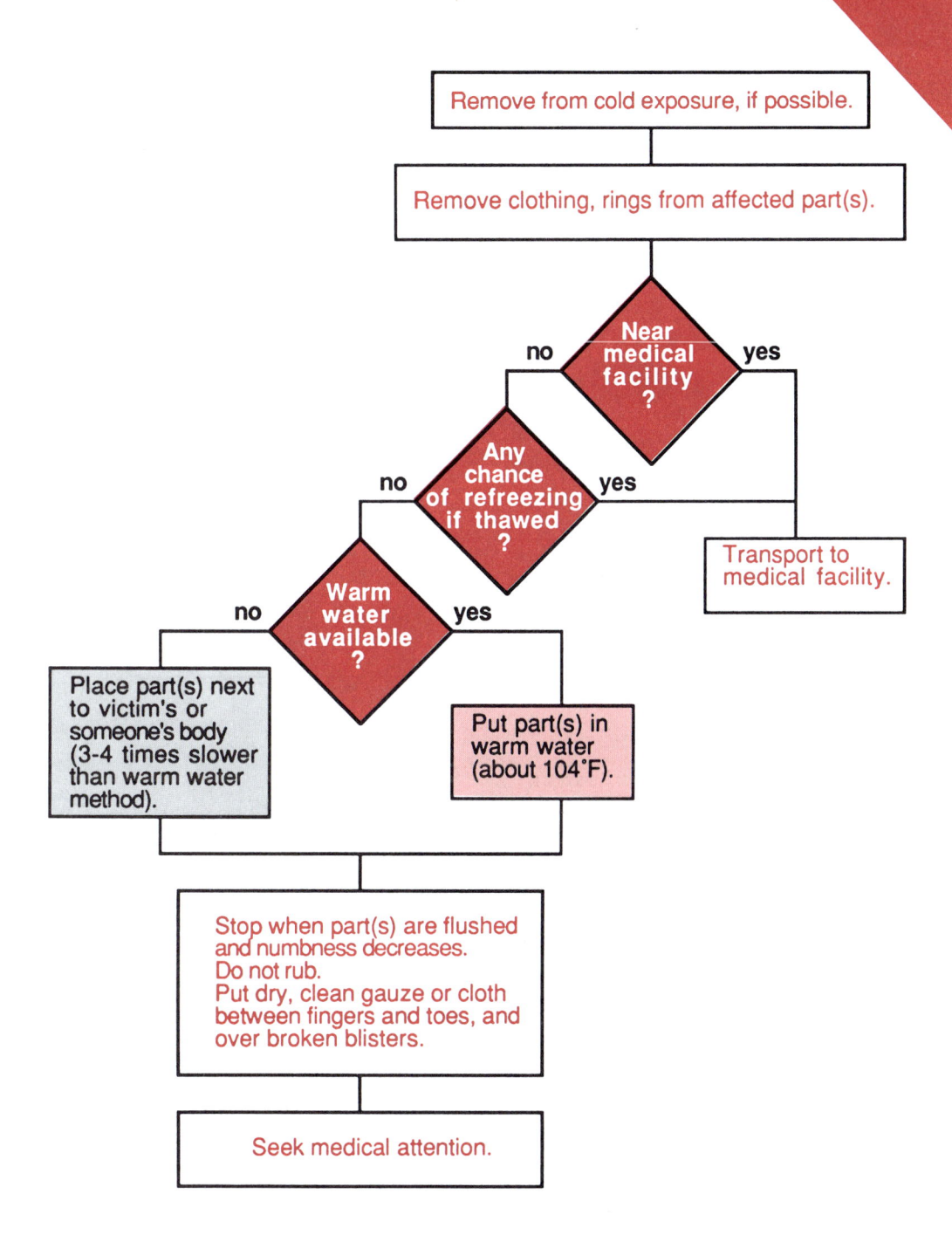

```
Remove from cold exposure, if possible.
              │
Remove clothing, rings from affected part(s).
              │
       Near medical facility?
       no ←──────────→ yes
       │                │
   Any chance of        │
   refreezing if        │
      thawed?           │
   no ←────→ yes        │
   │          │         │
Warm water    └─────────┤
available?              │
no ←──→ yes             │
 │       │              ▼
 │       │      Transport to medical facility.
 │       │
Place part(s) next    Put part(s) in
to victim's or        warm water
someone's body        (about 104°F).
(3-4 times slower
than warm water
method).
       │       │
       └───┬───┘
           ▼
Stop when part(s) are flushed
and numbness decreases.
Do not rub.
Put dry, clean gauze or cloth
between fingers and toes, and
over broken blisters.
           │
           ▼
   Seek medical attention.
```

Hypothermia

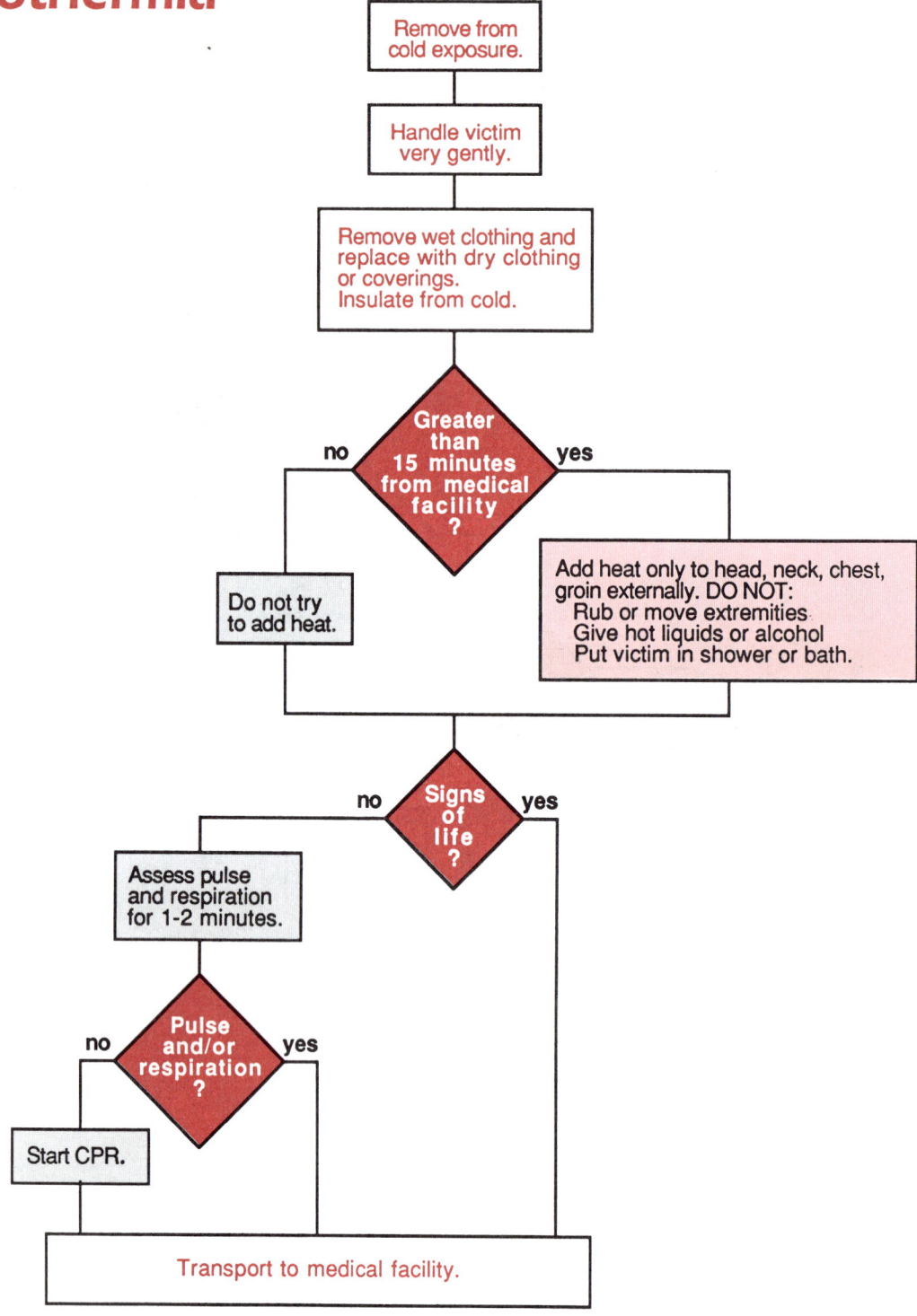

```
Remove from cold exposure.
          ↓
Handle victim very gently.
          ↓
Remove wet clothing and replace with dry clothing or coverings.
Insulate from cold.
          ↓
   Greater than 15 minutes from medical facility?
   ├── no → Do not try to add heat.
   └── yes → Add heat only to head, neck, chest, groin externally. DO NOT:
               Rub or move extremities
               Give hot liquids or alcohol
               Put victim in shower or bath.
          ↓
   Signs of life?
   ├── no → Assess pulse and respiration for 1-2 minutes.
   │         ↓
   │      Pulse and/or respiration?
   │      ├── no → Start CPR.
   │      └── yes ↓
   └── yes ↓
Transport to medical facility.
```

Cold Water Drowning

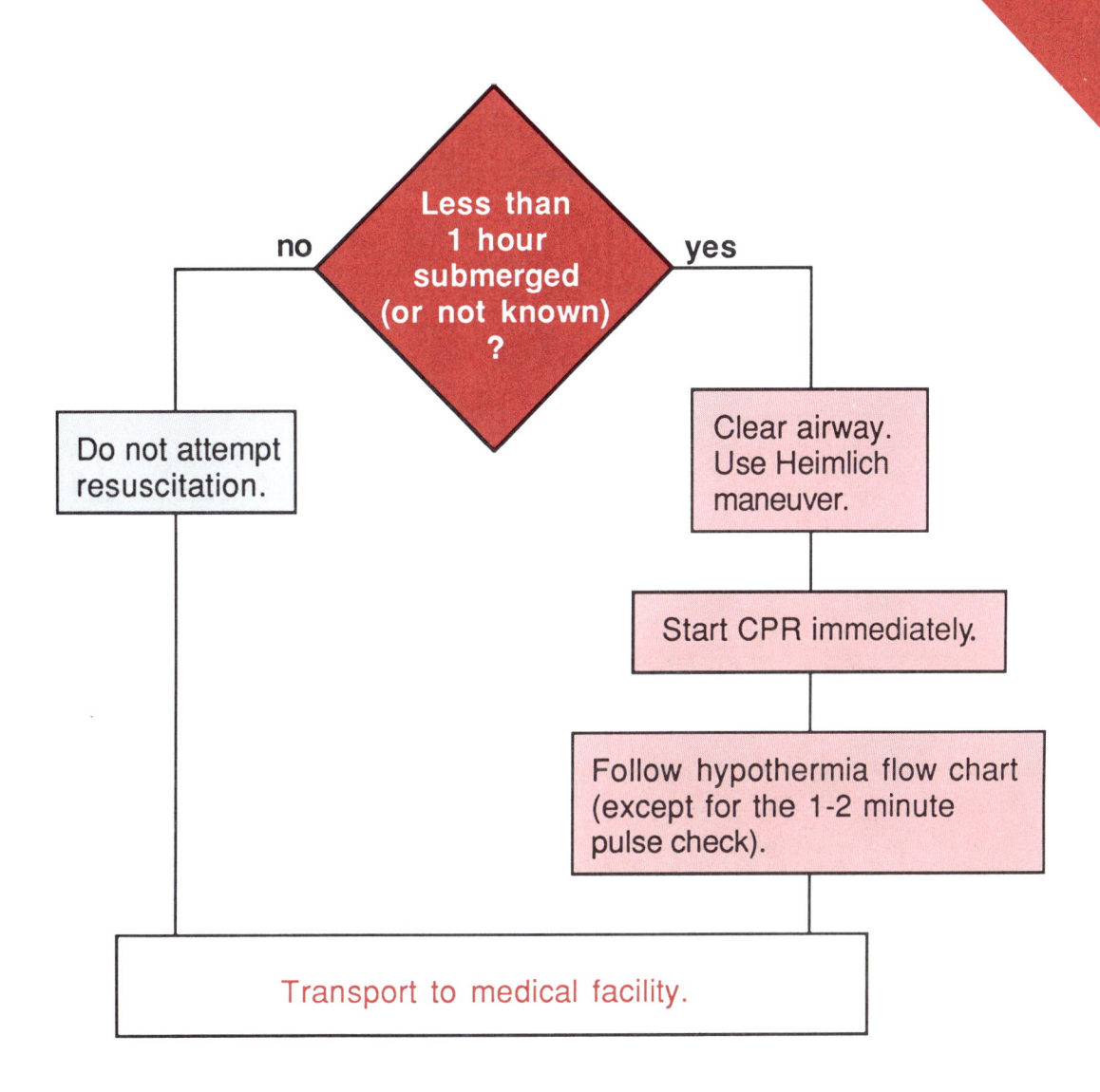

Less than 1 hour submerged (or not known)?

- **no** → Do not attempt resuscitation.
- **yes** →
  - Clear airway. Use Heimlich maneuver.
  - Start CPR immediately.
  - Follow hypothermia flow chart (except for the 1-2 minute pulse check).

Transport to medical facility.

Heat-Related Injuries

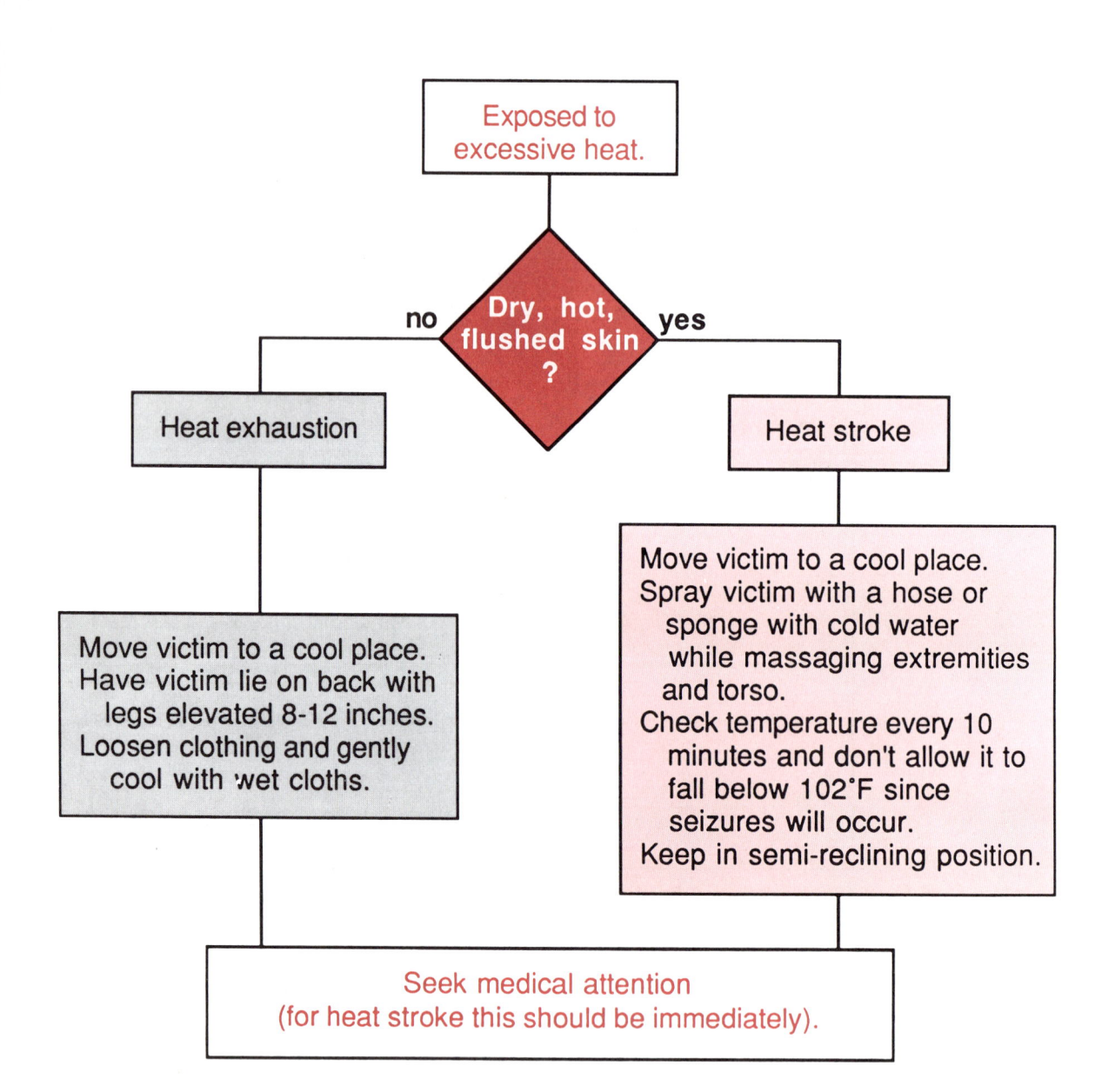

```
                    Exposed to
                    excessive heat.
                         │
                         ▼
              no    ◇ Dry, hot,    yes
           ┌────── flushed skin ──────┐
           │           ?              │
           ▼                          ▼
    Heat exhaustion              Heat stroke
           │                          │
           │                          ▼
           │              Move victim to a cool place.
           │              Spray victim with a hose or
           │                 sponge with cold water
           ▼                 while massaging extremities
  Move victim to a cool place.   and torso.
  Have victim lie on back with Check temperature every 10
  legs elevated 8-12 inches.      minutes and don't allow it to
  Loosen clothing and gently      fall below 102°F since
  cool with wet cloths.           seizures will occur.
           │              Keep in semi-reclining position.
           │                          │
           └──────────┬───────────────┘
                      ▼
           Seek medical attention
  (for heat stroke this should be immediately).
```

SELF-CHECK QUESTIONS

Activity 1: Frostbite

Which of the following actions represent proper first aid for frostbite?

Yes No
1. ☐ ☐ Rewarm a frostbitten part by exposing it to a fire or open flame.
2. ☐ ☐ Rewarm a frostbitten part by using warm water (102–106°F).
3. ☐ ☐ Placing frostbitten hands in another person's armpits is slow but can be effective.
4. ☐ ☐ Rub the frostbitten part to restore circulation.
5. ☐ ☐ Rub the frostbitten area with snow.
6. ☐ ☐ A victim with frozen lower extremities should be carried, if possible, to the nearest medical facility.
7. ☐ ☐ If a victim with a severely frostbitten foot cannot be carried to medical aid, keep the part frozen and assist him in walking.
8. ☐ ☐ Break any blisters that have formed.

Activity 2: Hypothermia

Which of the following actions represent proper first aid for hypothermia?

Yes No
1. ☐ ☐ Add heat to the head, neck, chest, and groin (i.e., hot water bottles, etc.).
2. ☐ ☐ Give hot coffee or chocolate to rewarm the victim.
3. ☐ ☐ Treat the victim gently.
4. ☐ ☐ Rewarm the arms and legs first since they are the most accessible.
5. ☐ ☐ If less than 15 minutes from a medical facility, add heat gradually.
6. ☐ ☐ If no pulse or respiration, start CPR.
7. ☐ ☐ Check breathing and pulse for at least one full minute.
8. ☐ ☐ Remove wet clothing.

Activity 3: Heat-Related Injuries

A. On a hot day a golfer complains of pain in his legs and arms. Which of the following should you do?

Choice 1   *Choice 2*

1. ☐ Make a salt water drink by mixing 1 teaspoon of salt to 1 quart of water.   OR   ☐ Make a salt water drink by adding 1 teaspoon of salt to 1 glass of water.

2. ☐ Give him ½ glassful of salted water every 15 minutes for one hour.   OR   ☐ Give him sips of salted water to wet his lips and tongue.

3. ☐ Massage the painful area.   OR   ☐ Gently stretch the painful area.

B. Match the following signs with the right heat-related emergency.

1. ☐ skin: hot, dry
2. ☐ skin: cool, clammy
3. ☐ sweating excessively
4. ☐ sweating absent
5. ☐ unconsious

1. heat exhaustion
2. heat stroke

C. A neighbor has hot, dry, red skin.

Which two of the following cooling techniques could you use to quickly reduce his body temperature?

1. ☐ Apply cold towels to his chest and back.
2. ☐ Place his feet and hands in buckets of cold water.
3. ☐ Place him in a large tub filled with cool water.
4. ☐ Apply cold, wet towels to the neck, armpits, head, and groin.
5. ☐ Apply cold, wet towels around his wrists and ankles.

10
Bone, Joint, and Muscle Injuries

- Fractures • Spinal Injuries
- Joint Injuries: Shoulder, Knee, Finger, Ankle
- Muscle Injuries

To evaluate a person with possible musculoskeletal damage you must examine the scene of the accident to determine what caused the injury, obtain an accurate victim history, and give a thorough physical examination.

Most victims with significant musculoskeletal injury will complain of pain. Usually the pain is well localized to the area of injury. Sometimes the person who has sustained a fracture will report having felt something snap.

With rare exceptions, fractures and other orthopedic injuries are not life threatening. In the victim with multiple injuries, fractures may be the most obvious and dramatic, but may not necessarily be the most serious. Therefore, the first aider should do the primary survey and manage any life threatening conditions first. Management of orthopedic injuries fit in their appropriate place in the secondary survey.

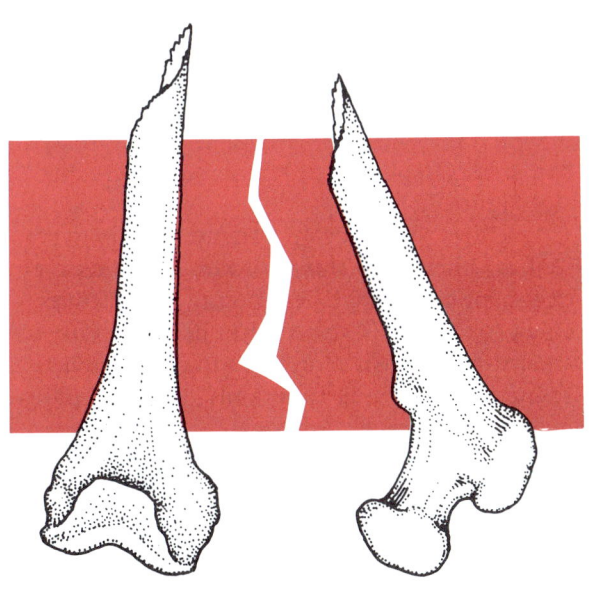

Look
Swelling and a black-and-blue mark indicate escape of blood into the tissues. Shortening or angulation between joints, deformity, or angulation in unusual direction around the joints, shortening of the extremity, and internal or external rotation when compared with the opposite extremity indicate a bony defect. Lacerations or even small puncture wounds near the site of the bony fracture are considered open fractures.

Feel
Feeling (palpation) along the length of a bone can help detect deformities, bony protuberances, or angulation that is not visible.

Always take the person's pulse below the fracture both before and after application of splints. In the arm, you should test the radial arteries, and in the leg, the pedal pulses. If there is no pulse, try to restore the blood flow with two or three gentle manipulations of the extremity. Do not make prolonged attempts.

It is difficult many times to distinguish between fractures and sprains without x-ray. If

158 FIRST AID ESSENTIALS

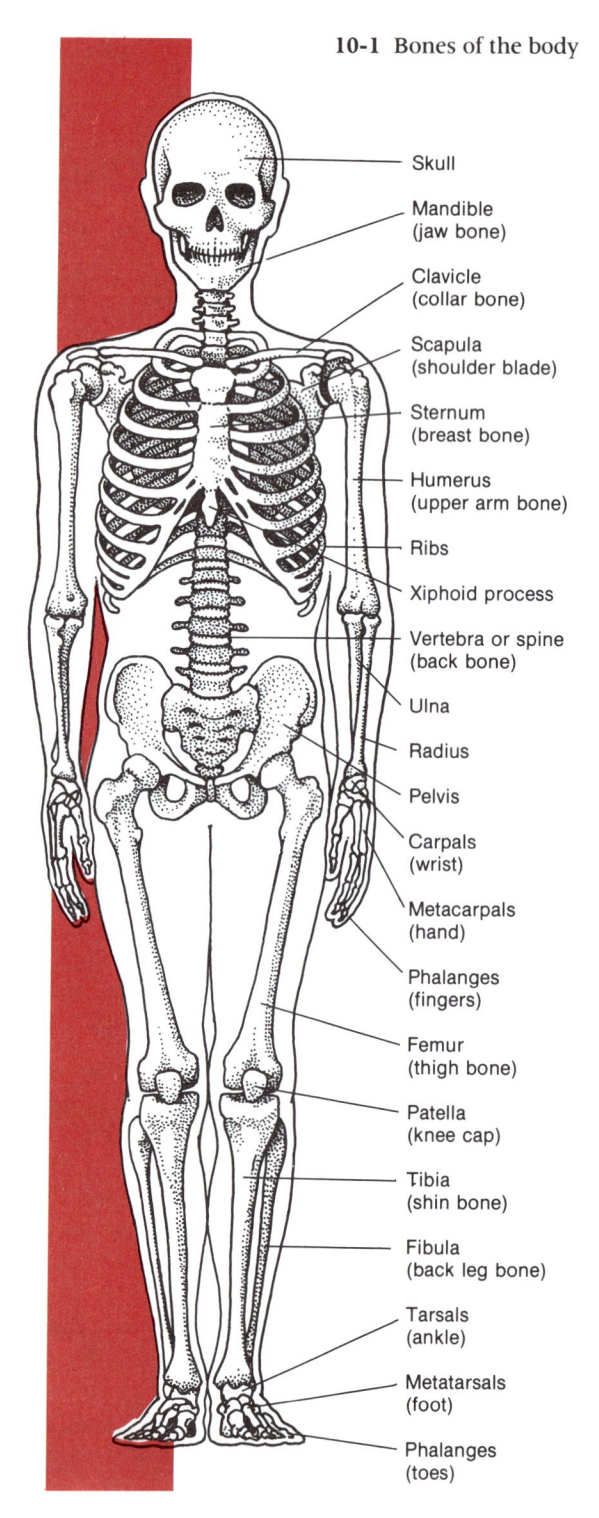

10-1 Bones of the body

- Skull
- Mandible (jaw bone)
- Clavicle (collar bone)
- Scapula (shoulder blade)
- Sternum (breast bone)
- Humerus (upper arm bone)
- Ribs
- Xiphoid process
- Vertebra or spine (back bone)
- Ulna
- Radius
- Pelvis
- Carpals (wrist)
- Metacarpals (hand)
- Phalanges (fingers)
- Femur (thigh bone)
- Patella (knee cap)
- Tibia (shin bone)
- Fibula (back leg bone)
- Tarsals (ankle)
- Metatarsals (foot)
- Phalanges (toes)

there is a question, immobilize and treat the injury as if it were a fracture. In general, the pain produced by a fracture will cause muscular spasm. The victim, therefore, will guard or not move that fractured bone at all.

Table 10-1 gives the signs and symptoms of common orthopedic injuries—fractures, dislocations, and sprains.

FRACTURES

A *fracture* is a break in a bone. It may either be closed, in which case the overlying skin is intact, or open, in which case there is a wound over the fracture site. (*See* Figure 10-2). In an open fracture, bone may protrude through the wound. Open fractures are more serious than closed fractures because the risks of contamination and infection are greater.

A *transverse* fracture cuts across the bone at right angles to its long axis. The fracture line of an *oblique* fracture crosses the bone at an oblique angle, or in a slanting direction. The *greenstick* fracture is an incomplete fracture that commonly occurs in children, whose bones (like green sticks) are still pliable. *Spiral* fractures usually result from twisting injuries, and the fracture line has the appearance of a spring. In *impacted* fractures, the broken ends of the bone are jammed together and may function as if no fracture were present. A *comminuted* fracture is one in which the bone is fragmented into more than two pieces (splintered, shattered, or crushed). (*See* Figure 10-3.)

Fractures—even open fractures—seldom present an immediate threat to life, and thus their treatment should be deferred until any life threatening conditions have been handled, for example, an airway established or hemorrhage controlled.

Immobilization is commonly done by splinting for the following reasons:

- To prevent a closed fracture from becoming an open one
- To prevent damage to surrounding nerves, blood vessels, and other tissues by the broken bone ends

TABLE 10-1. Common Orthopedic Injuries — Signs and Symptoms

Fracture	Dislocation	Sprain
Pain, tenderness	Pain	Pain on movement; tenderness
Deformity or shortening	Deformity	No deformity
Loss of use	Loss of movement	Painful movement
Swelling	Swelling	Swelling
Black-and-blue mark	Black-and-blue mark	Redness
Grating	Located at joint	
Guarding		
Exposed bone ends		

- To lessen bleeding and swelling
- To diminish pain

You should remember the following splinting and immobilization principles:

- Straighten severely angulated fractures of long bones before splinting. Explain to the victim that straightening the fracture may cause momentary pain, but that it will abate significantly once the fracture is straightened and splinted. Any overlying clothing should be cut away. Do not manipulate a fracture. If deformed but there is circulation, do not attempt to straighten it; splint in the position found. If circulation is absent, then attempt to restore the part to normal position. To reposition, apply steady increasing traction; don't use quick, forceful motions.
- Do not straighten dislocations and any fractures involving the spine, shoulder, elbow, wrist, or knee.
- The adage "splint them as they lie" should be changed to "immobilize them where they lie."
- In open fractures, do not attempt to push bone ends back beneath the skin surface. Simply cover them with a sterile dressing.
- Immobilize the joints above and below the fracture (e.g., at the wrist and elbow for fractures of the radius and ulna).
- Splinting should be done firmly, but not so tightly as to hinder circulation. Check pulses (radial or pedal) after the splint is in place to be certain that the circulation is still adequate. If the pulse disappears, loosen the splint until you feel the pulse again.
- For fractures of the femur or about the hip, a traction splint is best.
- All fractures should be immobilized before moving the victim.
- The fingers and toes should be exposed even though they are included within a splint.

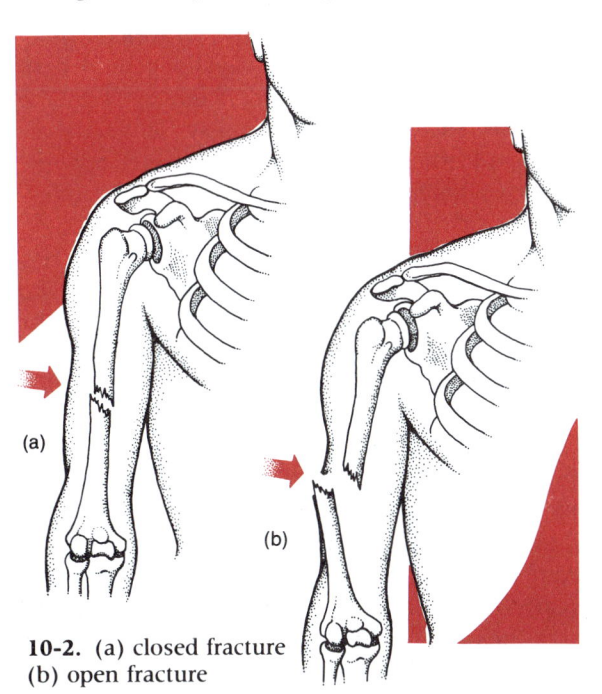

10-2. (a) closed fracture (b) open fracture

Types of Splints

Any device used to immobilize a fracture or dislocation is a splint. This device may be improvised, such as a rolled newspaper, pillow, or virtually any other object that can provide stability; or it may be one of the several commercially available splints.

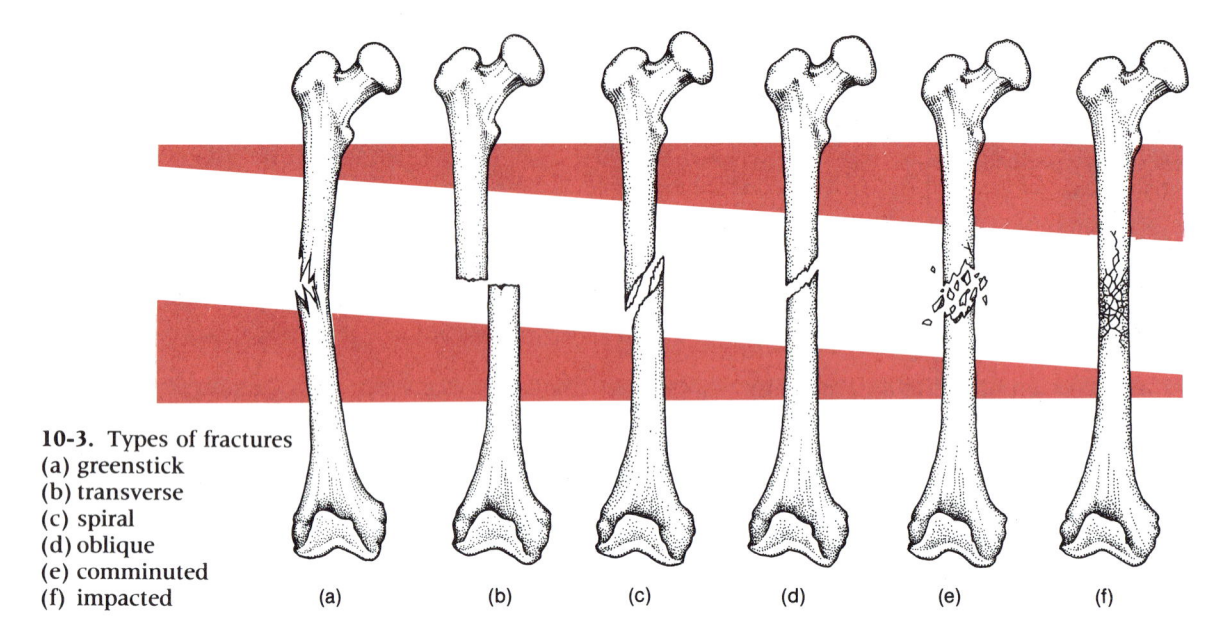

10-3. Types of fractures
(a) greenstick
(b) transverse
(c) spiral
(d) oblique
(e) comminuted
(f) impacted

A rigid splint is an inflexible device attached to a limb to maintain stability. It may be a padded board or a piece of heavy cardboard. Whatever its construction, it must be long enough to be secured well above and below the fracture site.

To apply a rigid splint, grasp the extremity above and below the fracture site and apply gentle traction. While one first aider maintains traction, the other wraps the limb and splint with bandages, tight enough to hold the splint firmly to the extremity but not so tight as to hinder circulation.

Refer to chapter 12 for illustrations and an explanation on splinting various body parts.

SPINAL INJURIES

The incidence of spinal cord injuries has been escalating for many reasons. One is the increased use of motorcycles. Another is the change Americans have made to smaller motor vehicles that provide less protection in an accident. Even the increase in participation in recreational sports is partly responsible for more spinal cord injuries. A mistake in handling such victims may mean the victim spends the rest of his or her life in a wheelchair or bed.

When a person has damage that paralyzes the legs only, he or she is called a paraplegic and will probably be confined to a wheelchair. If the spinal cord damage is farther up, causing paralysis in all four limbs, the person is said to be a quadriplegic and may require a device that is activated by mouth to move the wheelchair.

A first aider can tell if spinal damage may have occurred by first checking the circumstances of the accident, such as bent steering wheel and shattered windshield glass. Victims suspected of spine damage should not be moved except by professionally trained personnel with special equipment.

A second clue is a head injury. If a victim has been hit hard enough to cause head injury, the head has probably snapped suddenly in one or more directions. This endangers the spine. About 15% to 20% of victims with head injuries also have neck and spinal cord injuries.

The position of the victim's body may also suggest spinal damage. If the victim's head is at an unnatural angle or deformity along the spine is noticed, these are other clues to possible spine damage. Also, pain in the neck may be another symptom. Other symptoms of spinal damage may include loss of bowel or bladder control or paralysis.

If you are involved as a first aider at an accident scene and you are evaluating the victim for a possible spinal cord injury, ask the following questions:

1. *Is there pain?* A conscious victim should be asked about the presence of pain. Neck injuries (cervical) radiate pain to the arms; upper back injuries (thoracic) radiate pain around the ribs into the chest; and lower back injuries (lumbar) usually radiate pain down the legs. Often the victim describes the pain as "electric"—much like the pulsating pain that occurs when a dentist's drill exposes the nerve root of a tooth.

2. *Can you move your feet and legs?* Ask the victim to move his foot upward against the force of your hand. If the victim cannot perform this movement or if the movement is extremely weak against the pressure of your hand, the victim may have injured his spinal cord; the injury may be present anywhere along the spinal column.

3. *Can you move your fingers?* Moving the fingers is a sign that nerve pathways are intact. Ask the victim to grip your hand in his. Note the force of the grip. A strong grip indicates that a spinal cord injury is unlikely. If any one of these signs or symptoms is positive, spinal injury must be suspected. If you are not sure, assume that the victim has a spinal cord injury until proved otherwise.

First aiders should normally wait for paramedics or other rescue squads to transport the victim because of their training and equipment. Whatever you do, stabilize the victim against any movement. Never move the neck to reposition it.

If you determine that the victim may have spinal damage, the victim must be immobilized. Sometimes this just means telling the victim not to move. On other occasions, when the victim is unconscious, place objects on either side of the head to prevent it from rolling from side to side. If the victim is unconscious, determine if he or she is breathing and has a pulse.

If the victim is not breathing, give mouth-to-mouth resuscitation in the position in which the victim was found. The head tilt cannot be used because it would move the neck. Instead, jut the jaw forward by placing the fingers on the corners of the jaw and pushing forward. Keep the head and neck still and give mouth-to-mouth with the jaw held forward.

Victims with potential neck or back injury who are in water must be floated gently to shore. Before removal from the water, the victim must be secured to a backboard.

First aiders should remember to move the victim only if further injury is likely—such as in a smoking car or burning building. Bring help to the victim, not the victim to the help.

JOINT INJURIES

Shoulder Injuries

Assessment

The shoulder region is one of the most difficult areas of the body to evaluate.

It is essential to know whether the condition was produced by sudden trauma or was of slow onset. The following questions can help determine the nature of the injury:

1. Can the radial pulse be felt for impaired circulation?

2. What is the duration and intensity of the pain? Where is the pain located?

3. Is there grating sensation (crepitus) on movement, numbness, or distortion in temperature, such as a cold or warm feeling? A cold temperature can be an indication of blood vessel constriction, whereas an overly warm temperature may indicate an inflammatory condition.

4. Is there a feeling of weakness?

5. What movement or body positions seem to aggravate or relieve the pain?

6. If the complaint has happened before, what, if anything, provides pain relief (e.g., cold, heat, massage, or analgesic medication)?

Shoulder Separation/Dislocation

The extreme range of all its possible movement makes the shoulder joint highly susceptible to dislocations.

First Aid: Emergency care is to immobilize the injured part and adjacent joints by keeping the upper arm close to the body (not all shoulder dislocations allow this) and limiting further movement. Place a pillow between the arm and chest, and then place the arm in a sling with a swathe. Use ice and some compression if it relieves the victim's pain and discomfort. The physician will generally reset the dislocation (first aiders should never try to reset) and, depending on the severity, strap the injured arm so that no further harm comes to it. After a period of rest and rehabilitation (about three weeks), the victim can return to normal activity.

Fracture of the Clavicle
The clavicle is one of the most frequently fractured bones in the body. Fractured clavicles are caused by either a direct blow or a transmitted force resulting from a fall on the outstretched arm.

The victim usually supports the arm on the injured side and tilts his or her head toward that side, with the chin turned to the opposite side. The injured side appears a little lower than the uninjured side. Palpation may also reveal swelling and mild deformity.

First Aid: Care for this fracture immediately by applying a sling and swathe bandage and by treating the victim for shock, if necessary. Refer the victim to a physician, who will perform an x-ray examination of the area and continue to immobilize the injured area.

Contusions, Strains, and Tendonitis
Contusions: Blows about the shoulder that produce injury are most prevalent in collision and contact sports. Bruises of this area result in pain and restricted arm movement.

The most vulnerable part of the clavicle is the enlarged end near the shoulder. Contusions of this type are often called "shoulder pointers" and may cause the victim severe discomfort.

Strains: Throwing and swimming place great stress on the shoulder rotating mechanisms and can lead to an injury.

Tendonitis or Painful Shoulder: A painful shoulder is any irritation of the tendons or muscles surrounding the shoulder area. The cause of the painful shoulder is generally continuous overuse. Sports that involve repeated arm movement, like many of the throwing sports (e.g., baseball) or any other sports in which the shoulder is used extensively (e.g., swimming), often report painful shoulders.

Emergency care for contusions, strains, tendonitis: Begin cold therapy immediately after an injury. The best results are achieved if ice is applied for twenty minutes about three or four times during the first twenty-four hours after the injury. Continue this for twenty-four hours after the injury. After applying ice, you should immobilize the joint. Resting the joint is important.

The use of ice for extended periods is discouraged. Thermal damage, including damage to local blood vessels, may occur with prolonged applications of ice. The initial application of heat in an acute injury is not recommended because it increases swelling, thereby complicating the inflammatory process.

Post-Emergency Care
Topical analgesics: Some pain relief during the few days after the ice treatment may be necessary. External analgesics such as menthol, camphor, and eucalyptus oil act as counter-irritants and decrease the pain associated with minor muscle and joint injuries. Examples of brand names are Ben-Gay™ lotion, Mentholatum™ rub, and Infra-Rub™ cream.

These analgesics are applied to the skin over the source of the pain. The feeling of warmth from the topical analgesic has been proposed to crowd out pain perception and therefore divert the victim's attention. Be careful to avoid swelling and blistering of the skin. The recommended topical dosage to the affected area is no more than three to four times a day.

Analgesics and anti-inflammatory agents: For the pain and swelling of many injuries, the use of analgesics with anti-inflammatory properties may be appropriate. Aspirin is both inexpensive and as effective as any of the other currently available non-steroidal anti-inflammatory agents. Ibuprofen, an over-the-counter drug, provides an alternative anti-inflammatory analgesic for musculoskeletal pain.

Because of its lack of anti-inflammatory ability, acetaminophen is usually not as effective as aspirin for injuries producing inflammation, such as those found in joint injuries.

Knee Injuries

Knee injuries can be serious and consist of many types. There are many reasons for the large number of injuries to the knee, with automobile crashes and athletic participation leading the list.

Assessment of the Injured Knee

A physician is responsible for diagnosing the severity and exact nature of a knee injury. Usually a first aider is the first person to observe the injury and may be responsible for the initial assessment and immediate care of an injured knee. Also the first aider often relates pertinent information to a physician.

To determine the history and major complaints involved in a knee injury, use the following questions:

1. Was it a contact or noncontact injury? If contact, from what direction was the force applied?
2. In what direction did the knee go?
3. Did you hear a noise or feel any sensation at the time of injury, such as a pop or crunch?
4. Could you move the knee immediately after the injury? If not, was it locked in a bent or extended position? After being locked, how did it become unlocked?
5. Did swelling occur? If yes, was it immediate or did it occur later?
6. Where was the pain? Was it local, all over, or did it move from one side of the knee to the other?
7. Have you hurt the knee before?

You have probably seen a physician or an athletic trainer performing stress tests on a knee on the sidelines at a football game. There is still controversy as to the exact meaning and interpretation of many of the ligament stress tests. First aiders should not perform such testing due to lack of training and experience.

Various Knee Injuries

Fractured knee: A fracture of the knee generally occurs as a result of a fall or a direct blow. There will be an inability to kick the leg forward, and the leg will drag if an attempt is made to walk.

Fractures involving the knee may happen at the end of the femur, the end of the tibia, or in the patella. Such fractures may be confused with dislocations if deformity appears or with ligament damage if swelling and tenderness accompanies the injury.

To prevent further damage to nerves and blood vessels, immobilize the leg in the position found. If the leg is straight, use a padded board splint under the leg to keep it straight, or place two board splints (one on the inside and the other on the outside) on the leg. If bent, the knee should be immobilized in the bent position. When splints are not available, use a pillow or a blanket to immobilize the knee.

Check the pedal pulse for signs of circulatory impairment. If there is no pulse, try moving the leg (only once or twice) to a straight anatomical position. Do not force the leg. Stop if there is any resistance or an increase in pain.

Dislocation of the knee: This is a very serious injury. Deformity will be grotesque. Most concern should be for injury to the major artery supplying the leg below the knee (popliteal artery just behind the knee joint) rather than for ligament damage. Always check the pedal pulse for circulation before taking any other steps.

If pedal pulses are absent, the first aider should make an attempt to realign the limb in order to reduce the pressure on the artery. This is done by gently straightening the deformity with gentle traction along the axis of the limb. Continue to do this if no additional pain occurs. During straightening the joint may be relocated and the blood supply restored. Immobilize the limb with a rigid splint or pillow.

One attempt at gently straightening the knee should be attempted and no more. Then the knee should be immobilized in the position of deformity. No attempt to straighten any knee injury should be made when strong pedal pulses are present or when one attempt to realignment produce severe pain. In these cases, immobilize the knee in the position found.

Waiting longer than eight hours to reduce a knee dislocation can ultimately result in loss of the leg.

Dislocated patella: A dislocated patella most often is due to a blow or a very forceful unnatural contraction. Youth and young adults are most often the victims because of their participation in athletics where such injures are most often found.

The kneecap moves to the side of the joint. It can be a very painful injury and must be treated immediately. Some people have repeated kneecap dislocations, just as others have a tendency for shoulder dislocations.

The first aid for a dislocated patella is to reduce the dislocation as quickly as possible. Sometimes the victim can attempt to straighten the knee. Splint the leg so it cannot bend at the knee, and seek medical attention. The first aider should attempt to straighten the knee gently if additional pain is not produced. Sometimes the kneecap will relocate itself as the knee is straightened. If pain results while straightening the leg, immobilize the leg and knee in the deformed position.

Ligament injuries: The knee is quite prone to ligament injury from mild sprain to complete tearing. These injuries are quite common in athletics.

There are many tests to determine the stability of the knee after it has been hit. Some of these tests involve attempting to move the knee and applying certain stresses in different directions in an attempt to determine which ligament has been stretched or ruptured. Such testing should be reserved for physicians and experienced athletic trainers, not first aiders. In fact, some physicians and athletic trainers should not stress test a knee due to inexperience and lack of training.

Very often pain and tenderness are present in the area, and normal movement is not allowed because of the pain. Locking of the knee joint may also occur. These are all indications of serious ligament damage to the knee. Check the pedal pulse for signs of circulatory impairment.

First Aid is the ICE procedure: I stands for ice or cold application; C means compression with elastic bandage; E represents elevation of the knee. The first aider can gently straighten the knee to apply a splint. If pain occurs, the knee should be immobilized in the position as it is. A qualified physician should be sought to determine if a ligament injury has taken place and, if so, if a cast should be applied, followed by rest, or if surgery is needed.

Cartilage injuries: Cartilage injuries in the knee can be incapacitating. Such injuries can result from a traumatic event or long-term wear and tear of the cartilage. A trained orthopedic physician should be sought.

Though knee injuries are not life threatening, they are common and pose a concern for the victim and the first aider. The first aider will not be able to identify the type of injury, yet the first aid for most knee injuries is quite similar.

Finger Injuries

Finger Dislocation

Dislocations of the fingers have a high rate of occurrence in sports and are caused mainly by being hit on the tip of the finger by a ball.

First aid: The victim of a dislocated finger often attempts to pull the joint back in place. This is not recommended. The dislocation should be reduced by a physician after x-rays are taken to see that no other injury is involved. Broken bone chips can also be seen in the x-rays.

Taping to prevent another occurrence of the injury should be considered. The finger that was dislocated may be splinted to an adjacent, good finger to immobilize and protect it in future activity. To ensure the most complete healing, splinting should be maintained for about three weeks with the fingers flexed because inadequate immobilization could cause an unstable joint and/or excessive scar tissue and, possibly, a permanent deformity.

Since the thumb is necessary for hand dexterity, any traumatic injury to the thumb should be considered serious. Special consideration must be given to dislocations of the thumb.

Fractures of the Fingers

The presence of swelling and tenderness are involved in fractures of the fingers.

One of the most useful ways to differentiate between a contusion and a fracture is by using the "percussion" or "hammer" test. In this test the victim holds the fingers in full extension. The ends of the fingers are firmly "hammered" toward the hand transmitting the force down the shaft of the metacarpal and producing pain if a fracture is present.

Finger alignment should also be checked, but most important is nail alignment. If the normal fingernail alignment is disturbed, you should suspect a fracture. An x-ray will conclusively determine a broken bone.

First aid: Immediately place cold, apply compression, and elevate the arm. Seek medical attention. See Figure 12-16 for a recommended splinting technique.

Fingernail Avulsion

When a nail is partly torn loose, do not trim away the loose nail. Instead, secure the damaged nail in place with an adhesive bandage. If part or all of the nail has been completely torn away, apply an adhesive bandage coated with antibiotic ointment. Alleviate the victim's fears by telling him that a new nail will appear but it will take a month or more.

Ankle Injuries

A sprained angle is a very common injury. Because of the frequency of this injury, anyone trained to render emergency care should understand the nature of the injury itself and how to deal with it effectively. A sprained ankle should not be handled casually. It can have consequences that include a lifelong disability. In some cases, the damage requires surgical correction.

It is usually impossible for a first aider to determine the exact nature of an ankle injury. The injury could be a sprain, dislocation, or fracture. Identification cannot be made on the basis of appearance or the amount of pain. A mild sprain often is considerably more painful than a severe one. A severe sprain frequently presents very little swelling.

The first aider can ask the victim three important questions:

1. Which way did the ankle turn? Most (over 80%) ankle sprains are of the lateral or inverted type.
2. At the time of the injury, did you hear or feel anything snap or pop?
3. Have you ever had problems with this ankle before?

It is often difficult to distinguish between a severe sprain and a fracture. The injury should be treated as a fracture until the advice of a physician can be obtained.

First aid: Initial care consists of elevating the ankle, applying cold compresses or ice packs to the injury site, and supporting the ankle with an elastic bandage. Remembering the mnemonic ICE—*I*ce, *C*ompression, *E*levation—is a guide to sprained ankle injuries.

The application of cold initially causes vasoconstriction of blood vessels. This decreases blood flow, thereby diminishing the amount of bleeding in the injured ankle. Cryotherapy (use of cold) is effective in diminishing bleeding and edema (accumulation of fluid) by the combined effect of a decrease in blood flow and reduction in metabolic function of the cell.

Cold is available from ice, commercially prepared ice packs, frozen food cans, drinking fountains, etc. The earlier cold is applied, the better.

Never place ice directly on the skin except for intermittent ice massage because it can cause frostbite. Provide a towel between the ice bag and skin.

Applying cold for short periods of time does not cool deeper tissues—it only lowers skin temperature. Thus, the application of cold should be continued for at least twenty, and preferably thirty, minutes. This should occur about three times during the first twenty-four hours after the injury. Cold application will not only decrease the swelling, but also relieve the pain.

Some precautions about the use of cold, other

than never applying cold directly to the skin, include the warning not to use salt water (it is too cold) or chemical ice (liquid nitrogen or solid carbon dioxide, also called dry ice). Be aware that some victims may have rheumatic conditions, Raynaud's phenomenon, or cold allergy which can be adversely enhanced in a victim to whom cold is applied.

A common error is the early use of heat. Heat results in swelling and pain if applied too early. A minimum of twenty-four hours, and preferably even seventy-two hours, should pass before any heat is applied to the injured ankle.

Swelling is like glue and can lock up a joint within a matter of hours. It is vitally important not only to prevent swelling by using cold promptly, but it is even more important to make the swelling recede as quickly as possible with a compression bandage (elastic bandage).

Experts disagree on the use of elastic bandages. Some believe that elastic bandages are often misused, especially in ankle injuries. The bandage should be applied firmly, but not too tightly. Toes should be checked periodically for blue or white discoloration, indicating that the bandage has been applied too tightly. Comparing the toes of the injured foot with those of the uninjured foot is also suggested. Pain, tingling, loss of sensation, and loss of pulses indicate impaired circulation. The elastic bandage should be loosened if any of these signs or symptoms are present.

To counteract swelling, take any soft pliable material (i.e., a sock, T-shirt, etc.) and either fold or cut it into the shape of a horseshoe. Place this "horseshoe" around the ankle bone knob on the injured side with the curved part down. Then place a figure-of-eight wrap around the ankle covering the "horseshoe" and foot with an elastic bandage. This technique applies compression to the soft tissue areas, not just the ankle bone and tendon. Apply the elastic bandage (3 or 4 inch width) carefully to avoid hindering circulation.

Check the pulse at the juncture of the big toe and the second toe. When in doubt as to the extent of the injury, splint the foot as you would a fracture by immobilizing the ankle with a pillow splint and then refer the victim to a physician.

To further reduce swelling and curtail bleeding, instruct the victim to elevate his or her ankle on two or three pillows for the first 24 to 48 hours. Some medical specialists say, "Keep the foot higher than the knee and the knee higher than the heart." Avoid any weight on the ankle. Some experts recommend crutches for the victim.

Swelling and pain should begin to subside within forty-eight hours, and the ankle should be nearly normal within ten days. If the injury is not healing on schedule, see a physician.

If a fracture is suspected, immobilize the foot using a pillow splint.

MUSCLE INJURIES

Muscle injuries are hard to explain because little solid information is available, and there are misconceptions and disagreement on proper emergency care. Though muscle injuries pose no real emergency, first aiders have ample opportunities to care for them.

Muscle Strains

Another term often used for muscle strain is muscle pull. Skeletal muscles have the capability to stretch and contract. However, if the muscle is stretched while attempting to contract or stretched beyond its normal range of motion, a tear of the muscle fibers may occur. There are various degrees of severity of muscle strains, depending on the degree of the actual muscle tear.

Signs of muscle strain include:

• The victim may have heard a snap when the tissue was torn.
• A sharp pain may have been felt immediately after the injury.
• There was a spasmodic muscle contraction of the affected part.
• Extreme joint tenderness occurs upon palpation.

- Disfigurement may be seen either in the form of an indentation or cavity where tissues have separated, or a bump indicating contracted tissue.
- There is a severe weakness and loss of function of the injured part.

Muscle Contusions

Another category of muscle injury is the blow to the muscle, or contusion. This injury is also known as a "charley horse."

First Aid of Muscle Strains and Contusions

Muscle injuries must receive proper and early care to avoid delay in recovery. This is especially true of muscle strains. It is well known that a severely injured muscle does not regenerate itself. Healing is by scar formation.

Even though the ice, compression, and elevation (ICE) procedure is used univerally for immediate care of acute muscle strains and contusions, many first aiders and even emergency room personnel continue to treat new muscle injuries erroneously with heat packs.

Ice: The first initial in the acronym ICE stands for ice. Ice is applied to the injured area. Methods of applying cold include the use of crushed ice, immersion in ice water, or the application of cold towels. The application of ice should continue for twenty to thirty minutes of each hour for the first day, if possible. This procedure may be done into the second day of injury.

Placing towels or elastic wraps between the ice packs and the body insulates against the full effects of the cold. Frostbite will not occur if cold packs are applied for limited time periods. Constant use of an ice pack is not necessary because of the lasting effect of cold. For example, it takes two to four hours for the forearm and ankle to gradually return to pre-application temperatures.

The use of cold to an injured area reduces pain, hemorrhage, swelling, and muscle spasm following a muscle strain or contusion.

Compression: The second initial, C, stands for compression. In an attempt to limit internal bleeding, a compression bandage is applied to the injured area. Often, the compression bandage is applied directly to the site, ice is placed over the first layer of elastic bandage wrap, and more compression elastic wrap is put over the ice. The ice, together with the compression, serves to limit internal bleeding, which is associated with all acute muscle injuries. Compression of the injured area may also aid in squeezing some fluid and debris out of the injury site. The victim should wear the elastic wrap continuously for eighteen to twenty-four hours.

Elastic bandages may be applied too tightly, thus inhibiting circulation. Leave fingers and toes exposed to allow observation of possible color change. Pain, pale skin, numbness, and tingling are all signs of a bandage that is too tight.

Elevation: The E stands for elevation. Elevating the injured area limits circulation to that area and, hence, further limits internal bleeding. It is simple to prop up an injured leg or upper extremity to limit bleeding. The aim of this step is to get the injured part up to about the level of the heart, if possible. This should aid venous blood return to the heart.

Muscle Cramps

Another category of muscle injuries is the muscle cramp, in which the muscle goes into uncontrolled spasm and contraction, resulting in severe pain and a restriction or loss of movement. Muscle cramps can occur in any skeletal muscle that is overworked.

When the cramp occurs in the leg or hand muscles, the victim may attempt to relieve the spasm or cramp by gradually stretching of the muscle. Since a muscle cramp is really an uncontrolled spasm or contraction of the muscle, a gradual lengthening of the muscle may help to lengthen those muscle fibers and relieve the cramp. Other experts have implicated diet or lack of fluids as some of the possible reasons that an individual suffers from muscle cramps.

Pinching the upper lip (an accupressure technique) has been advocated for reducing calf muscle cramping.

Fractures

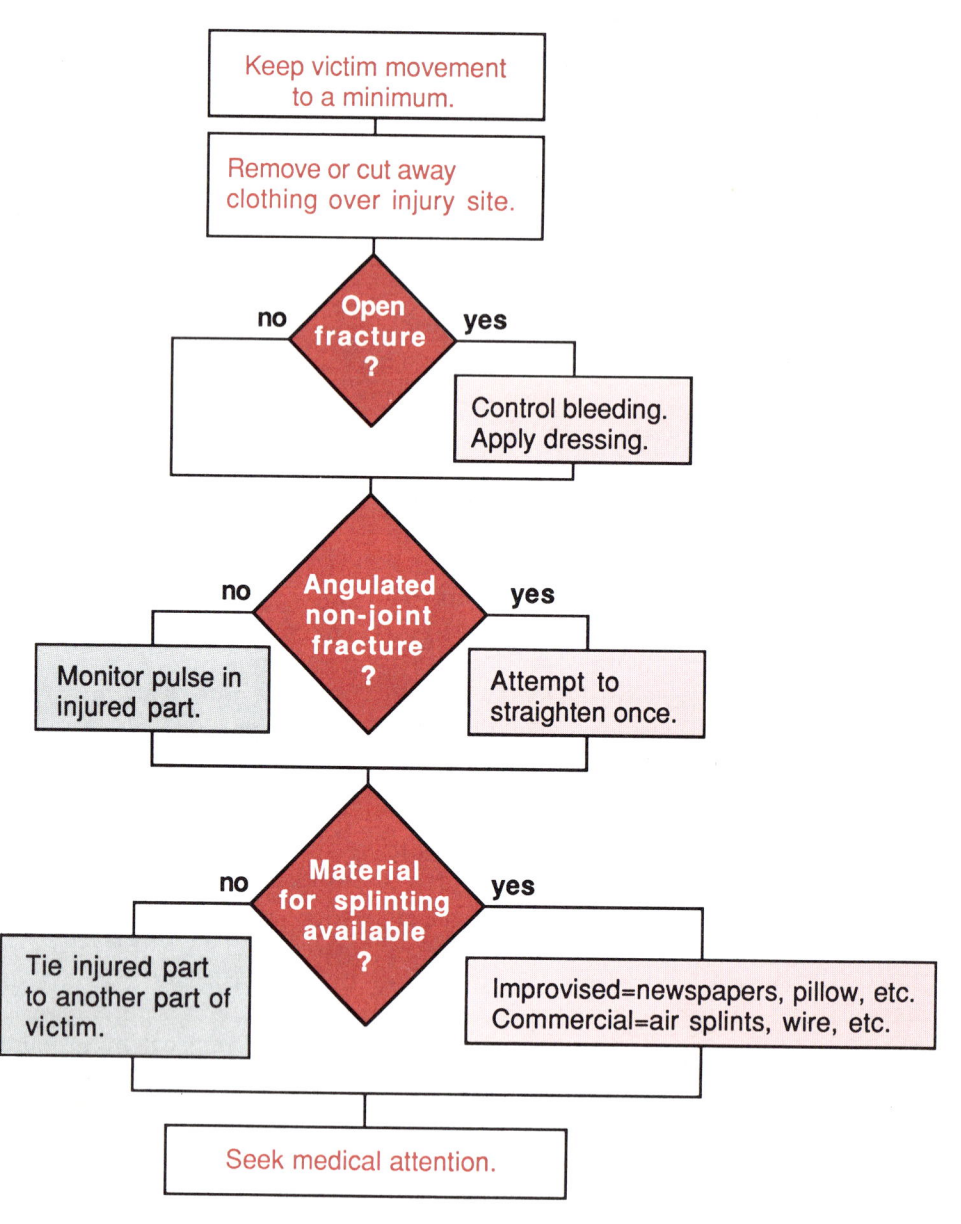

```
Keep victim movement to a minimum.
          ↓
Remove or cut away clothing over injury site.
          ↓
      Open fracture?
   no ←         → yes → Control bleeding. Apply dressing.
          ↓
   Angulated non-joint fracture?
   no → Monitor pulse in injured part.
   yes → Attempt to straighten once.
          ↓
   Material for splinting available?
   no → Tie injured part to another part of victim.
   yes → Improvised=newspapers, pillow, etc.
         Commercial=air splints, wire, etc.
          ↓
   Seek medical attention.
```

If a back or neck injury is suspected, immobilize victim in the exact position found by placing rolled blankets, clothing, etc. next to victim's head, neck, torso. Do not move unless victim is in immediate danger. In most cases, wait for trained rescuers with special equipment.

Spinal Injury

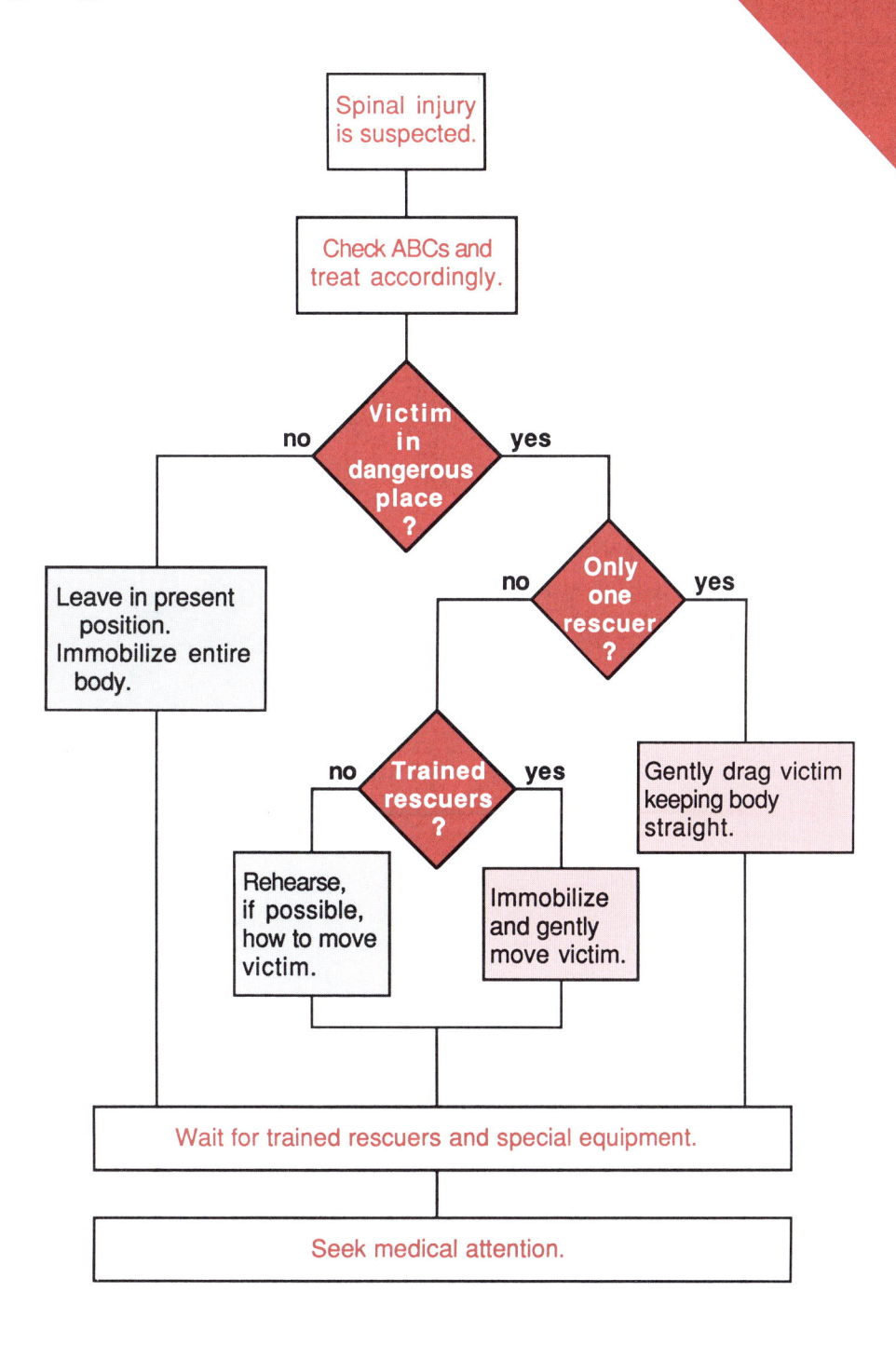

```
Spinal injury is suspected.
        │
Check ABCs and treat accordingly.
        │
   Victim in dangerous place?
   ├── no ──> Leave in present position. Immobilize entire body.
   └── yes ──> Only one rescuer?
              ├── yes ──> Gently drag victim keeping body straight.
              └── no ──> Trained rescuers?
                        ├── yes ──> Immobilize and gently move victim.
                        └── no ──> Rehearse, if possible, how to move victim.

Wait for trained rescuers and special equipment.

Seek medical attention.
```

Shoulder Injuries

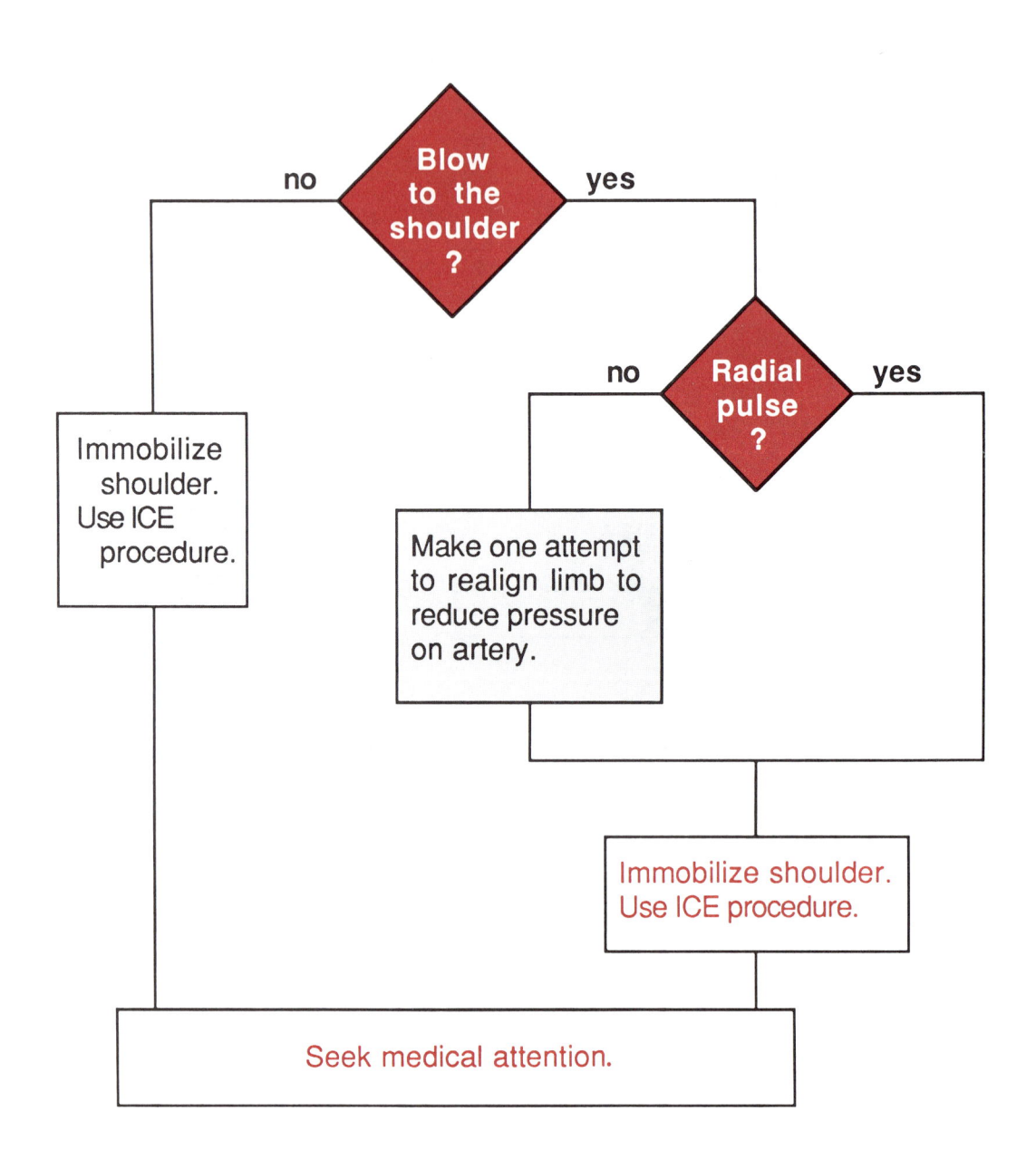

Blow to the shoulder?
- no → Immobilize shoulder. Use ICE procedure. → Seek medical attention.
- yes → **Radial pulse?**
  - no → Make one attempt to realign limb to reduce pressure on artery. → Immobilize shoulder. Use ICE procedure. → Seek medical attention.
  - yes → Immobilize shoulder. Use ICE procedure. → Seek medical attention.

Knee Injuries

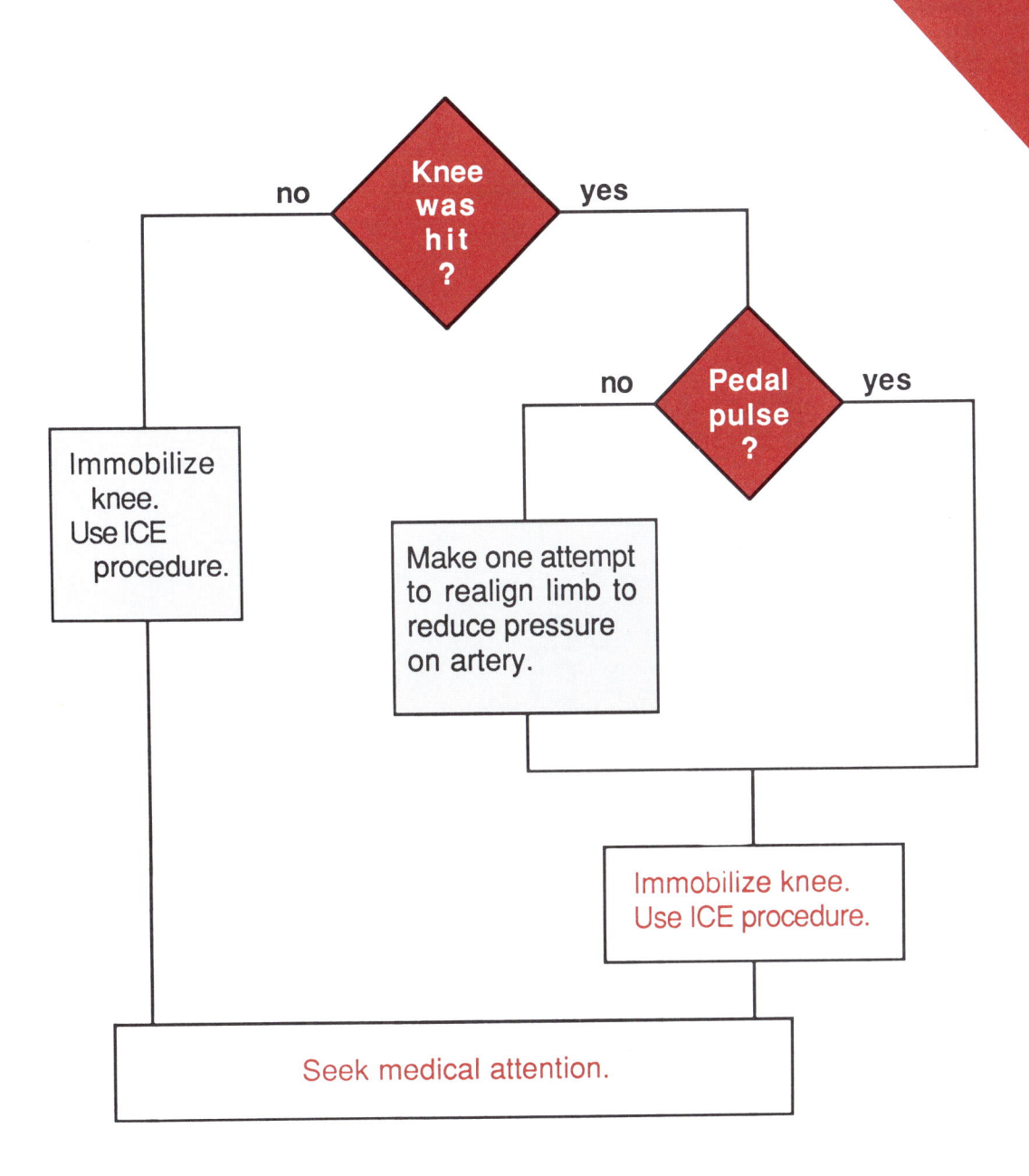

- **Knee was hit?**
  - **no** → Immobilize knee. Use ICE procedure. → Seek medical attention.
  - **yes** → **Pedal pulse?**
    - **no** → Make one attempt to realign limb to reduce pressure on artery. → Immobilize knee. Use ICE procedure. → Seek medical attention.
    - **yes** → Immobilize knee. Use ICE procedure. → Seek medical attention.

Ankle Injuries

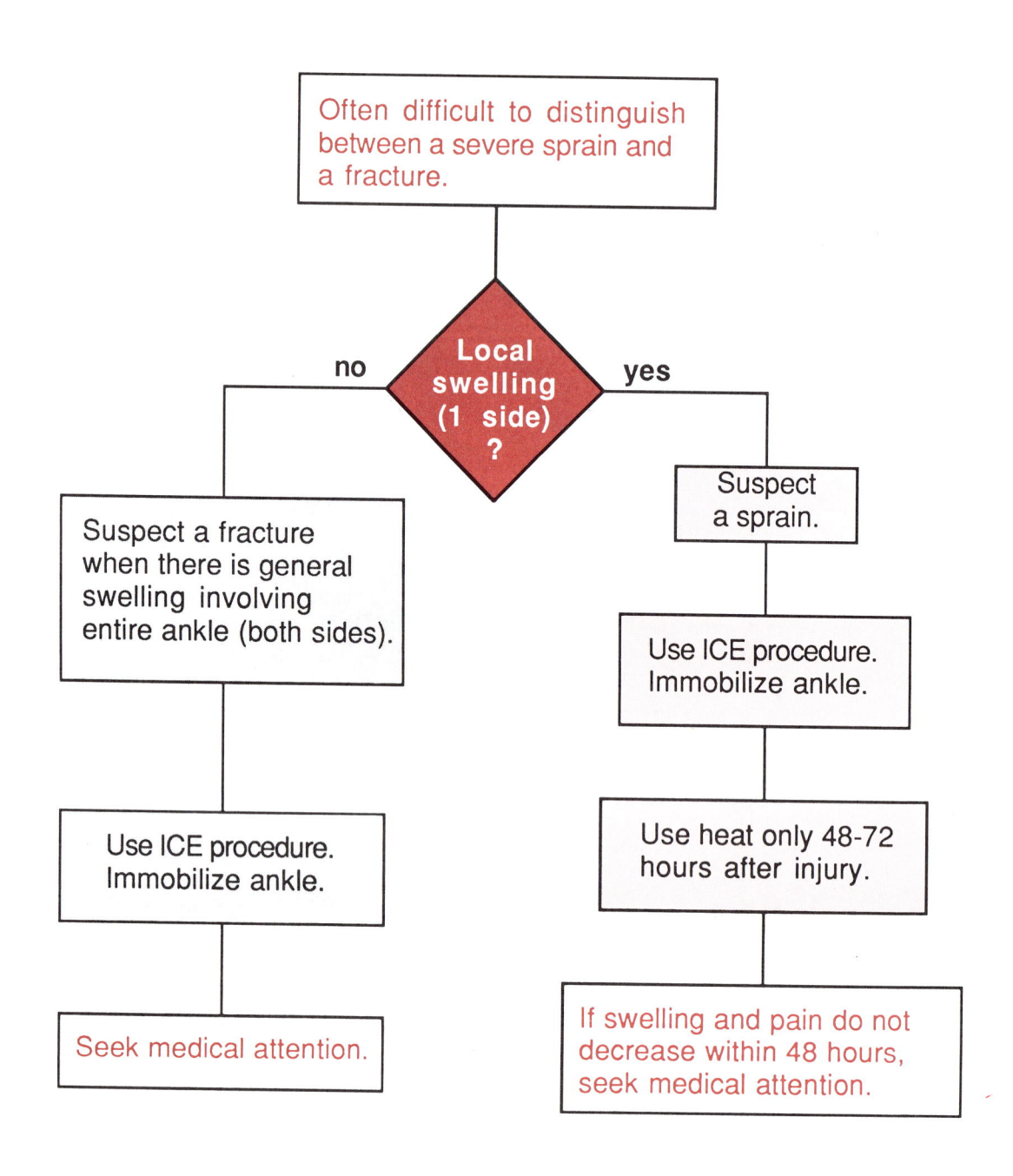

Often difficult to distinguish between a severe sprain and a fracture.

Local swelling (1 side)?

no → Suspect a fracture when there is general swelling involving entire ankle (both sides).

Use ICE procedure. Immobilize ankle.

Seek medical attention.

yes → Suspect a sprain.

Use ICE procedure. Immobilize ankle.

Use heat only 48-72 hours after injury.

If swelling and pain do not decrease within 48 hours, seek medical attention.

Muscle Injuries

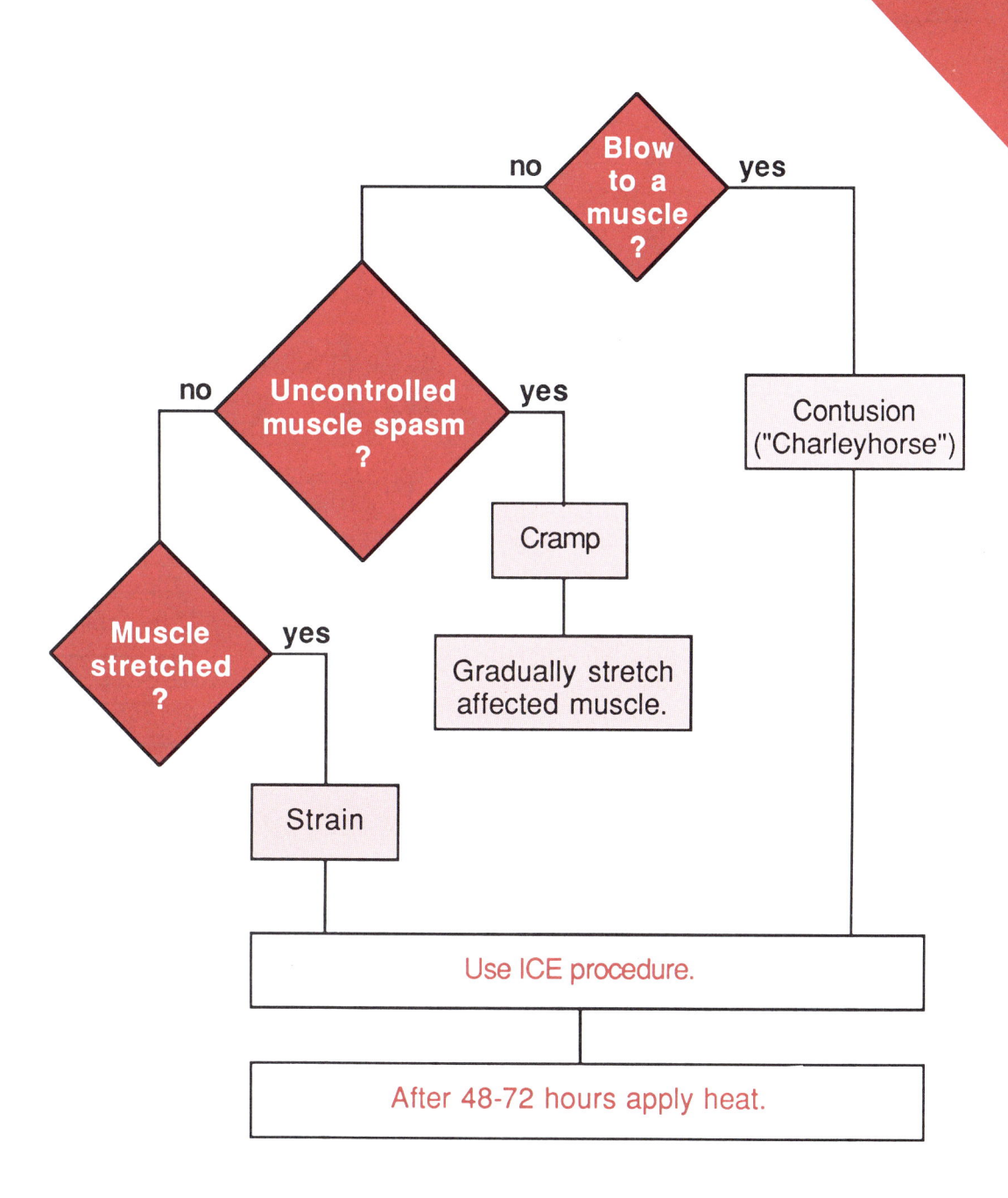

```
                    Blow
              no    to a    yes
                   muscle
                     ?

         Uncontrolled
    no   muscle spasm   yes          Contusion
              ?                     ("Charleyhorse")

                         Cramp

   Muscle      yes
  stretched
      ?                Gradually stretch
                       affected muscle.

         Strain

              Use ICE procedure.

         After 48-72 hours apply heat.
```

Sprains, Strains, Contusions, Dislocations

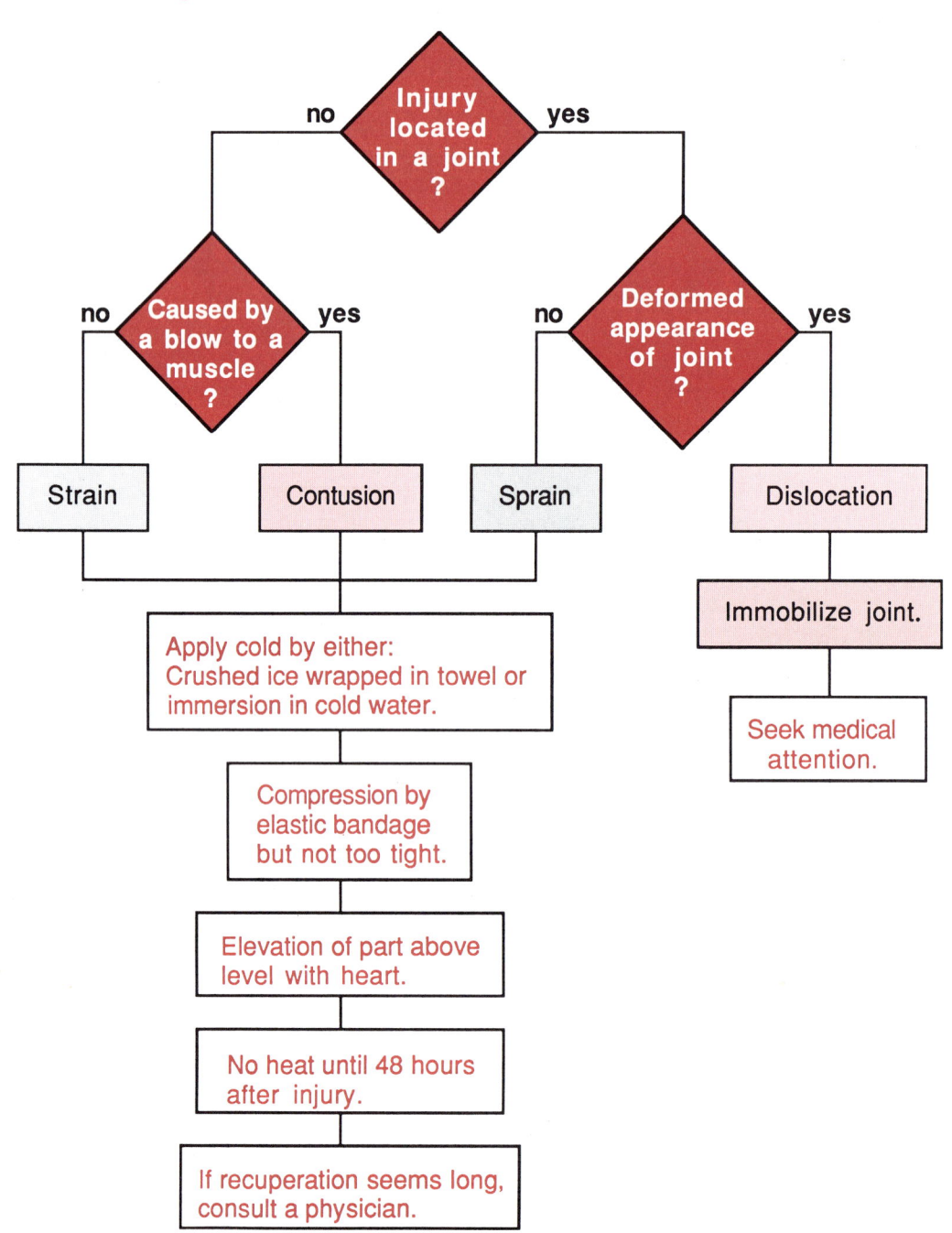

```
                    Injury
              no   located    yes
                  in a joint
                      ?

     Caused by                    Deformed
  no  a blow to  yes         no  appearance  yes
      a muscle                    of joint
         ?                           ?

  Strain    Contusion      Sprain         Dislocation

                                        Immobilize joint.

           Apply cold by either:
           Crushed ice wrapped in      Seek medical
           towel or immersion in        attention.
           cold water.

           Compression by
           elastic bandage
           but not too tight.

           Elevation of part above
           level with heart.

           No heat until 48 hours
           after injury.

           If recuperation seems long,
           consult a physician.
```

SELF-CHECK QUESTIONS

Activity 1: Fractures

Which of the following represent proper first aid procedures for fractures?

    Yes No
1. ☐ ☐ Immobilize all fractures and suspected fractures before moving the victim.
2. ☐ ☐ Check pulses periodically to be certain the circulation is adequate.
3. ☐ ☐ Splint the joints above and below the fracture.
4. ☐ ☐ In open fractures, attempt to push the bone ends back beneath the skin surface.
5. ☐ ☐ Straighten fractured joints (wrist, elbow, knee, etc.)

Activity 2: Spinal Injuries

A. Which of the following signs and symptoms may indicate a spinal injury?
1. ☐ Tells about pain down his arms or legs
2. ☐ Is able to strongly grip your hand and move his foot against your hand pressure
3. ☐ Has a severe head injury
4. ☐ Cannot move his fingers and toes when asked to do so

B. Mark each statement true (T) or false (F).
1. ☐ Do not move a victim unless extreme hazards exist (i.e., burning building or car).
2. ☐ Careless moving of a victim may permanently confine him to a wheelchair.
3. ☐ Move a spinal cord injured victim as quickly as possible to a medical facility.
4. ☐ The head tilt can be used for nonbreathing spinal cord injured victims.

Activity 3: Joint Injuries

Mark the following statements true (T) or false (F).
1. ☐ First aiders can try to reset or reduce a dislocation.
2. ☐ Use a sling and swathe for a broken clavicle (collarbone).
3. ☐ Use heat application followed by cold when treating joint or muscle injury.
4. ☐ A pillow serves well as a splint on the foot.
5. ☐ Elastic bandage, if used correctly, can effectively be used on joint and muscle injuries.
6. ☐ When using ice, place it directly on the skin.
7. ☐ The initials ICE represent the treatment for joint and muscle injuries.
8. ☐ Telling the difference between a broken ankle and a sprained ankle can be difficult.

Activity 4: Muscle Injuries

Mark the following statements true (T) or false (F).
1. ☐ Muscle injuries represent a real emergency.
2. ☐ Muscle strains and muscle pulls describe the same injury.
3. ☐ A muscle strain can involve the tearing of a muscle.
4. ☐ A blow to the muscle is also known as a "charley horse."
5. ☐ Heat packs can initially be placed on a muscle injury to reduce pain.
6. ☐ An application of cold should be left on the muscle injury for at least 20 to 30 minutes.
7. ☐ Apply the cold or ice directly on the skin to reduce swelling and bleeding.
8. ☐ Elastic bandages can be applied too tightly.

11

Medical Emergencies

- Heart Attack • Stroke • Diabetic Emergencies
- Epilepsy • Asthma

HEART ATTACK

Sudden death from heart attack is the most important medical emergency today. "Heart attack," though not a scientific term, is commonly used to describe the symptoms of an acute myocardial infarction (AMI) and of several other heart conditions. A heart attack occurs when the blood supply to some portion of the heart is either cut off or reduced to such low levels that cells in the area cannot survive.

Signs and Symptoms

Difficulty in determining a heart attack from the character of the pain is understandable because as many as one third of all myocardial infarctions are either painless or produce so little discomfort that the pain is ignored. The character of heart pain is highly variable and there are a number of medical conditions that produce similar pain patterns. The typical forms of heart pain are usually easily recognized, but heart pain or similar pain from another cause may tax the skills of the most expert cardiologist. Because treatment at the onset of a heart attack is vital to survival and how well a person recovers, the rule to follow is that if you suspect a heart attack for any reason, seek medical attention at once rather than delaying a decision.

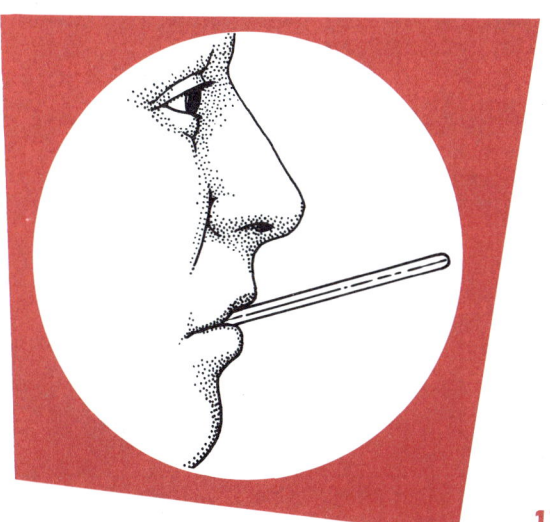

The classic symptom is often described as a pressure rather than a pain, or a sensation of a clenched fist. The pressure, squeezing sensation, or dull pain is usually located in the center of the chest, sometimes a little to the left of the sternum, but usually not confined to the left side of the chest near the nipple. The pain may be in the pit of the stomach and may even be present as abdominal pain causing the person to think he has indigestion. That symptom, along with vomiting which sometimes occurs with the onset of a heart attack, often leads to an initial suspicion of indigestion rather than of acute heart attack.

The pain may be in the upper sternum, traveling into the left or right shoulder or both, into the neck and jaw, and down the arm (more often the left arm), and it may follow a course along the inner aspect of the arm into the ring and little finger. It does not go into the thumb and index finger. The discomfort may rarely radiate into the back.

The main difference between the pain of angina and that of heart attack is its duration (refer to Table 11-1). If the pain persists over fifteen to thirty minutes, it is more likely to be a heart attack. The pain of heart attack may last for hours and may be more severe. Also, the pain of heart attack can occur at rest. Many such attacks occur at night, waking a person from sleep. Heart attack pain can and does occur during exertion as well as at rest.

The medical disorder that is perhaps the most difficult to separate from myocardial pain is spasm of the esophagus. The muscular cramp of the esophagus causes a squeezing pain behind the sternum so similar to heart pain that only medical tests can really separate the two. Pleurisy causes chest pain, but it is sharp, not dull, and it occurs with respiration and movement of the chest wall. A variety of musculoskeletal pains resemble heart pain but they, too, are associated with chest wall movement.

Besides chest pain, other symptoms are commonly associated with a heart attack. These include the following:

1. Sweating, often quite profuse (The victim may soak through his clothing and complain of a "cold sweat.")
2. Respirations are usually normal but may be rapid and shallow.
3. Nausea and/or vomiting.
4. Weakness may be profound.
5. Dizziness.
6. Palpitations are sometimes experienced by victims with irregular heart rhythms as a sensation that the heart is "skipping a beat."

First Aid

If warning signs make you suspect a heart attack, immediate care and action may mean the difference between life and death. The importance of what happens in the first few hours after an attack is emphasized by the fact that about 40% of all people with a heart attack die during this time outside the hospital because they do not receive emergency medical care at once. This is by far the most dangerous period after a heart attack has occurred.

Emergency care should be designed to create as little stress on the victim as possible. Medical care should be obtained at once. The sooner the victim can be placed in a coronary care unit and supervised by trained personnel, without endangering the victim in transit, the better.

For victims suspected of having a heart attack, the Metropolitan Insurance Company has developed these useful guidelines:

You can best help — possibly save a life — if you know in advance:

1. The nearest hospital equipped to handle heart attack emergencies.
2. How to do cardiopulmonary resuscitation (CPR).

TABLE 11-1. Chest Pain — Differences Between Angina and Heart Attack

Signs and Symptoms	Angina Pectoris	Acute Myocardial Infarction
Pain intensity	Mild to moderate	Very severe, intense.
Duration	3 to 5 minutes	30 minutes to several hours.
Precipitating factors	Physical or emotional stress	None.
Relieving factors	Rest Nitroglycerin	None.
Associated symptoms	May be none	Profuse perspiration; nausea and vomiting; fear of impending doom

Adapted from National Highway Traffic Safety Administration, *Emergency Medical Care* (Washington, D.C.: U.S. Government Printing Office).

3. How to quickly call a doctor, the hospital and/or an ambulance.

4. The fastest route to the hospital.

Knowing these things, you should:

1. Help the victim to the least painful position—usually sitting with legs up and bent at knees. Loosen clothing around the neck and midriff. Be calm and reassuring.

2. Quickly call an ambulance to get the victim to the hospital via local rescue squad, police, fire, or other available service. Once the ambulance is on the way, notify the family physician, if you have one.

3. If the ambulance is coming, comfort the victim while waiting. Otherwise, help the victim to a car, trying to keep the victim's exertion to a minimum. If possible, take another CPR-trained person with you. The victim should sit up.

4. Drive cautiously to the hospital. Watch the victim closely (or have other passenger do so). If he or she loses consciousness, check for breathing and feel for neck pulse under the side angle of the lower jaw to check for circulation. If there is no pulse, start CPR. Continue CPR until trained help arrives to take over.

5. If the victim retains consciousness to the hospital, make sure he or she is carried, not walked, to the emergency room.

Obviously, for cardiac arrest cardiopulmonary resuscitation (CPR) is performed.

STROKE

Stroke is the third most common cause of death, and in the middle-aged and older Americans it is a frequent cause of disability.

A stroke in medical terms is known as a cerebrovascular accident (CVA). The person who has a stroke may die shortly after the onset. However, in many cases the person survives the initial stroke to be left with a neurologic deficit or may even recover completely.

Causes of Stroke

Strokes can be divided into two broad categories. One category of stroke is the result of *infarction*, which occurs when the blood supply to a limited portion of the brain is inadequate and death of nerve tissue follows. Infarction may be caused by embolism or by blood vessel occlusion due to atherosclerosis. Emboli are usually small blood clots arising from diseased blood vessels (carotid) in the neck or from clots or material arising from the heart. Other types of emboli that may cause occlusion of cerebral blood vessels are air, tumor tissue, and fat. An infarction can also occur when there is marked narrowing of the blood vessels in the neck or within the skull due to atherosclerosis.

The second category is *hemorrhages*. The development of the hemorrhage is usually sudden and marked by a severe headache and stiff neck.

Signs and Symptoms

The signs and symptoms of a stroke depend, of course, on the area of the brain involved. Among the most common are:

- Impaired speech
- Confusion and/or dizziness
- Paralysis of one side of the body
- Unequal pupil size
- Seizures
- Temporary loss of speech or trouble in speaking or understanding speech
- Temporary dimness or loss of vision, particularly in one eye
- Mouth drawn to one side of the face or drooping on one side; paralysis of facial muscles, resulting in loss of expression. (Eyelid droops on affected side.)
- Loss of bladder or bowel control
- Sudden severe headache
- Nausea and/or vomiting

First Aid

The initial care of the stroke victim should include careful attention to the victim's airway. If the victim is semiconscious or unconscious, he or she should be placed on one side, preferably with the paralyzed side down. This position frees the victim's useful extremities. The paralyzed side should be adequately cushioned. Positioning on the side will permit the pooling of secretions in the cheek rather than the throat.

Because of the impairment of blood flow to the brain, keep the victim's head propped up about fifteen degrees to allow for adequate venous drainage.

Remove dentures. Also remove any mucus and food debris from the mouth in a swabbing motion with a piece of cloth wrapped around a finger. Do not give any liquids—the throat may be paralyzed.

The first aider must often rely on the family to obtain an accurate history of the problem because the victim may be unable to provide meaningful input.

The victim may have unusual behavior. This may be manifested in being combative and using abusive and profane language.

If an eye has been affected by stroke, consider protecting the eye by closing the lid and taping the eyelid down to prevent drying, which can result in loss of vision.

Avoid doing or saying anything that will increase the victim's anxiety. Do not overly handle the victim because it may aggravate the stroke. Calm reassurance of the victim and the family is one of the best things a first aider can do. Transportation to the medical facility must be as gentle and prompt as possible.

The first few minutes of care are critical in avoiding further injury, and the care is reassuring to the victim. Learning to recognize the signs and symptoms of stroke and providing proper emergency care until medical help arrives can help cope with this major killer and disabler.

DIABETIC EMERGENCIES*

With nearly 11 million Americans having diabetes, most of us have a friend or relative who has diabetes.

Diabetes is the inability of the body to appropriately metabolize carbohydrates. The islets of Langerhans of the pancreas fail to produce enough of a hormone called insulin. The function of insulin is to take glucose (sugar) from the blood and carry it into the cells to be used. The excess glucose remains in the blood, and the body cells must rely on fat as fuel. Since glucose is a major body fuel, when it cannot be metabolized, serious consequences can develop.

When the glucose level becomes too high, diabetic coma, or ketoacidosis, may occur; and the body tries to eliminate the excess urine, which can result in dehydration. Meanwhile, the cells, deprived of glucose, begin to metabolize fats for fuel. Metabolism of fat results in the production of acids and ketones as wastes. The ketones cause the victims' breath to have a fruity odor. As dehydration increases and the body is robbed of fuel, the person comes closer and closer to coma.

The opposite condition, insulin shock, can result when a person with diabetes has taken too much insulin or not eaten. The glucose level in the blood drops dangerously low and the victim becomes weak and disoriented, or unconscious.

Both of these conditions can be fatal unless something is done to reverse them.

Diabetic Coma (Ketoacidosis or Hyperglycemia)

Victims of diabetic coma often behave similarly to people who are intoxicated. The victim is in need of insulin to restore the sugar balance, but a first aider should not administer it. You can give the victim water if it can be kept down, but you should seek medical care immediately. If the victim is unconscious, maintain an open airway and be alert for vomiting. Turn the victim on his side to prevent choking. Look for a medic alert tag on the victim's wrist or neck that will indicate that the victim is diabetic. Take the victim to the hospital.

Insulin Shock (Hypoglycemia)

This condition can develop because the victim has taken too much insulin, too little food, or both. Unlike diabetic coma, insulin shock develops very rapidly and can cause bizarre behavior, which may be mistaken for mental illness.

---
*Copyright by the American Diabetes Association. Reprinted with permission from the Emergency Personnel Program manual.

11 / MEDICAL EMERGENCIES

In an emergency
THINK

LOW Blood Sugar
(Insulin reaction or Hypoglycemia)

Symptoms

Sudden Onset
Staggering, poor coordination
Anger, bad temper
Pale color
Confusion, disorientation
Sudden hunger
Sweating
Eventual stupor or unconsciousness

Action to take:

Provide sugar! If the person can swallow without choking, offer any food or drink containing sugar, such as soft drinks, fruit juice, or candy. Do not use diet drinks when blood sugar is low.

If the person does not respond in 10 to 15 minutes, take him/her to the hospital.

HIGH Blood Sugar
(Hyperglycemia or Acidosis)

Symptoms

Gradual Onset
Drowsiness
Extreme thirst
Very frequent urination
Flushed skin
Vomiting
Fruity or wine-like breath odor
Heavy breathing
Eventual stupor or unconsciousness

Action to take:

Take this person to the hospital. If you are uncertain whether the person is suffering from high or low blood sugar, give some sugar-containing food or drink. If there is no response in 10–15 minutes, this person needs immediate medical attention.

DIABETES!

Warning: A diabetic emergency may resemble alcohol or drug intoxication. Know the symptoms of low and high blood sugar. **THINK DIABETES!**

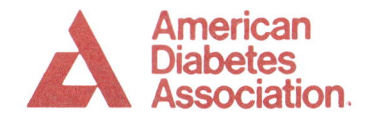

American Diabetes Association.

First aid for insulin shock includes giving the victim something containing sugar, such as a soft drink, candy, or fruit juice. Do not use diet drink when blood sugar is low. Often, the victim will recover amazingly fast. If the person does not feel better in ten to fifteen minutes, take him or her to the hospital. For an unconscious victim, a cube of sugar or loose sugar may be placed under the tongue of the victim because some sugar is absorbed through the lining of the mouth.

Telling the difference between the two conditions, diabetic coma and insulin shock, can be difficult. If the victim is awake, the victim can often direct the first aider as to what to do. If the victim has eaten but not taken insulin, the problem is most likely diabetic coma. If the victim has not eaten but has taken insulin, the problem is most likely insulin shock.

If the first aider cannot distinguish between the two conditions and sugar is available, have the victim take it. If the condition is insulin shock, there will be noticeable improvement. If it is diabetic coma, there is little danger that a small amount of sugar will worsen the victim's condition. Do not give liquids to an unconscious victim. These procedures may save the life of a victim or avoid brain damage.

EPILEPSY*

Epilepsy is a common neurological condition. It is sometimes called a seizure disorder. It takes the form of brief, temporary changes in the normal functioning of the brain's electrical system. These brief malfunctions occur when more than the usual amount of electrical energy passes between cells.

You cannot see what is happening inside a person's brain. But you can see the unusual body movements, the effects on consciousness, and the changed behavior that the malfunctioning cells are producing. These changes are what we call epileptic seizures.

Source: Epilepsy Foundation of America. Reprinted with permission.

Recognition of epilepsy and knowledge of first aid is important because it is very easy to mistake epilepsy for some other condition.

Types of Seizures

Epileptic seizures may be convulsive or nonconvulsive in nature, depending on where in the brain the malfunction takes place and on how much of the total brain area is involved.

Convulsive seizures are the ones that most people generally think of when they hear the word "epilepsy." In this type of seizure the person undergoes convulsions that usually last from two to five minutes, with complete loss of consciousness and muscle spasm.

Nonconvulsive seizures may take the form of a blank stare lasting only a few seconds, an involuntary movement of arm or leg, or a period of automatic movement in which awareness of one's surroundings is blurred or completely absent.

Since these seizure types are so different, they require different kinds of action from the public, and some require no action at all. Table 11-2 describes seizures in detail and how to handle each type.

Should Medical Attention Be Called?

An uncomplicated convulsive seizure due to epilepsy is not a medical emergency, even though it looks like one. It stops naturally after a few minutes without ill effects. The average victim is able to resume normal activity after a rest period and may need only limited assistance, or no assistance at all, in getting home.

However, several medical conditions other than epilepsy can cause seizures. These require immediate medical attention and include:

encephalitis	poisoning	hypoglycemia
meningitis	pregnancy	high fever
heat stroke		head injury

The following guidelines are designed to help people with epilepsy avoid unnecessary and expensive trips to the emergency room and to help you decide whether or not to call an ambulance when someone has a convulsive seizure.

TABLE 11-2. Seizure: Recognition and First Aid

Seizure Type	What It Looks Like	What It Is Not	What To Do	What Not To Do
Generalized Tonic-Clonic (Also called Grand Mal)	Sudden cry, fall, rigidity, followed by muscle jerks, shallow breathing or temporarily suspended breathing, bluish skin, possible loss of bladder or bowel control, usually lasts 2 minutes. Normal breathing then starts again. There may be some confusion and/or fatigue, followed by return to full consciousness.	Heart attack. Stroke. Unknown but life threatening emergency.	Look for medical identification. Protect from nearby hazards. Loosen tie or shirt collars. Place folded jacket under head. Turn on side to keep airway clear. Reassure when consciousness returns. If single seizure lasted less than 10 minutes, ask if hospital evaluation wanted. If multiple seizures, or if one seizure lasts longer than 10 minutes, take to emergency room.	Don't put any hard implement in the mouth. Don't try to hold tongue. It can't be swallowed. Don't try to give liquids during or just after seizure. Don't use oxygen unless there are symptoms of heart attack. Don't use artificial respiration unless breathing is absent after muscle jerks subside, or unless water has been inhaled. Don't restrain.
Absence (Also called Petit Mal)	A blank stare, lasting only a few seconds, most common in children. May be accompanied by rapid blinking, some chewing movements of the mouth. Child having the seizure is unaware of what's going on during the seizure, but quickly returns to full awareness once it has stopped. May result in learning difficulties if not recognized and treated.	Daydreaming. Lack of attention. Deliberate ignoring of adult instructions.	No first aid necessary, but medical evaluation should be recommended.	
Simple Partial (Also called Jacksonian)	Jerking begins in fingers or toes, can't be stopped by patient, but patient stays awake and aware. Jerking may proceed to involve hand, then arm, and sometimes spreads to whole body and becomes a convulsive seizure.	Acting out, bizarre behavior.	No first aid necessary unless seizure becomes convulsive, then first aid as above.	
Simple Partial (Also called Sensory)	May not be obvious to onlooker, other than patient's preoccupied or blank expression. Patient experiences a distorted enviornment. May see or hear things that aren't there, may feel unexplained fear, sadness, anger, or joy. May have nausea, experience odd smells, and have a generally "funny" feeling in the stomach.	Hysteria. Mental Illness. Psychosomatic illness. Parapsychological or mystical experience.	No action needed other than reassurance and emotional support.	
Complex Partial (Also called Psychomotor or Temporal Lobe)	Usually starts with blank stare, followed by chewing, followed by random activity. Person appears unaware of surroundings, may seem dazed and mumble. Unresponsive. Actions clumsy, not directed. May pick at clothing, pick up objects, try to take clothes off. May run, appear to be afraid. May struggle or flail at restraint. Once pattern established, same set of actions usually occur with each seizure. Lasts a few minutes, but post-seizure confusion can last substantially longer. No memory of what happened during seizure period.	Drunkenness. Intoxication of drugs. Mental Illness. Indecent exposure. Disorderly conduct. Shoplifting.	Speak calmly and reassuringly to patient and others. Guide gently away from obvious hazards. Stay with person until completely aware of environment. Offer to help getting home.	Don't grab hold unless sudden danger (such as a cliff edge or an approaching car) threatens. Don't try to restrain. Don't shout. Don't expect verbal instructions to be obeyed.
Atonic Seizures (Also called Drop Attacks)	The legs of a child between 2–5 years of age suddenly collapse under him and he falls. After 10 seconds to a minute he recovers consciousness, and can stand and walk again.	Clumsiness. Lack of good walking skills. Normal childhood "stage."	No first aid needed (unless he hurt himself as he fell), but the child should be given a thorough medical evaluation.	
Myoclonic Seizures	Sudden brief, massive muscle jerks that may involve the whole body or parts of body. May cause person to spill what they were holding or fall off a chair.	Clumsiness. Poor coordination.	No first aid needed, but should be given a thorough medical evaluation.	
Infantile Spasms	Starts between 3 months and two years. If a child is sitting up, the head will fall foward, and the arms will flex forward. If lying down, the knees will be drawn up, with arms and head flexed forward as if the baby is reaching for support.	Normal movements of the baby, especially if they happen when the baby is lying down.	No first aid, but prompt medical evaluation is needed.	

Source: © Epilepsy Foundation of America. Reprinted with permission.

Do not call an ambulance if:

1. Medical I.D. jewelry or card identified the person as epileptic, *and*
2. The seizure ends in under *ten minutes, and*
3. Consciousness returns without further incident, *and*
4. There are no signs of injury, physical distress, or pregnancy.

Call an ambulance if:

1. The seizure has happened in water.
2. There is no medical I.D. and no way of knowing whether the seizure is caused by epilepsy, *and*
3. The seizure continues for more than *five* minutes. Setting a five-minute limit on a seizure of unknown origin before calling for emergency assistance (against ten minutes if medical I.D. is worn) is a precaution based on the possibility that a seroius condition other than epilepsy may be causing the convulsion.

If an ambulance arrives after the person has regained consciousness, you should ask the person whether the seizure was associated with epilepsy and whether emergency room care is wanted. The same questions should be asked of a person without medical I.D. whose seizure lasts less than five minutes and for whom an ambulance has not yet been called.

ASTHMA

The sight of a person suffering an acute asthmatic attack is most distressing and, to first aiders inexperienced with this form of illness, very frightening.

All asthmatics have hyperirritable airways, making the bronchial tree sensitive and overreactive to substances and conditions that do not normally adversely affect other people.

Although asthma is precipitated by various "triggers," the result is the same—an airway obstruction due to:

- Bronchospasm
- Swelling of mucous membranes in the bronchial walls
- Plugging of bronchi by thick, mucous secretions

Status asthmaticus is a severe, prolonged asthmatic attack that even a physician using epinephrine cannot break; it is a true emergency. The chest is greatly distended and the victim has great difficulty in moving air. There may be inaudible breath sounds and wheezes because of the little air movement. The victim is usually exhausted and dehydrated.

Signs and Symptoms

Asthma is characterized by a sudden narrowing of the smaller air passageways in the lungs. The victim becomes acutely short of breath and a wheezing will be heard during exhalation.

Wheezing is the most obvious sign of this condition. It is a whistling, high-pitched sound produced by air being forced through a constricted airway. The wheezing is usually quite audible, but it may be absent if the attack is very severe and there is very little movement of air. Not all wheezes are asthma.

Other important signs leading to suspicion of asthma include:

- A known history of severe allergies or a family history of allergies
- Previous attacks of shortness of breath
- A recent respiratory infection
- Prescription medications in the form of pills and/or inhaler
- An unproductive cough
- Rapid respiration rate

First Aid

The first aider may be called on to assist a person who is suffering from an acute asthmatic attack. In most cases, the first aider can do little other than recognize the nature of the ailment and, if needed, obtain medical assistance. Considerations during an emergency may include:

- The keystone of asthma care is adequate fluid intake. Doubling the intake of liquids will benefit the victim. Water given orally, if possible, is warranted.
- Often steam or vaporizer inhalations are beneficial.
- Inhalation of nebulized medication should not be done more than every one or two hours and rarely used for more than one day. Many asthmatics carry a nebulizer or inhaler or at least know which one is effective.
- Help the victim into a comfortable breathing position that he or she chooses. Do not make the victim assume a position you think will be comfortable. The best position is usually sitting straight up. The victim probably won't let you position him or her in any other way. He or she knows better than you what position enables him to breathe most comfortably.
- Place the victim in a room that is as free as possible of common allergens (e.g., dust, feathers, animals). It should also be free of odors (e.g., tobacco smoke, paint).
- Panic is often present in the acute asthmatic attack. A calm and caring attitude and a comforting voice can prevent panic from escalating.
- Keep all questions to the victim as brief and essential as possible. The victim may be struggling merely to breathe. Attempt to find out when the onset of the attack began and if previous attacks have occurred.
- Observe skin and nail bed color for cyanosis and note wheezing patterns.
- Home therapy may not be sufficient if the asthma has been present for several hours or if there have been recurrent attacks within a few days. Therefore, medical advice should be obtained.

Heart Attack

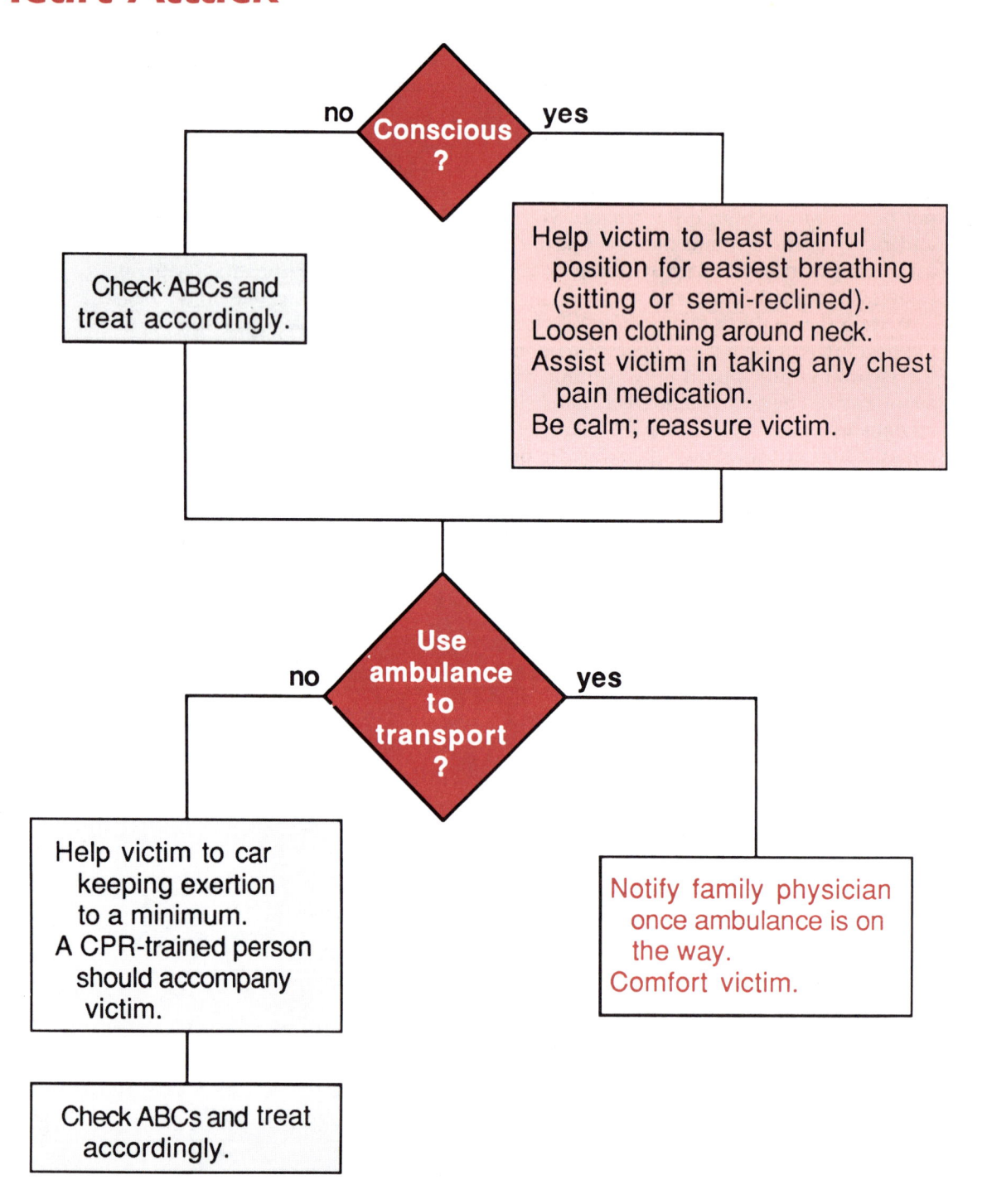

```
                    Conscious?
              no  /          \  yes
                 /            \
   Check ABCs and            Help victim to least painful
   treat accordingly.        position for easiest breathing
                             (sitting or semi-reclined).
                             Loosen clothing around neck.
                             Assist victim in taking any chest
                             pain medication.
                             Be calm; reassure victim.

                    Use ambulance to transport?
              no  /          \  yes
                 /            \
   Help victim to car         Notify family physician
   keeping exertion           once ambulance is on
   to a minimum.              the way.
   A CPR-trained person       Comfort victim.
   should accompany
   victim.

   Check ABCs and treat
   accordingly.
```

Stroke

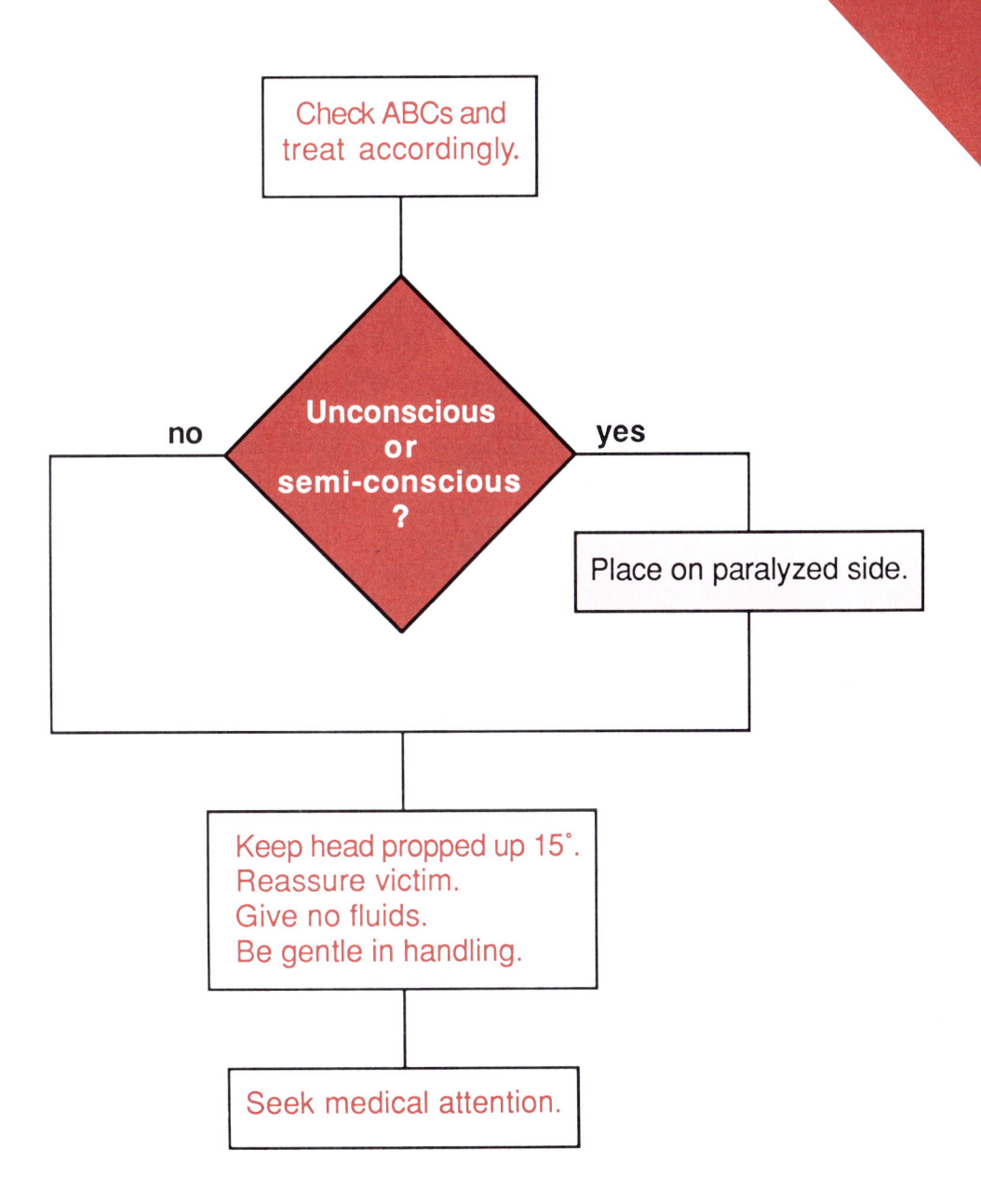

```
        Check ABCs and
        treat accordingly.
                │
                ▼
       ┌─────────────────┐
   no  │  Unconscious    │  yes
◄──────┤       or        ├──────►
       │ semi-conscious? │
       └─────────────────┘
                              │
                              ▼
                    Place on paralyzed side.

                │
                ▼
        Keep head propped up 15°.
        Reassure victim.
        Give no fluids.
        Be gentle in handling.
                │
                ▼
        Seek medical attention.
```

Diabetic Emergencies

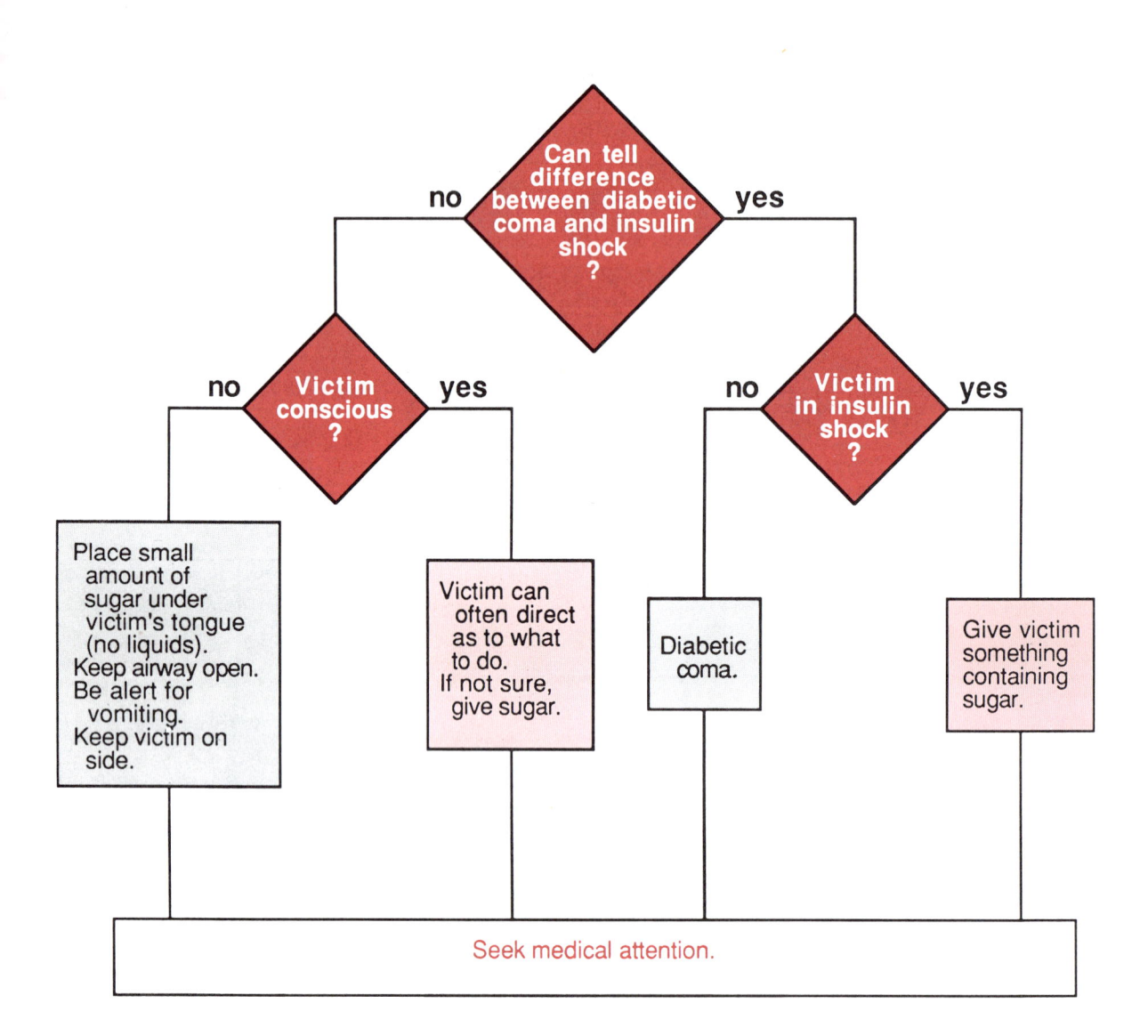

```
                    Can tell
                    difference
              no   between diabetic   yes
                   coma and insulin
                       shock
                         ?

         Victim                        Victim
    no   conscious    yes         no   in insulin   yes
           ?                           shock
                                         ?

 Place small        Victim can                    Give victim
  amount of         often direct                  something
 sugar under        as to what      Diabetic      containing
victim's tongue     to do.          coma.         sugar.
 (no liquids).      If not sure,
Keep airway open.   give sugar.
Be alert for
  vomiting.
Keep victim on
   side.

              Seek medical attention.
```

188

Seizures

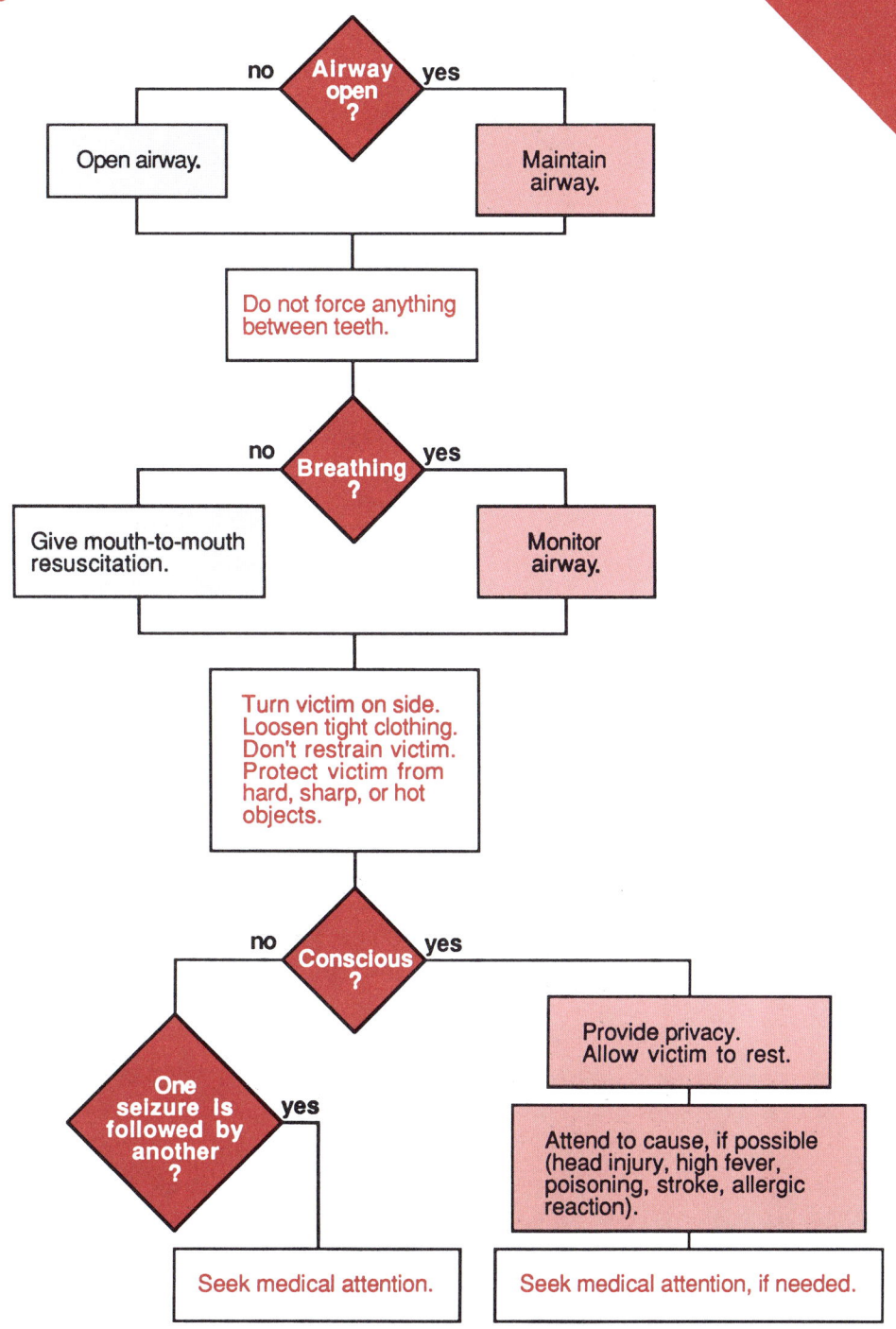

- **Airway open?**
  - no → Open airway.
  - yes → Maintain airway.
- Do not force anything between teeth.
- **Breathing?**
  - no → Give mouth-to-mouth resuscitation.
  - yes → Monitor airway.
- Turn victim on side. Loosen tight clothing. Don't restrain victim. Protect victim from hard, sharp, or hot objects.
- **Conscious?**
  - yes → Provide privacy. Allow victim to rest. → Attend to cause, if possible (head injury, high fever, poisoning, stroke, allergic reaction). → Seek medical attention, if needed.
  - no → **One seizure is followed by another?**
    - yes → Seek medical attention.

Asthma

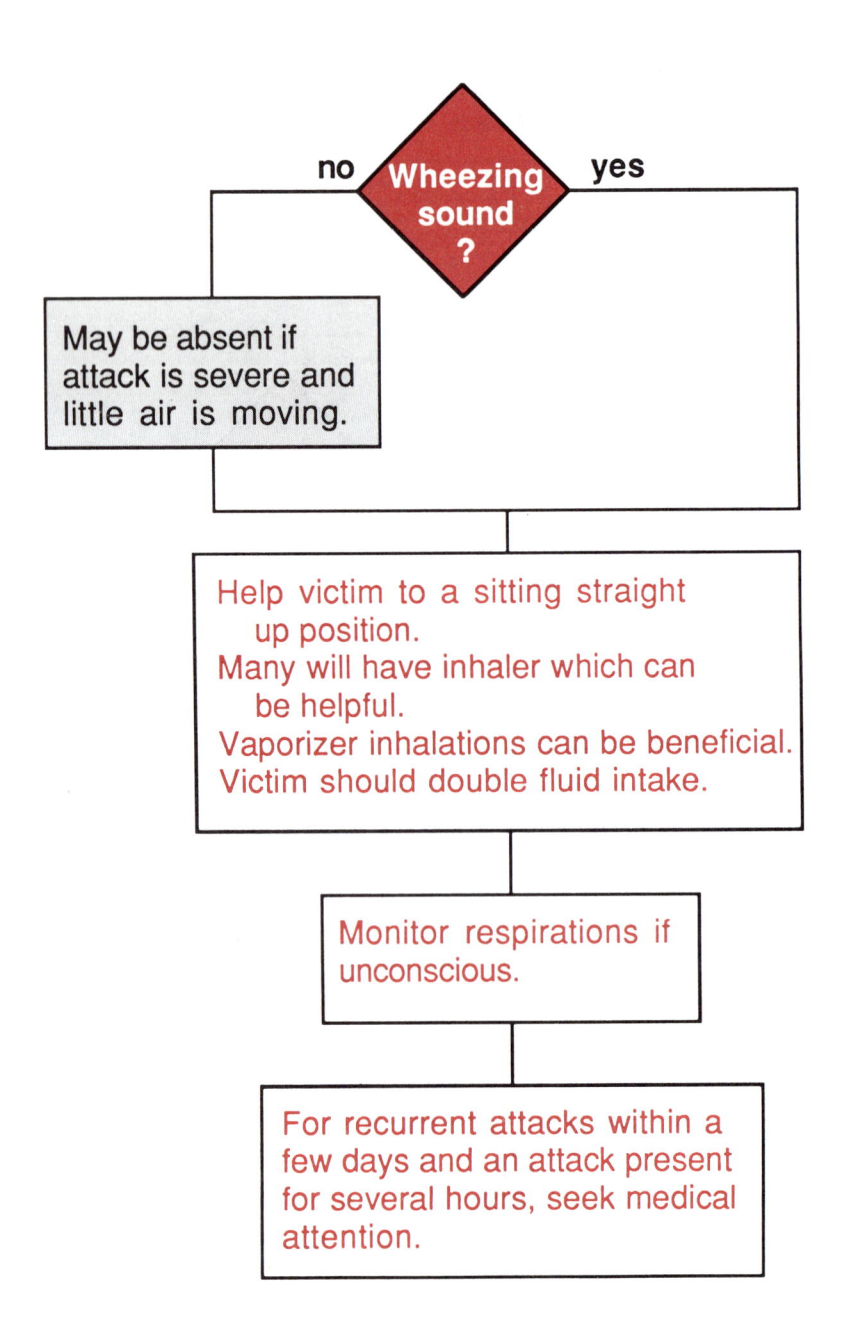

Wheezing sound?

- **no** → May be absent if attack is severe and little air is moving.
- **yes** →

Help victim to a sitting straight up position.
Many will have inhaler which can be helpful.
Vaporizer inhalations can be beneficial.
Victim should double fluid intake.

Monitor respirations if unconscious.

For recurrent attacks within a few days and an attack present for several hours, seek medical attention.

SELF-CHECK QUESTIONS

Activity 1: Heart Attack

A. A person having a heart attack may have which of the following signs and symptoms?

1. ☐ He complains of a squeezing chest pain.
2. ☐ He has leg cramping.
3. ☐ He sweats excessively.
4. ☐ He appears weak and complains of dizziness.

B. A co-worker complains about chest pain making you suspect a heart attack. Which of the following should you do?

    Yes No
1. ☐ ☐ Quickly call for an ambulance.
2. ☐ ☐ Help him move and stretch his arms.
3. ☐ ☐ Help the victim to a lying down position.
4. ☐ ☐ If the heart stops, a trained person should give CPR.
5. ☐ ☐ Loosen tight clothing at the neck and belt.
6. ☐ ☐ Place the victim in a semi-sitting position.

Activity 2: Stroke

A. Which of the following signs and symptoms may indicate a stroke has occurred?

    Yes No
1. ☐ ☐ A sudden, severe headache
2. ☐ ☐ The pupil of the one eye is larger than the pupil of the other eye
3. ☐ ☐ Chest pain and nausea complaints
4. ☐ ☐ No feeling exists in his left arm and leg
5. ☐ ☐ Swelling occurs in the left arm and leg
6. ☐ ☐ Talk is difficult to understand

192 FIRST AID ESSENTIALS

B. A partially paralyzed elderly man has difficulty speaking. You suspect a stroke has occurred. Which of the following should you do?

    Yes No
1. ☐ ☐ Relieve his anxieties by calmly being reassuring.
2. ☐ ☐ Give him a glass of water to drink.
3. ☐ ☐ Keep his head propped up.
4. ☐ ☐ If he is unconscious, place him on his paralyzed side.

C. Write the appropriate letter in each space below to specify whether the signs and symptoms described indicate

(a) A heart attack OR (b) A stroke.

1. ☐ ☐ Mouth drawn or drooping to one side
2. ☐ ☐ Sweating, nausea, and vomiting
3. ☐ ☐ Chest pain and feelings of nausea
4. ☐ ☐ Unequal size of the pupils of the eyes
5. ☐ ☐ Partial paralysis of the body

Activity 3: Diabetic Emergencies

Which of the following actions should you take when a diabetic emergency occurs?

    Yes No
1. ☐ ☐ Look for a medic alert tag on the person's wrist or neck.
2. ☐ ☐ Give a conscious diabetic several glasses of a diet drink.
3. ☐ ☐ Wait 30 minutes to see if his condition improves.
4. ☐ ☐ Give a conscious diabetic anything containing sugar if there is any doubt about which diabetic emergency he is experiencing.

Activity 4: Epilepsy

Which of the following actions should you take when a convulsive seizure happens?

Yes No
1. ☐ ☐ Put a "bite stick" or other hard implement between victim's teeth.
2. ☐ ☐ Hold the victim down.
3. ☐ ☐ Give some water during or just after a seizure.
4. ☐ ☐ Look for medical identification.
5. ☐ ☐ Loosen tight clothing around neck (i.e., tie).
6. ☐ ☐ Turn on side to prevent choking.
7. ☐ ☐ Person in a seizure lasting longer than 10 minutes should be taken to emergency room.
8. ☐ ☐ Take victim to emergency room if multiple seizures occur.

Activity 5: Asthma

Mark the statements true (T) or false (F).

1. ☐ In most asthma cases a first aider can do little except obtain medical assistance if needed.
2. ☐ Don't give water because of possible choking.
3. ☐ A vaporizer may be helpful.
4. ☐ Inhaling nebulized medication can be effective.
5. ☐ The best position for the victim is lying down on his side.
6. ☐ Keep the victim talking since it keeps the air moving into the lungs.

12
First Aid Skills
- Bandaging • Splinting

Dressings control bleeding and prevent contamination. Bandages hold dressings in place. Dressings come in many different forms. Sterile gauzes are most commonly used. When these cannot be found, nonsterile substitutes such as towels or handkerchiefs can be applied. Many different forms of bandages exist. Roller gauze, triangular, and cravat bandages make-up the bandages most often used by first aiders. However, self-adhering and formfitting bandages have become popular especially to emergency medical technicians.

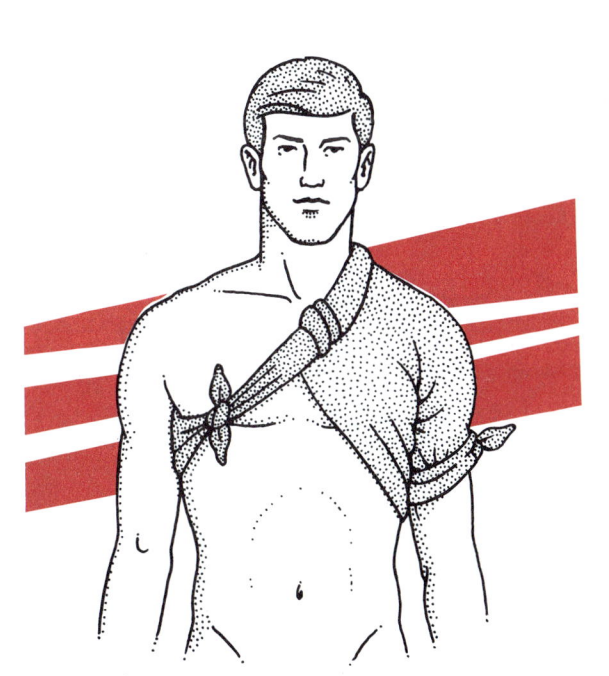

Bandages need not be textbook perfect as long as they hold the dressings in place. Care should be taken, however, so that bandages are not applied too tightly or too loosely. Too tightly applied bandages will restrict blood flow, and too loose bandages fail to hold the dressing in place. When extremities are bandaged, the fingers and toes should be left exposed so that any color changes in them can be noted. Such changes may indicate impaired circulation. Pain, color change, numbness, and tingling represent other signs of a too tight bandage.

Methods of applying dressings and bandages vary greatly and differ according to the types used and the injured part to which they are applied. Because of the variety of good bandaging techniques, the examples shown on the following pages represent a consensus among first aid experts as to the appropriate methods.

The following illustrations show suggested bandaging and splinting skills. This compilation represents the skills needed for most first aid situations likely to be encountered.

Triangular and Cravat Bandages

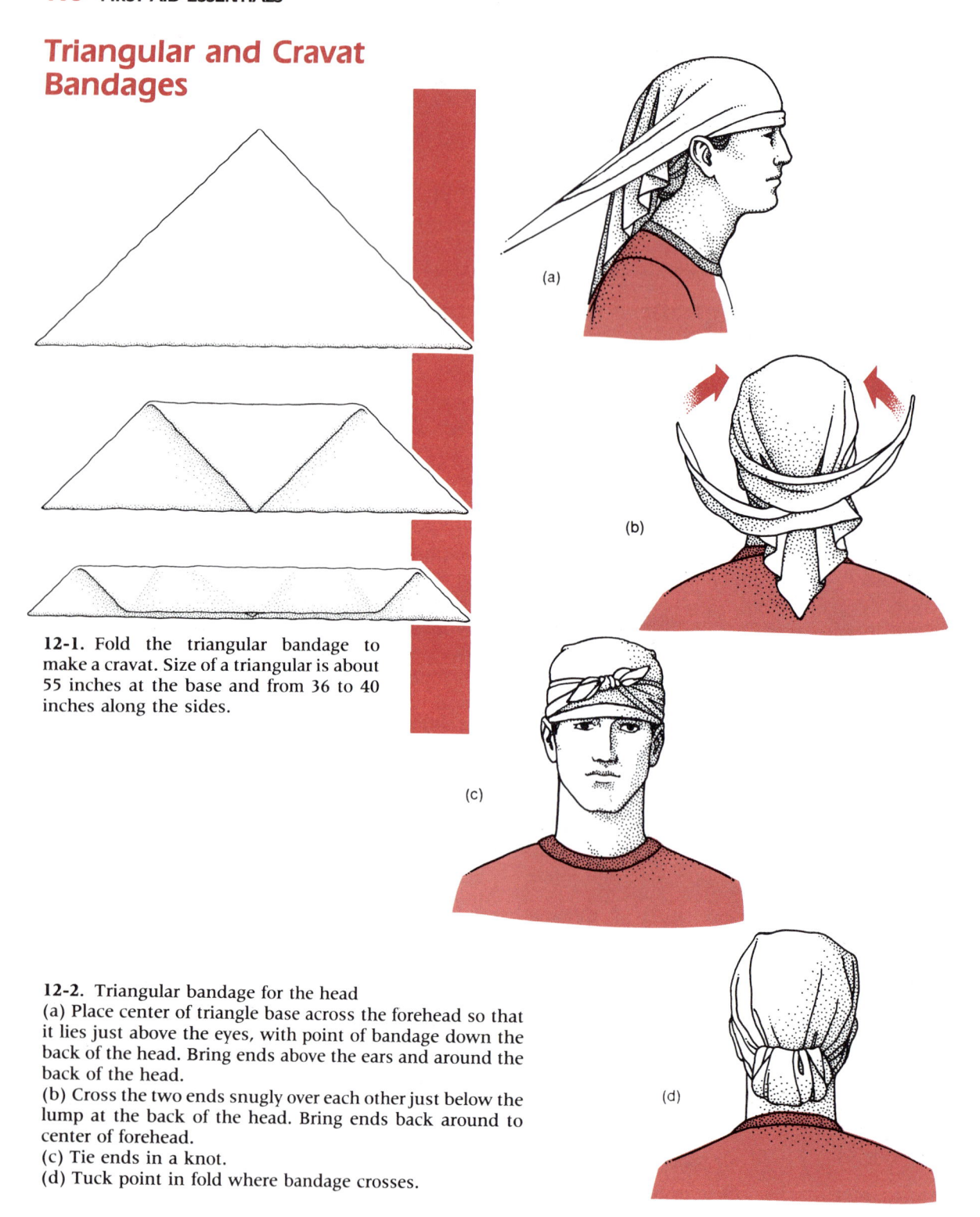

12-1. Fold the triangular bandage to make a cravat. Size of a triangular is about 55 inches at the base and from 36 to 40 inches along the sides.

12-2. Triangular bandage for the head
(a) Place center of triangle base across the forehead so that it lies just above the eyes, with point of bandage down the back of the head. Bring ends above the ears and around the back of the head.
(b) Cross the two ends snugly over each other just below the lump at the back of the head. Bring ends back around to center of forehead.
(c) Tie ends in a knot.
(d) Tuck point in fold where bandage crosses.

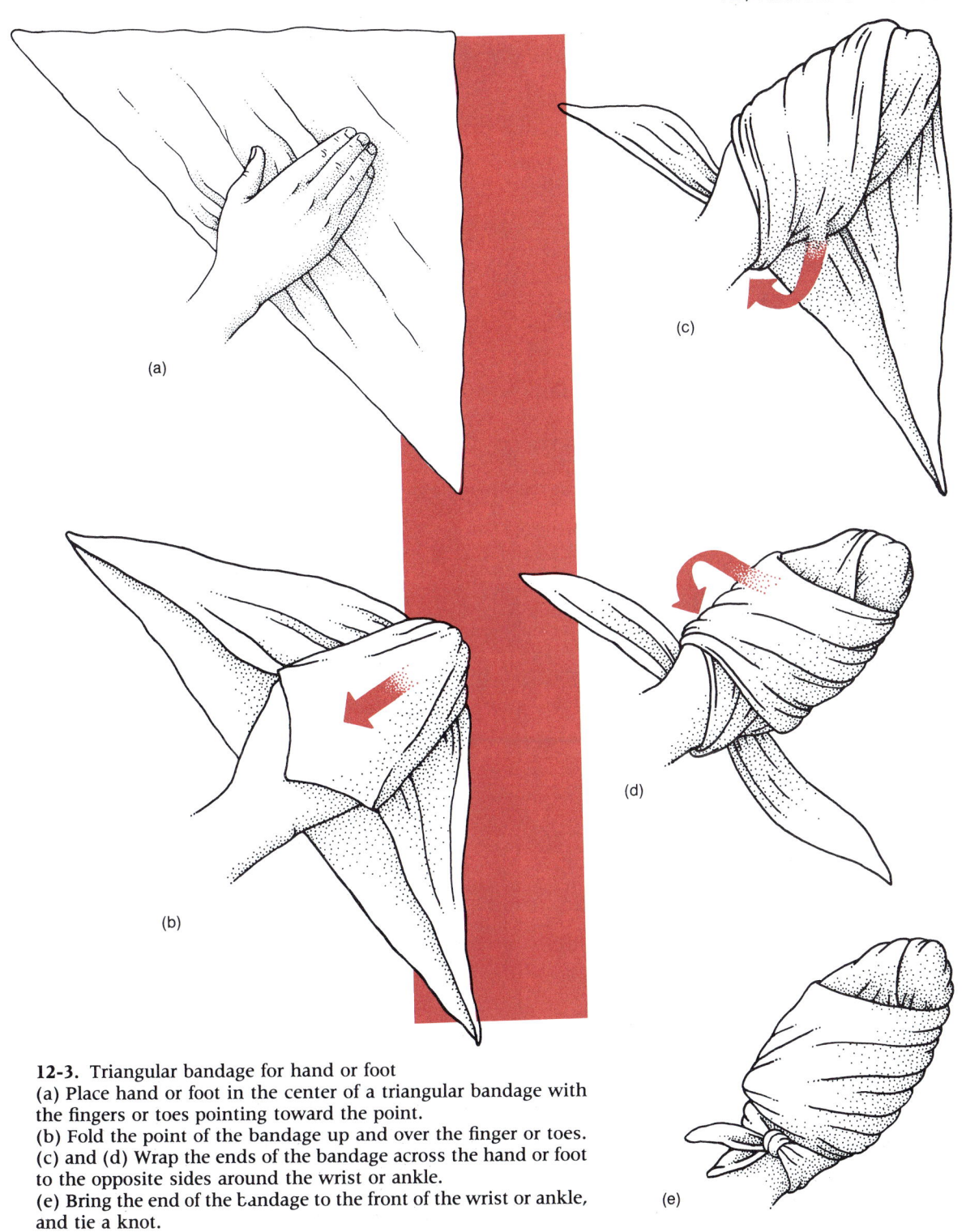

12-3. Triangular bandage for hand or foot
(a) Place hand or foot in the center of a triangular bandage with the fingers or toes pointing toward the point.
(b) Fold the point of the bandage up and over the finger or toes.
(c) and (d) Wrap the ends of the bandage across the hand or foot to the opposite sides around the wrist or ankle.
(e) Bring the end of the bandage to the front of the wrist or ankle, and tie a knot.

198 FIRST AID ESSENTIALS

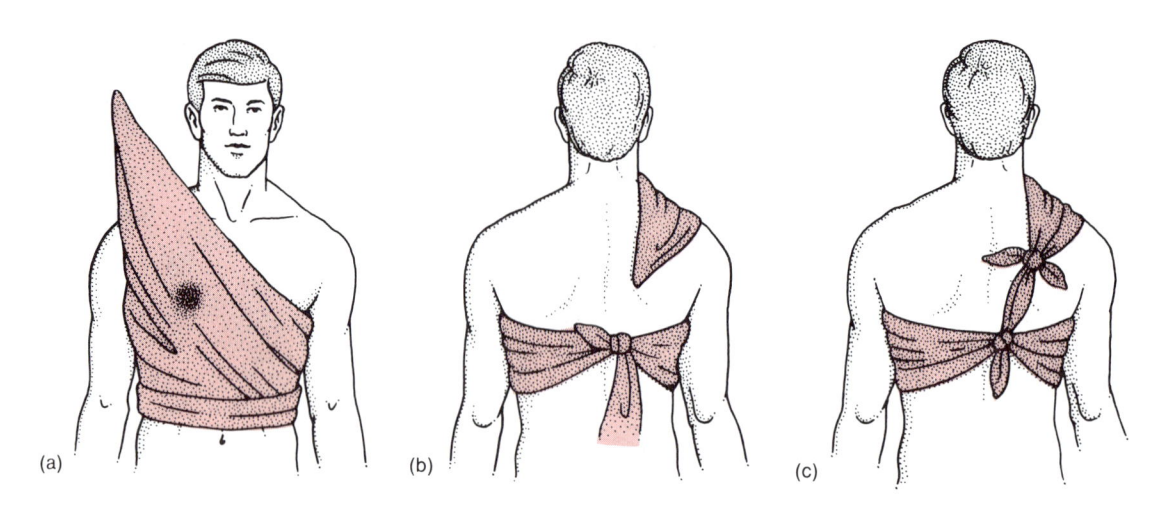

12-4. Triangular bandage for chest or back
(a) Fold the base of the bandage up far enough to secure the dressing and tie the ends around the torso. Tie so there is one long and one short and extra bandage will be left.
(b) Place the point of the bandage over the shoulder.
(c) Bring the long end up to the shoulder and tie it to the point of the triangle.

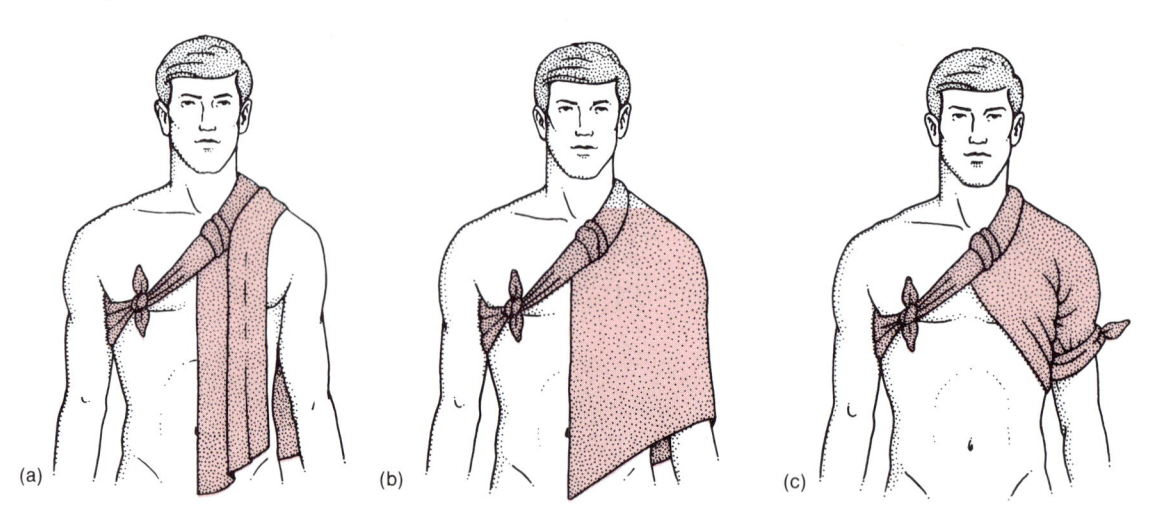

12-5. Triangular bandage for the shoulder
(a) Place a cravat bandage on the point of the triangular bandage and roll them together several times toward the triangle base. Place the cravat over the injured shoulder near the neck. Bring the cravat ends under the opposite armpit and tie slightly in front or back of it.
(b) Bring the base of the triangular bandage down and over the dressing on the shoulder.
(c) Fold up the base of the triangular bandage. Wrap the ends around the arm and tie on the outside.

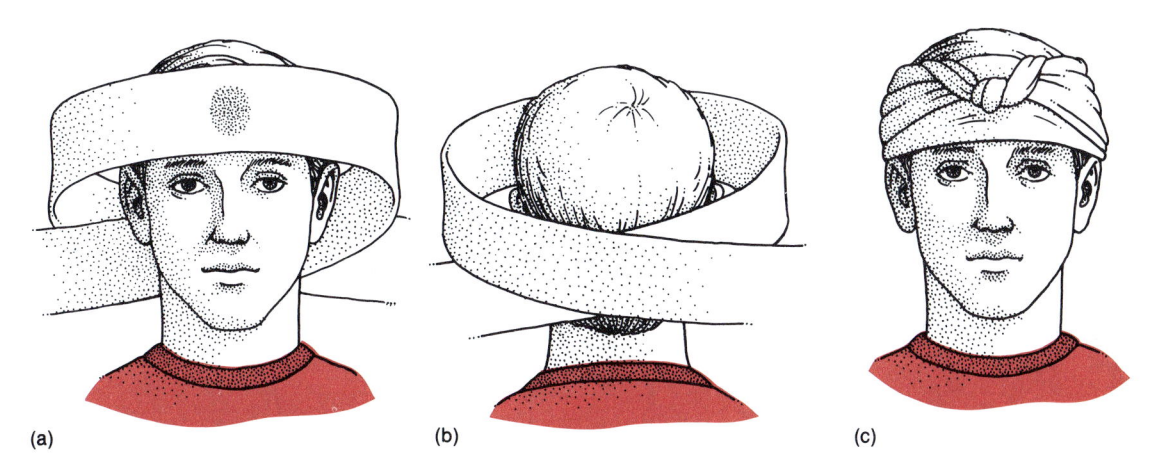

12-6. Cravat bandage for the head, ear, or eyes
(a) Place middle of bandage over the dressing covering the wound.
(b) Cross the two ends snugly over each other.
(c) Bring ends back around to where the dressing is and tie the ends in a knot.

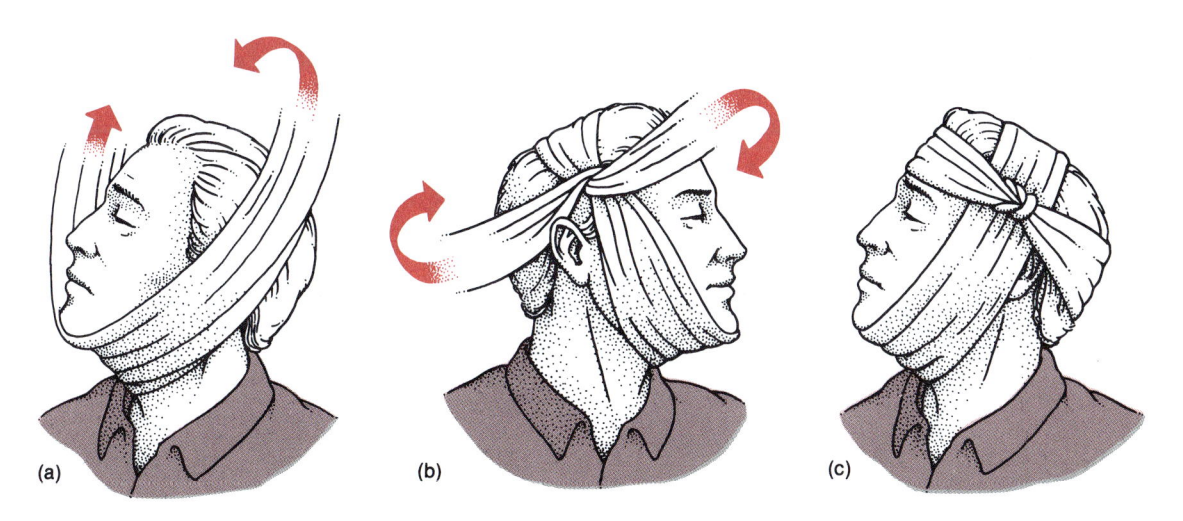

12-7. Cravat bandage for cheek, ear, or head
(a) Place bandage under chin and carry ends upward. Adjust bandage to make one end longer than the other.
(b) Take longer end over top of head to meet short end at temple. Cross ends.
(c) Take ends in opposite directions to other side of head and tie them over the part of bandage applied first.

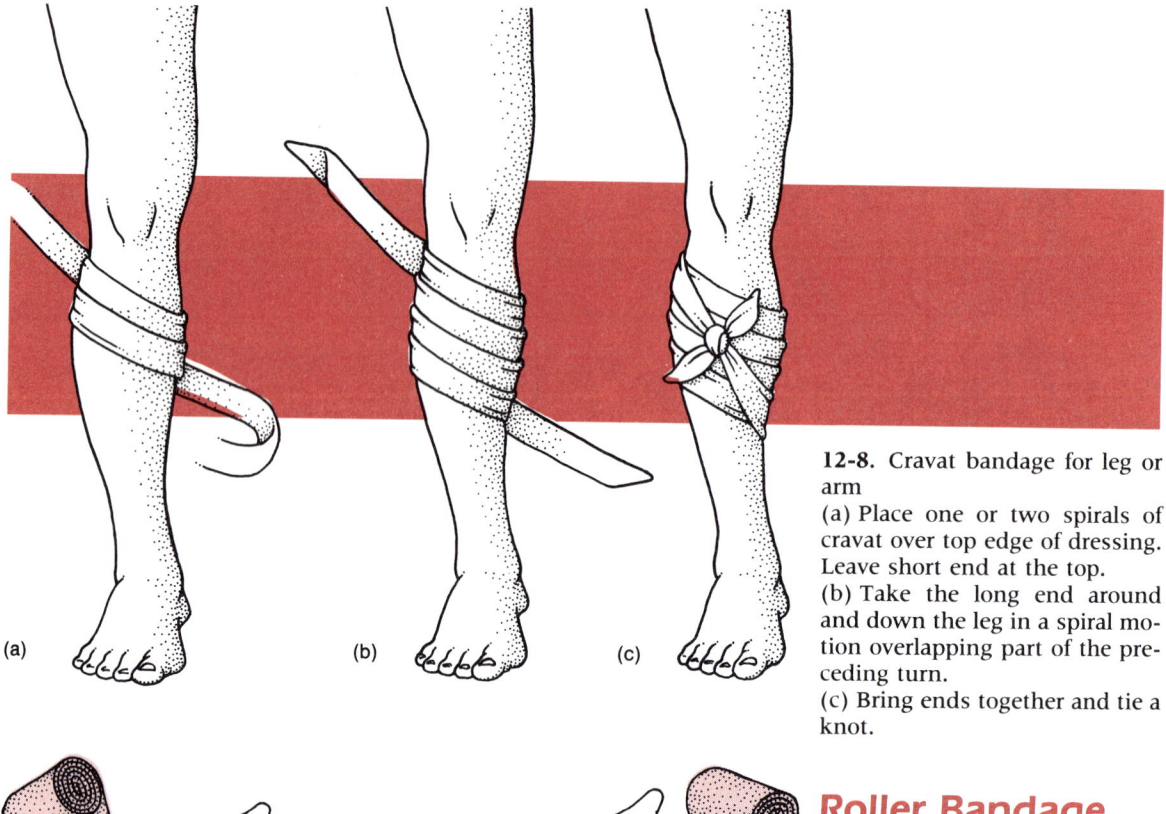

200 FIRST AID ESSENTIALS

12-8. Cravat bandage for leg or arm
(a) Place one or two spirals of cravat over top edge of dressing. Leave short end at the top.
(b) Take the long end around and down the leg in a spiral motion overlapping part of the preceding turn.
(c) Bring ends together and tie a knot.

Roller Bandage

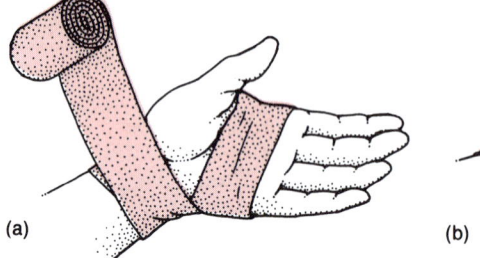

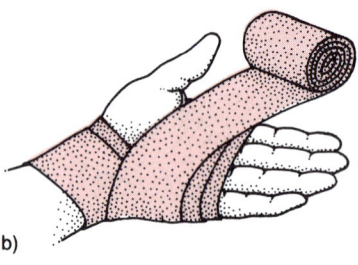

12-9. Roller bandage for hand
(a) Anchor the bandage with one or more turns around the palm of the hand. Then, carry it around the wrist.
(b) Repeat this figure-of-eight maneuver as many times as is necessary to fix the dressing properly.

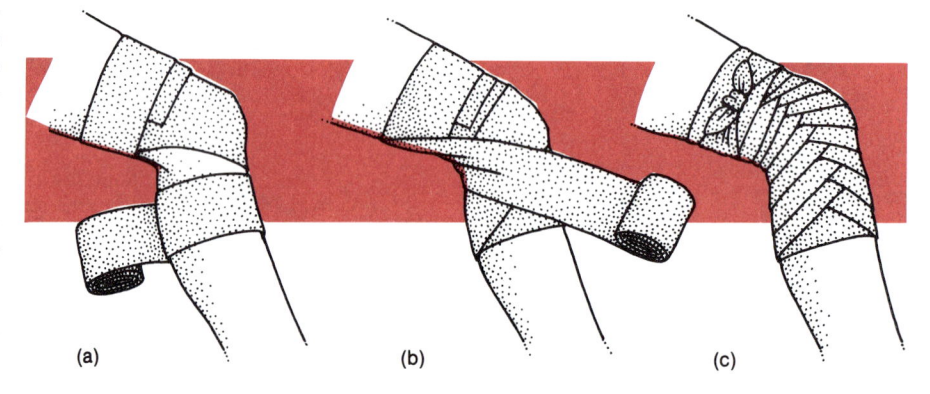

12-10. Roller bandage for knee
(a) Make several anchoring turns above the knee joint, overlapping the top edge of the dressing. Proceed diagonally downward across the dressing. Circle below the joint.
(b) Proceed diagonally upward across the dressing and downward across the dressing.
(c) Repeat the figure-of-eight process until the area is sufficiently covered.

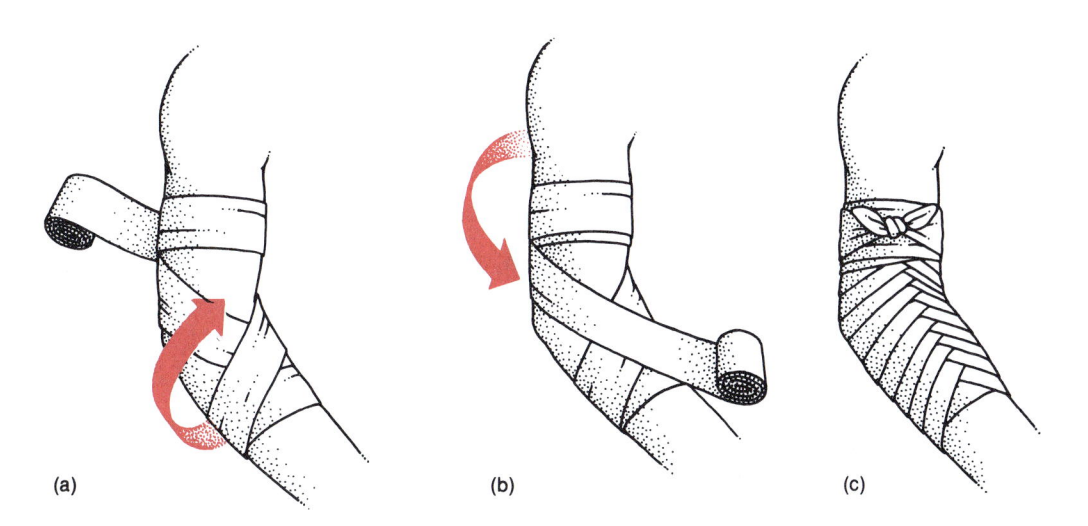

12 / FIRST AID SKILLS   201

(a)   (b)   (c)

12-11. Roller bandage for elbow
(a) Make several anchoring turns above the elbow joint, overlapping the top edge of the dressing. Proceed diagonally downward across the dressing. Circle below the joint and proceed upward diagonally.

(b) Proceed downward diagonally.
(c) Repeat the figure-of-eight process until the area is sufficiently covered.

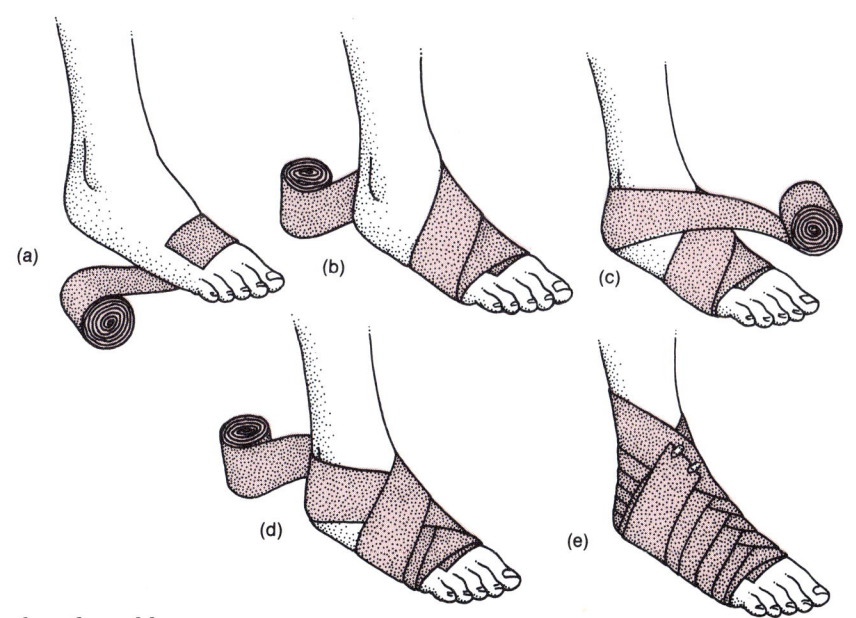

(a)   (b)   (c)
(d)   (e)

12-12. Roller bandage for ankle
(a) Anchor bandage with one or two circular turns around the foot.
(b) Bring bandage diagonally across the top of the foot and around the back of the ankle.
(c) Continue bandage down across the top of the foot and under the arch.

(d) Continue figure-of-eight turns, with each turn overlapping the last turn by about three-fourths of its width.
(e) Bandage until the foot (not toes) and lower leg are covered. Secure bandage with tape or clips.

12-13. *Recurrent Bandage* for fingers, toes, scalp, or stumps of limbs
(a) Anchor bandage at the bone with several circular turns.
(b) Hold bandage down at the base where it is anchored. Bring bandage up and over and down the back side to the base again.
(c) Hold down bandage at the base. Repeat the back-and-forth bandaging process until several layers are covered.
(d) To hold bandage in place, start at the base, and make circular turns up and back to the base.
(e) To secure bandage, apply piece of tape up and then down other side.

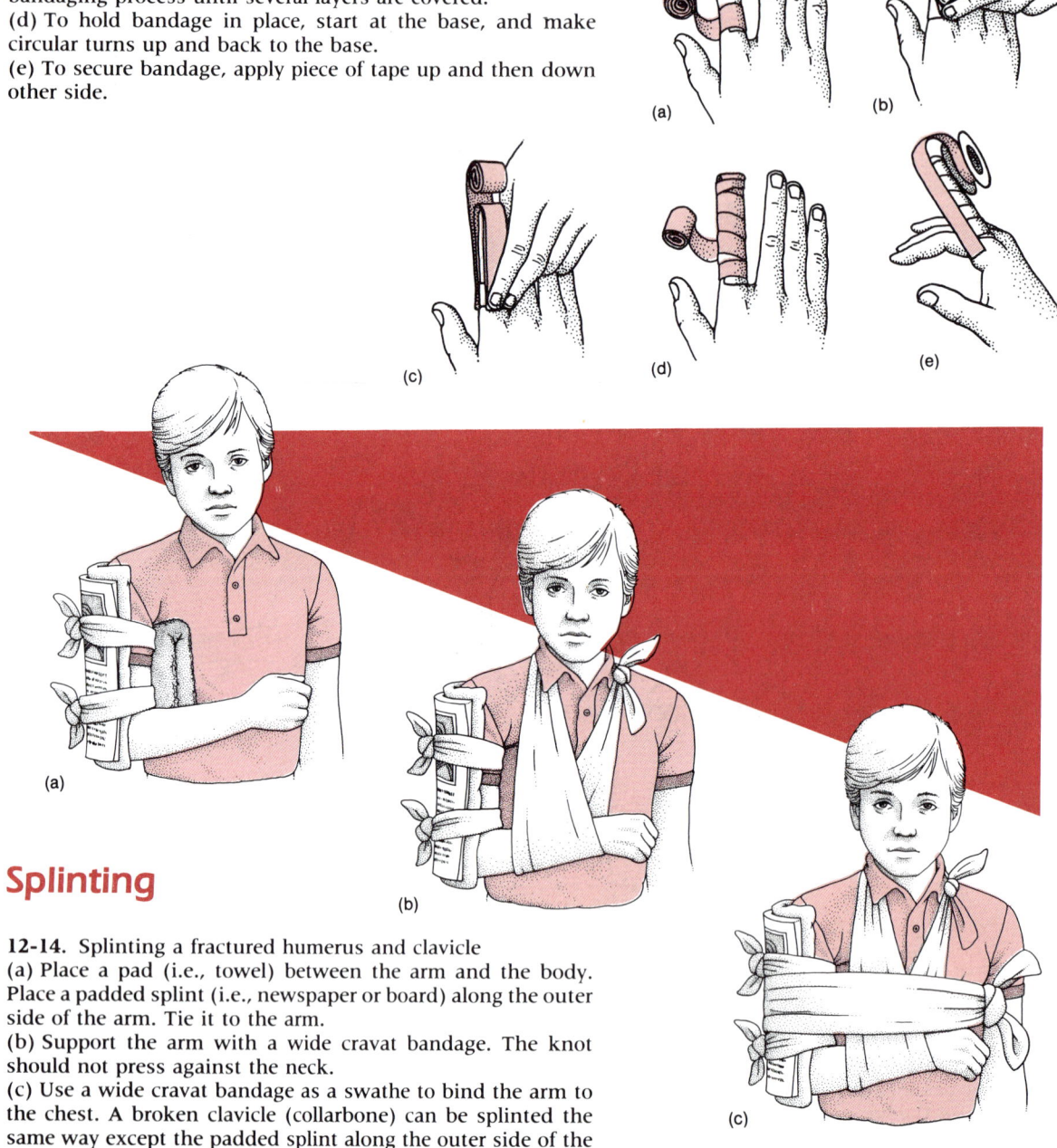

Splinting

12-14. Splinting a fractured humerus and clavicle
(a) Place a pad (i.e., towel) between the arm and the body. Place a padded splint (i.e., newspaper or board) along the outer side of the arm. Tie it to the arm.
(b) Support the arm with a wide cravat bandage. The knot should not press against the neck.
(c) Use a wide cravat bandage as a swathe to bind the arm to the chest. A broken clavicle (collarbone) can be splinted the same way except the padded splint along the outer side of the arm is not used.

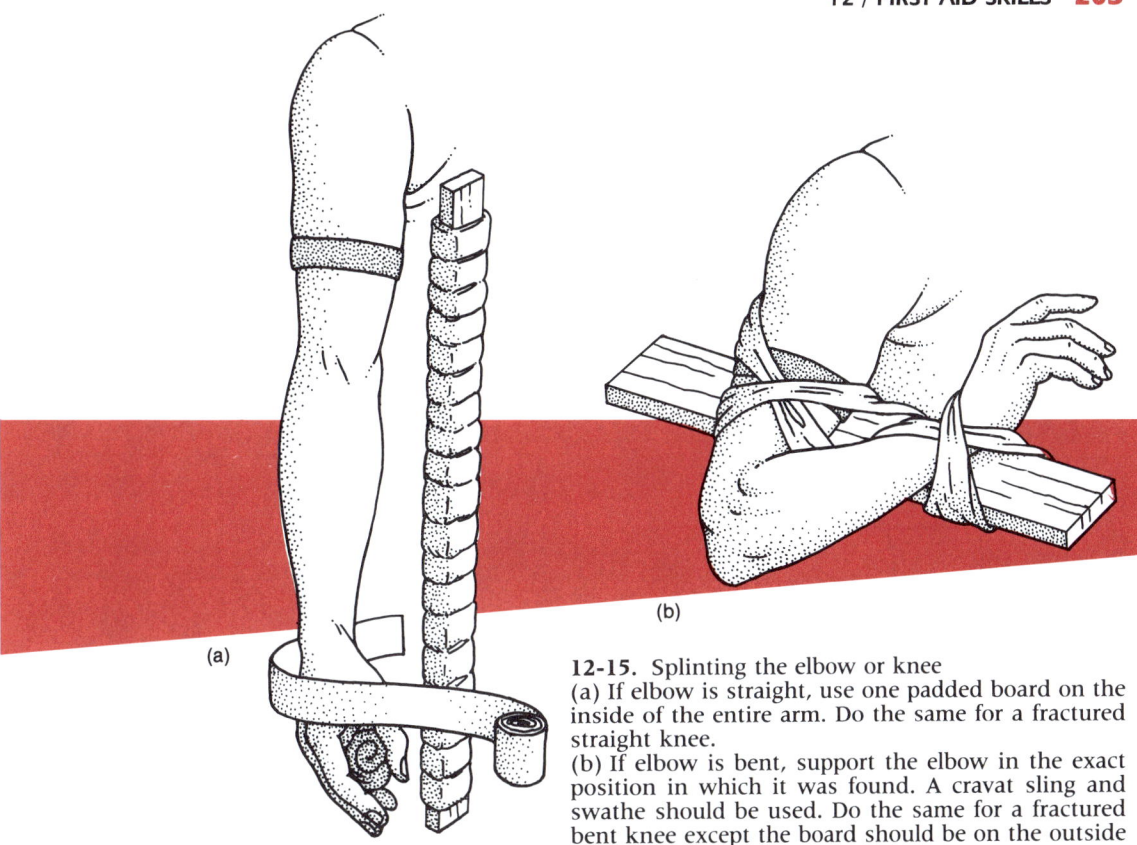

12-15. Splinting the elbow or knee
(a) If elbow is straight, use one padded board on the inside of the entire arm. Do the same for a fractured straight knee.
(b) If elbow is bent, support the elbow in the exact position in which it was found. A cravat sling and swathe should be used. Do the same for a fractured bent knee except the board should be on the outside of the leg.

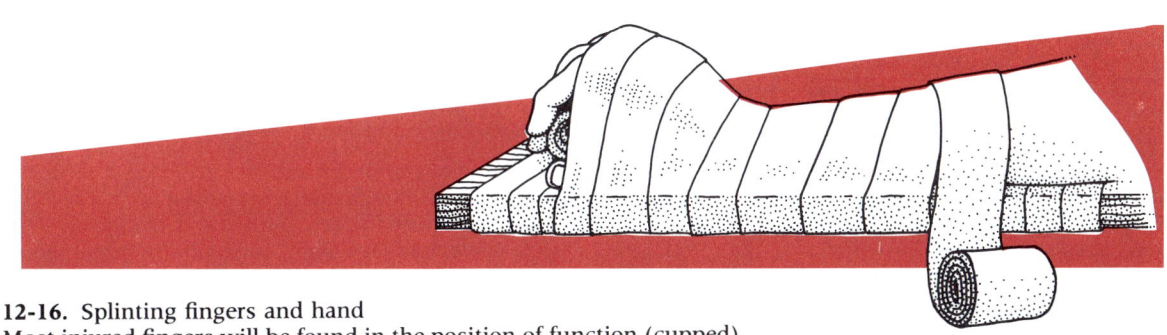

12-16. Splinting fingers and hand
Most injured fingers will be found in the position of function (cupped). Place a ball of gauze or cloth under the victim's fingers to hold them in a cupped position. Roller gauze, elastic bandage, or several cravat bandages may be used to secure the hand and fingers to the splint. Taping the injured finger to an adjacent finger or to a small piece of wood are other alternatives.

204 FIRST AID ESSENTIALS

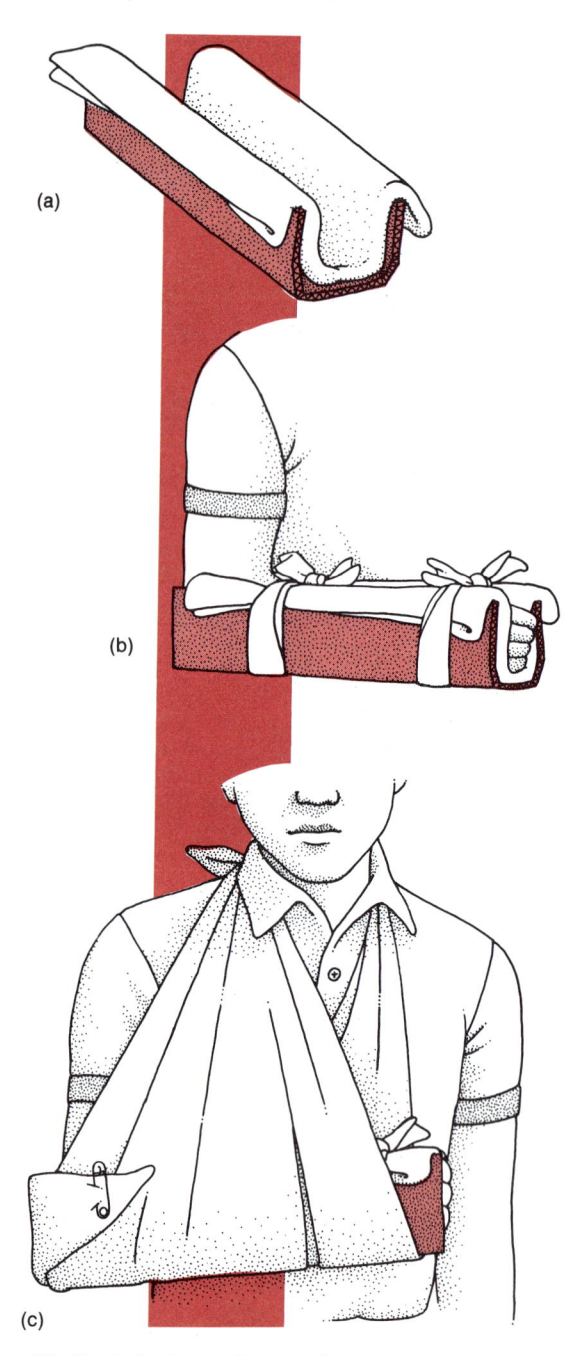

12-17. Splinting a fractured forearm
(a) Use padded splint made of cardboard, newspaper, or board.
(b) Tie the splint in place.
(c) Place the forearm in a sling. Not shown is the use of a wide cravat bandage as a swathe.

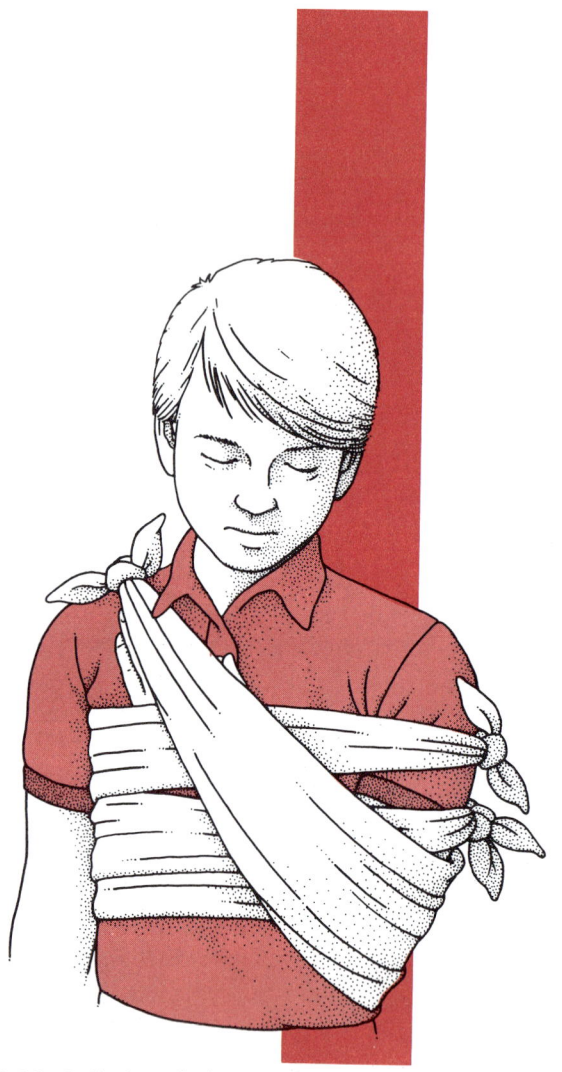

12-18. Splinting rib fractures
Place arm of injured side across chest.
Bind arm tightly to chest with cravat bandages.
Tie a cravat bandage along angle of arm for support.

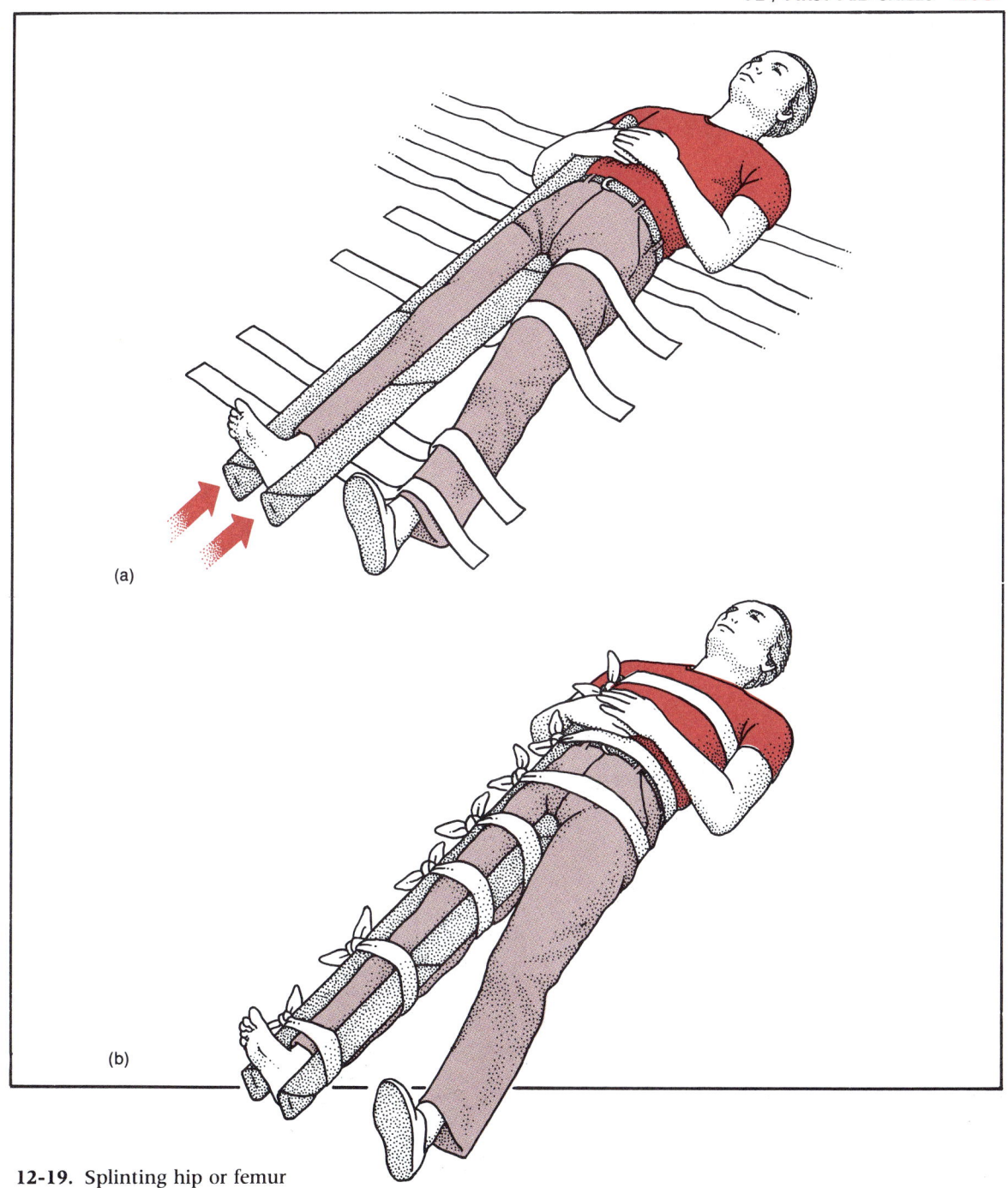

12-19. Splinting hip or femur
(a) Use a stick to slide cravat bandages or cloth strips into position. One splint should be long enough to reach from the crotch to past the heel. The other should reach from the armpit to past the heel.
(b) Tie the splints on snugly. The knots should not press the body.

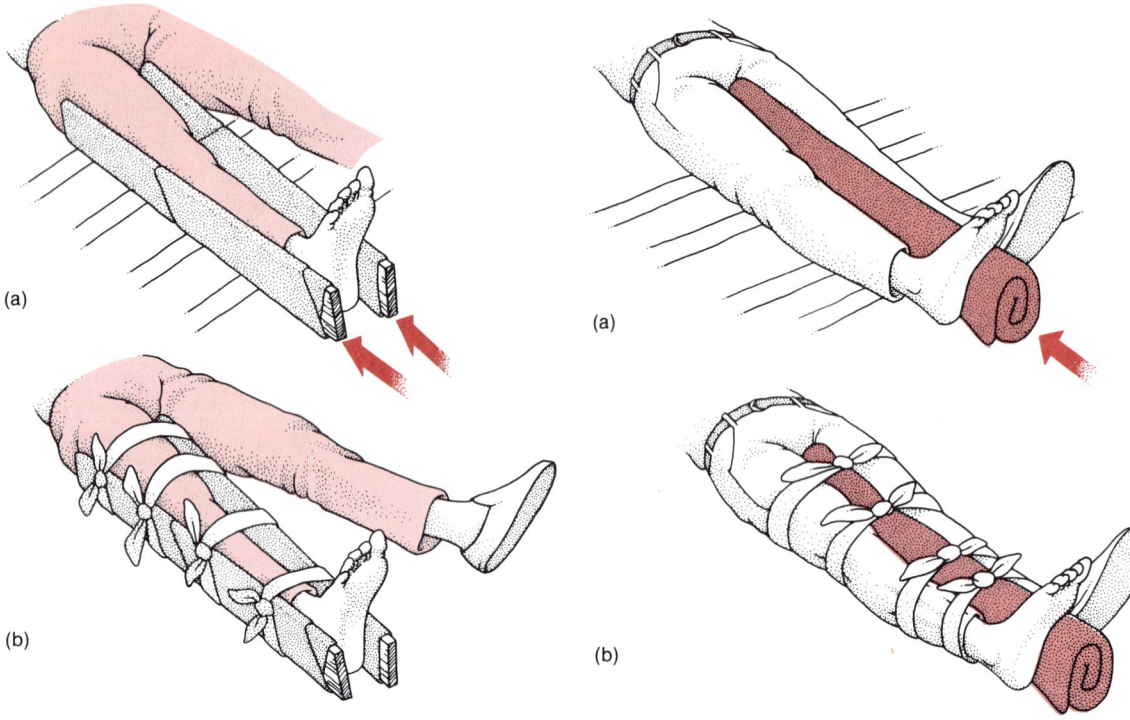

12-20. Splinting the lower leg
(a) Use a stick to push cravat bandages or cloth strips under the leg. Place padded boards or other suitable objects along the inner and outer sides and the injured leg. Both boards must reach from well above the knee to past the heel.
(b) Tie the splints in place. The knots should not press the body.

12-21. Improvise splinting of femur of the lower leg
(a) Use a stick to push cravat bandages or cloth strips under both legs. Place a folded blanket or similar thick padding between the person's legs.
(b) Tie the person's legs together so that the uninjured leg can immobilize the injured leg.

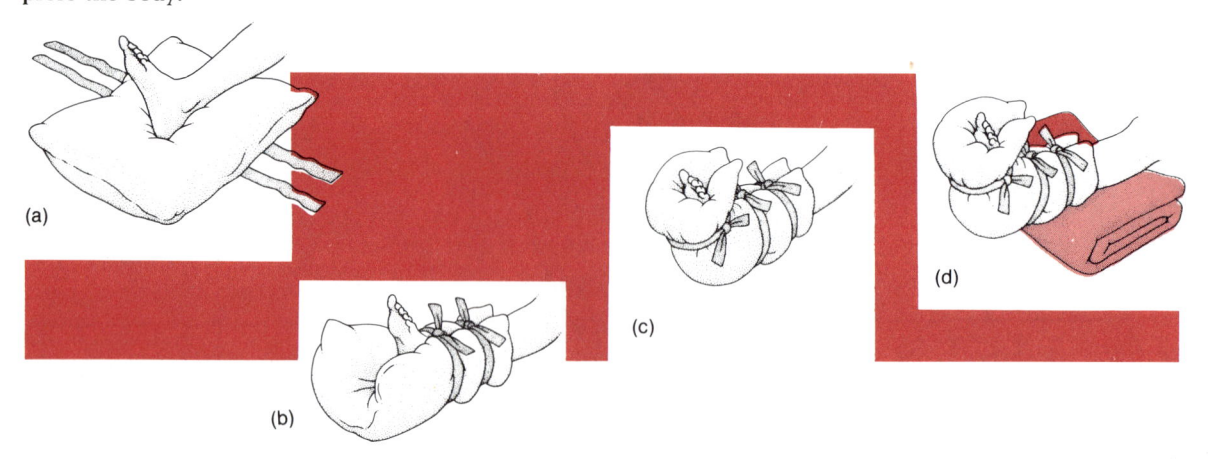

12-22. Splinting an ankle or foot
(a) Remove the shoe so that monitoring of the ankle or foot can occur. Place cravat bandages or cloth strips and a pillow under the lower calf and foot.
(b) Fold the upper part of the pillow around the ankle and tie it in place.
(c) Fold the lower part of the pillow and tie it in place, leaving the toes exposed.
(d) Elevate the foot to decrease swelling.

Traction Splints

Traction splints are used to provide constant pull on an extremity. They supply the traction that is always a part of the immobilization of a fracture, and they prevent broken bone ends from over-riding due to muscle contraction. They do not reduce the fracture but simply immobilize the bone ends and prevent further injury. Traction splints are generally used for fractures of the femur or the hip.

The most commonly used traction splints are the Thomas half ring splint and the Hare traction splint. The basic principles of application are the same for both:

- Traction is applied to the injured leg by grasping the ankle and calf and gently pulling.
- While the first rescuer maintains this traction, the second rescuer slides the splint under the leg and secures the half ring splint in position, pressing firmly against the ischial tuberosity—the rounded projection of the hipbone.
- When the half ring has been fastened, the second rescuer applies and secures the ankle hitch.
- Traction is developed by tightening the winding device, or windlass, until the victim experiences relief of pain.
- The splint is then elevated so that the victim's foot is clear of the ground and the leg is secured by cravats or Velcro straps at intervals along the splint.

A Hare traction splint is applied in much the same way as the Thomas half ring splint. But with the Velcro straps between the two longitudinal rods and the traction apparatus at the foot, the application of traction becomes much simpler and much faster.

Pulses, color, and capillary refilling must be checked every five to ten minutes after applying either splint.

13
Moving and Rescuing Victims

- Emergency Moves • Nonemergency Moves
- Water Rescue

In general, a victim should not be moved until he or she is ready for transportation to a hospital, if required. All necessary first aid should be provided first. A victim should be moved only if there is an immediate danger to him or others if he is not moved, that is:

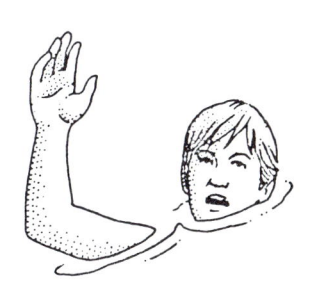

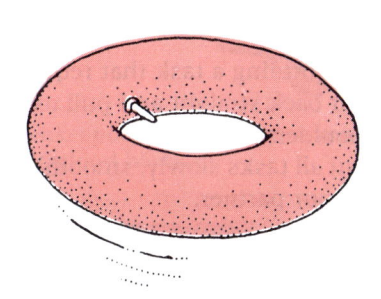

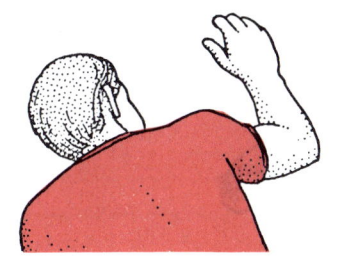

- There is a fire or danger of fire.
- Explosives or other hazardous materials are involved.
- It is impossible to protect the accident scene.
- It is impossible to gain access to other victims in a vehicle who need life-saving care.

Note that a cardiac arrest victim would typically be moved unless he is on the ground or floor because cardiopulmonary resuscitation must be performed on a firm surface.

If it is necessary to move a victim, the speed with which he is moved depends on the reason for moving him, for example:

- *Emergency move.* If there is a fire, pull the victim away from the area as quickly as possible.
- *Nonemergency move.* If the victim needs to be moved to gain access to others in a vehicle, give due consideration to his injuries before and during movement.

EMERGENCY MOVES

The major danger in moving a victim quickly is the possibility of aggravating spine injury. In an emergency, every effort should be made to pull the victim in the direction of the long axis of the body to provide as much protection to the spine as possible. If the victim is on the floor or

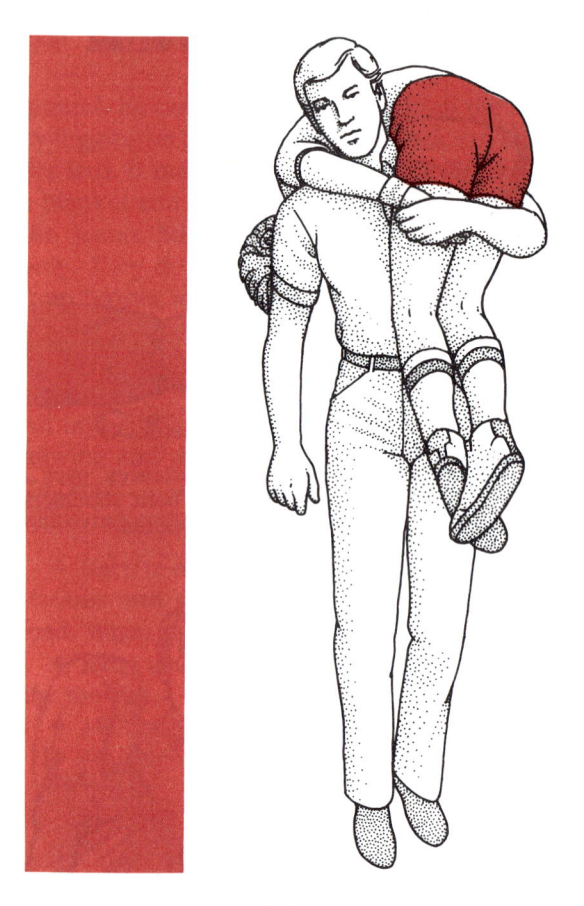

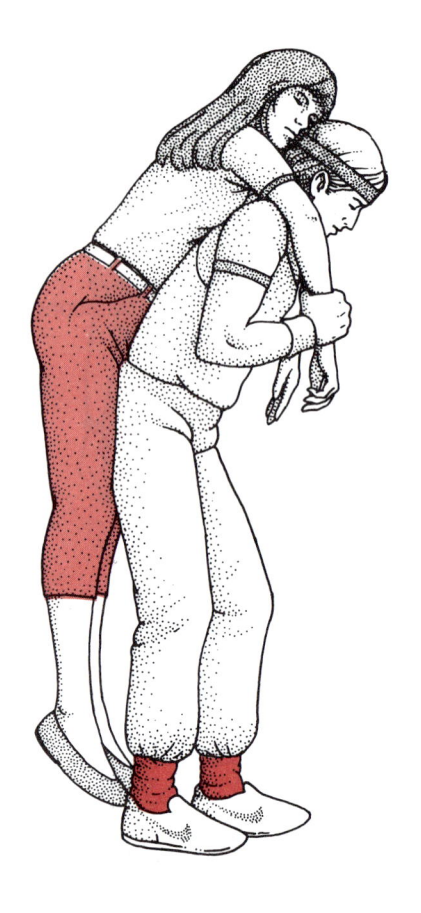

13-6. Fireman carry. If the person's injuries permit, longer distances can be traveled if the person is carried over your shoulder.

13-7. Pack-strap carry. When injuries make the fireman carry unsafe, this method is better for longer distances than the one-person lift.

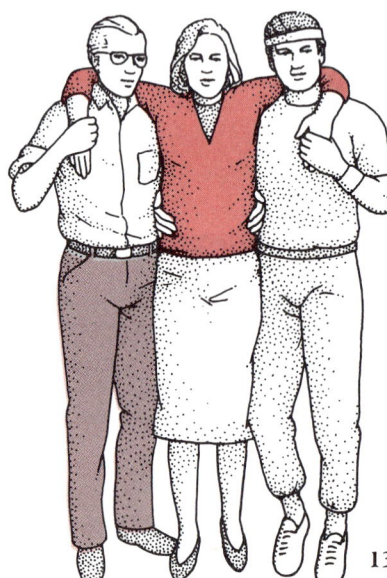

13-8. Helping the person to walk

13 / MOVING AND RESCUING VICTIMS 213

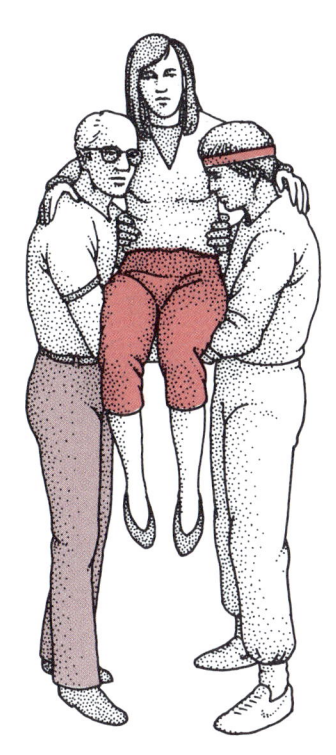

13-9. Two-handed seat carry

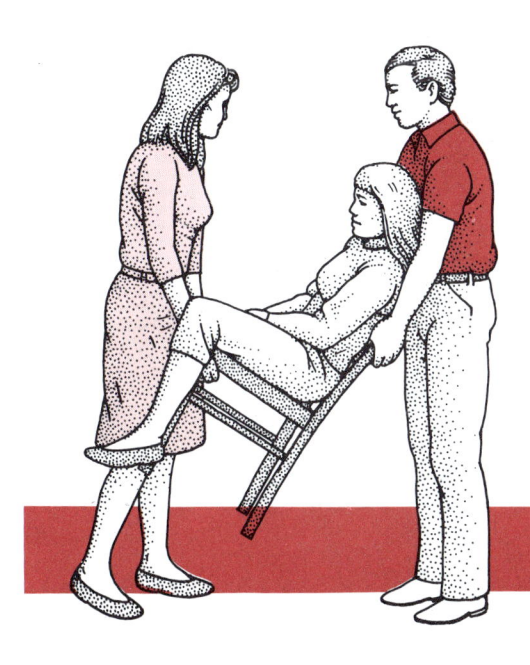

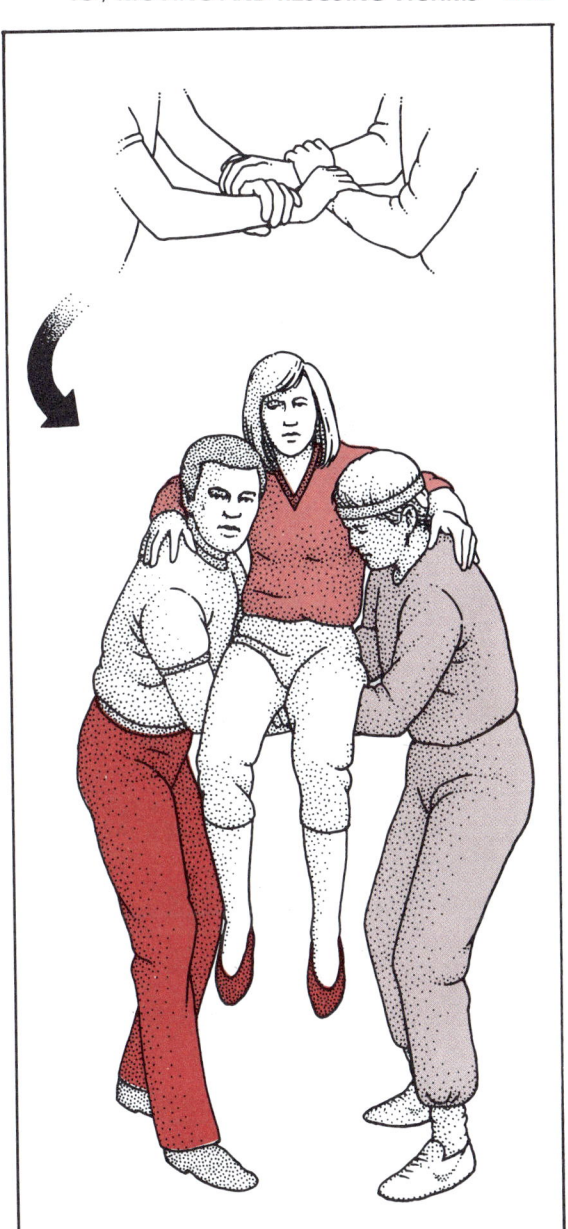

13-10. Four-handed seat carry. This is the easiest two-man carry when no equipment is available.

13-11. Chair carry

214 FIRST AID ESSENTIALS

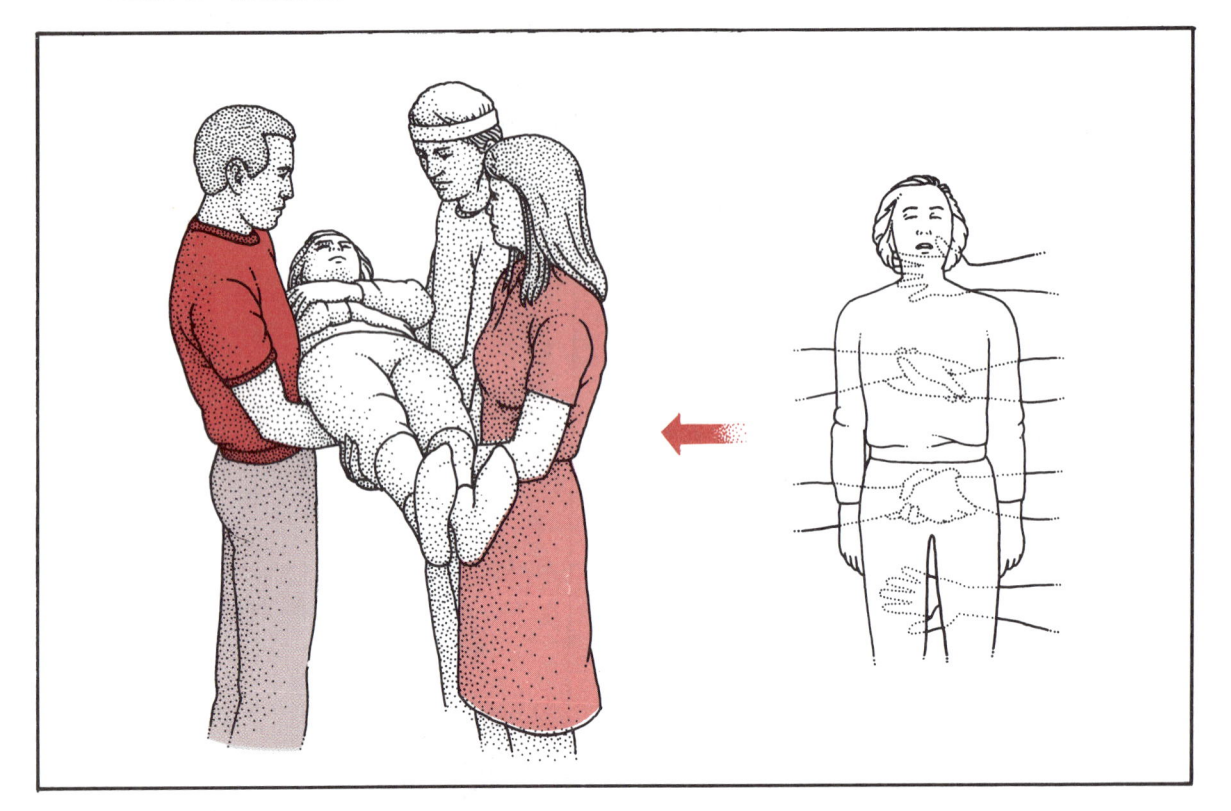

13-12. Hammock carry. Three to six people stand on alternate sides of the injured person and link hands beneath him.

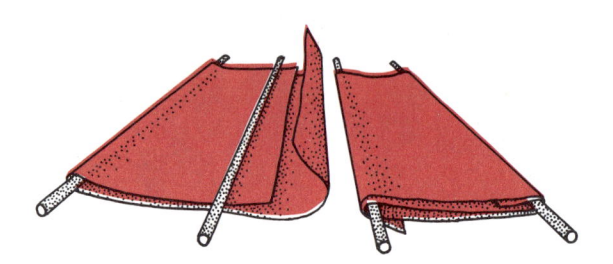

13-13. Blanket and pole improvised stretcher. If the blanket is wrapped as shown, the person's weight will keep it from unwinding.

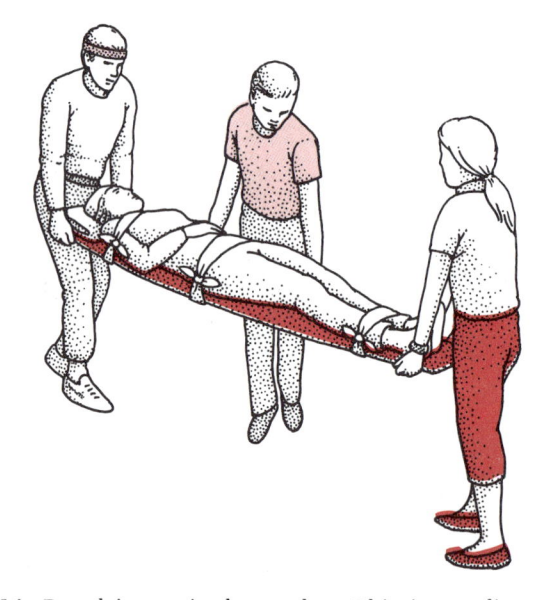

13-14. Board improvised stretcher. This is sturdier than a blanket-and-pole stretcher but heavier and less comfortable. Tie the person on to prevent rolling off.

WATER RESCUE

About 7,000 Americans die each year from drowning, making it the third leading cause of accidental death. Drowning statistics do not reflect the whole problem. An estimated 70,000 people are near-drowning victims each year. Even this figure does not give the entire picture because in many instances the victim recovers and the incident is not reported.

Since drowning situations seem to happen all the time, especially during the summer months, all adults and teenagers should be familiar with the basic rescue techniques available to poor swimmers or nonswimmers.

Reach-Throw-Row-Go

Reach-throw-row-go identifies the priority list for attempting a rescue.

Reach

The first and simplest rescue technique is the reach. This method is easily mastered, but it requires the ability to judge distance accurately and a lightweight pole, ladder, long stick, or any object that can be extended to the victim. (See Figures 13-15(a) and 13-15(b).)

Once you have your "reacher," secure your footing. Also have a bystander grab your belt or pants for stability. Make sure you are secure before reaching down to assist the victim. Keep talking; this not only calms the victim, it helps you think through each step.

Throw

Throwing is another elementary rescue. It provides a maximum range of about fifty feet for the average untrained rescuer. You can throw anything that floats — objects such as empty fuel or paint cans, plastic containers, life jackets or floating cushions, short pieces of wood — whatever is available. If there is rope handy, tie it to the object to be thrown because you can retrieve it in case you miss. (See Figure 13-15(c).)

Row

If the victim is beyond reach and you can find a nearby sailboard, boogie board, rowboat, canoe, or an outboard craft that can be started, you may attempt this form of rescue. Using these crafts requires skill only acquired through practice. In a life-or-death situation, however, even the inept use of these craft will be safer and faster than a swimming rescue. There is an element of danger for the rescuer that should be considered.

Craft powered by hand, paddle, or oar may be slower but they are safer than a motor-driven craft with which you are unfamiliar. Inexperienced hands on a throttle are more dangerous than inexperienced hands on an oar.

If rowing out to a victim, align with an object on the shoreline and in line with the victim. Fix this in your memory. Since you must row facing the opposite direction, you will need to turn your head every five or so strokes to check on the victim and your position.

Upon reaching the victim, never attempt to pull the victim in over the sides of a boat but over the stern or rear end. This has been the cause of countless double drownings. (See Figure 13-15(d).)

Go

If the previous "reach-throw-row" priorities are impossible to do, you must make an assessment, weighing the potential risk to yourself versus the reward to the victim. Entering even calm water to make a swimming rescue is difficult and hazardous. It takes skill, training, and excellent physical condition. All too frequently a would-be rescuer becomes a victim as well. (See Figure 13-15(e).)

After The Rescue

Once the victim is out of the water, protect yourself and the victim against the cold. Get into dry clothing as soon as possible. Be prepared to administer mouth-to-mouth or CPR resuscitation. All rescued victims should be seen by a physician and hospitalized because victims can die a few minutes or up to ninety-six hours or more after the incident of secondary complications. Aspiration pneumonia is a late complica-

216 FIRST AID ESSENTIALS

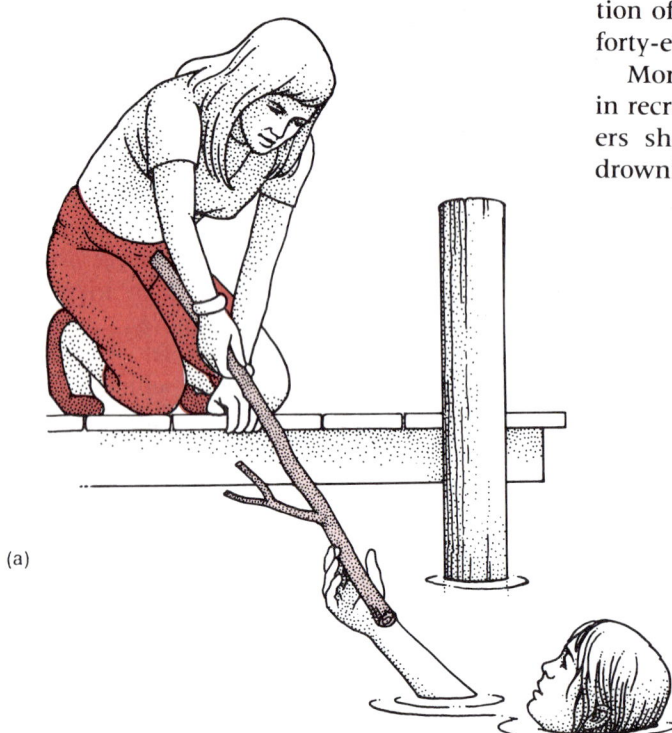

tion of near-drowning episodes, occurring after forty-eight to seventy-two hours have elapsed.

More and more people are taking to the water in recreational activities. All adults and teenagers should be prepared to rescue those in a drowning situation.

13-15. Water Rescue
(a) Reach the person from shore.
(b) If you cannot reach the person from shore, wade closer.
(c) If an object that floats is available, throw it to the person.
(d) Use a boat if one is available.
(e) If you must swim to the person, use a towel or board for him to hold onto. Do not let him grab you.

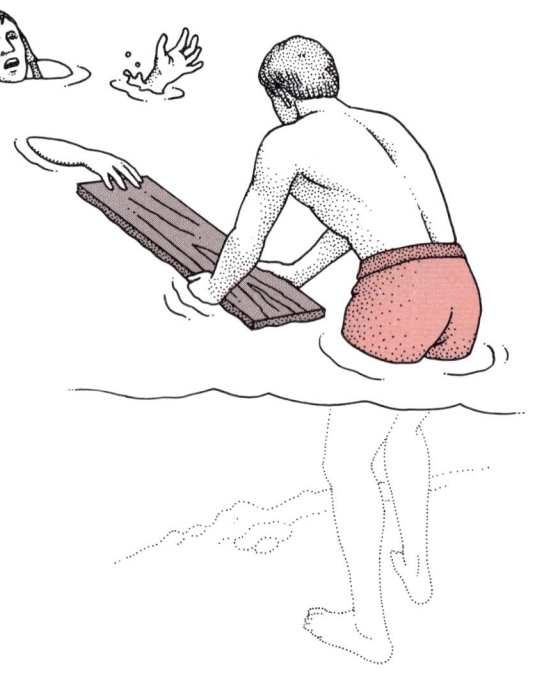

13 / MOVING AND RESCUING VICTIMS 217

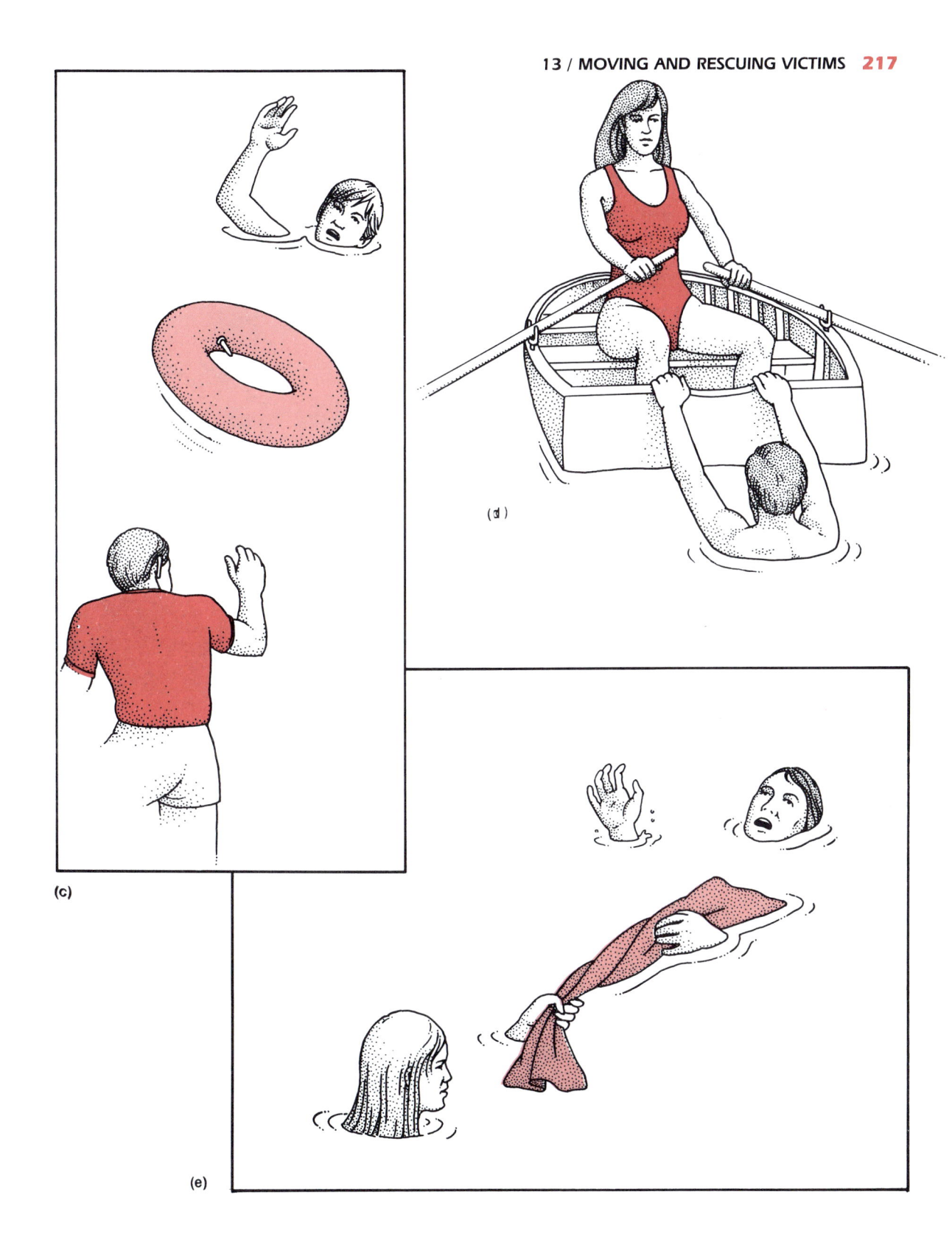

(c)

(d)

(e)

Ice Rescue

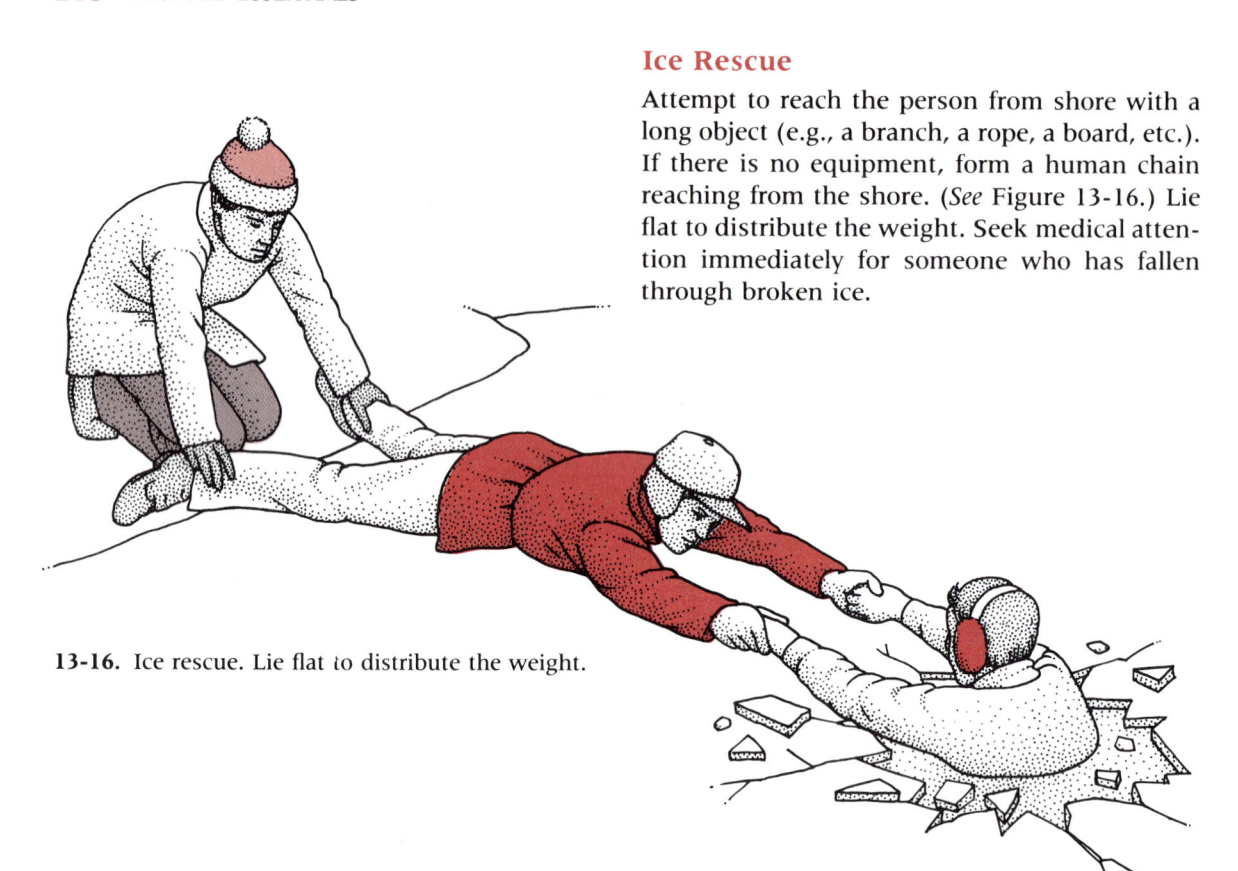

Attempt to reach the person from shore with a long object (e.g., a branch, a rope, a board, etc.). If there is no equipment, form a human chain reaching from the shore. (*See* Figure 13-16.) Lie flat to distribute the weight. Seek medical attention immediately for someone who has fallen through broken ice.

13-16. Ice rescue. Lie flat to distribute the weight.

Answers to Self-Check Questions

Page 4, *Activity 1:* 1. About 2 million; 2. About 100,000 (140,000 including accidents, homicides, and suicides); 3. About 9 million; 4a. heart disease; 4b. cancer; 4c. stroke; 4d. accidents; 5a. motor-vehicle; 5b. falls; 5c. drowning; 5d. fires and burns; 5e. poisoning by solids and liquids; 5f. suffocation; 6.1. Southeastern states; 6.2. Rocky Mountain states; 7. male; 8. teens and elderly; 9. home; 10. Saturday; 11. July, August.

Page 15, *Activity:* **A.** 1. F; 2. F; 3. T. 4. F; 5. T; 6. T; 7. T; 8. F; 9. T; 10. T; 11. T. **B.** 1. B; 2. B; 3. A; 4. B; 5. A; 6. A; 7. A; 8. A; 9. A; 10. A; 11. A; 12. A; 13. A; 14. A; 15. A.

Pages 28 and 29, *Activity 1:* 1. B; 2. B; 3. A; 4. A; 5. A; 6. B; 7. B; 8. B; 9. B; 10. B; 11. B; 12. A; 13. B.

Page 29, *Activity 2:* 1. B; 2. A; 3. B; 4. A; 5. A; 6. A; 7. B; 8. A; 9. B.

Page 30, *Activity 3:* 1. A; 2. B; 3. A; 4. A; 5. A; 6. B; 7. A; 8. D; 9. A.

Page 31, *Activity 4:* 1. D; 2. A; 3. B.

Page 50, *Activity 1:* **A.** 1. T; 2. F; 3. T. **B.** 1. Choice 1; 2. Choice 2; 3. Choice 2; 4. Choice 1; 5. Choice 2. **C.** 3, 5. **D.** 1. 4; 2. 1; 3. 1; 4. 3; 5. 3; 6. 3; 7. 2.

Page 51, *Activity 2:* **A.** 1, 2, 3, 4, 5. **B.** 1, 2, 3, 4, 5. **C.** 1. T; 2. T; 3. F; 4. F; 5. T.

Page 52, *Activity 3:* **A.** 1. T; 2. T; 3. T; 4. T; 5. F. **B.** 1. Yes; 2. Yes; 3. Yes; 4. No. **C.** 1. Choice 2; 2. Choice 1; 3. Choice 1; 4. Choice 2; 5. Choice 1.

Page 68, *Activity 1:* **A.** 1. F; 2. F; 3. T; 4. F; 5. T; 6. F; 7. T. **B.** 1. **C.** 1. F; 2. F; 3. T; 4. T; 5. T; 6. T; 7. T.

Page 69, *Activity 2:* **A.** 1. Yes; 2. Yes; 3. No; 4. No. **B.** 1. Yes; 2. No; 3. No; 4. No; 5. Yes. *Activity 3:* 1. T; 2. F; 3. F; 4. F; 5. T; 6. T.

Page 70, *Activity 4:* 1. T; 2. T; 3. F; 4. T.

Pages 98 and 99, *Activity 1:* **A.** 1. Yes; 2. Yes; 3. Yes; 4. Yes; 5. Yes. **B.** 1. Yes; 2. Yes; 3. Yes; 4. Yes; 5. Yes.
Activity 2: **A.** 1. Yes; 2. No; 3. Yes; 4. No. **B.** 1. T; 2. T; 3. F; 4. T. **C.** 1. No; 2. No; 3. No; 4. Yes; 5. No. **D.** 2, 2. **E.** 1, 2, and 4.

Page 100, *Activity 3:* 1. Choice 1; 2. Choice 2; 3. Choice 1; 4. Choice 2.
Activity 4: 1. T; 2. T; 3. F; 4. F.
Activity 5: **A.** 1. No; 2. No; 3. No; 4. Yes.

Page 101, *Activity 5:* **B.** 2. **C.** 1. Choice 2; 2. Choice 1. **D.** 1. Yes; 2. No; 3. Yes; 4. Yes; 5. No. **E.** 1. No; 2. Yes; 3. No; 4. Yes.

Page 102, *Activity 6:* **A.** 1. Choice 2; 2. Choice 2. **B.** Choice 2. **C.** 1. Choice 2; 2. Choice 1. *Activity 7:* 1. Yes; 2. Yes; 3. Yes; 4. No; 5. Yes; 6. Yes; 7. No.

Pages 103 and 104, *Activity 8:* **A.** 2, 3. **B.** 1. Yes; 2. No; 3. Yes; 4. Yes; 5. No. **C.** 3.
Activity 9: **A.** 3. **B.** 1. **C.** 2.

Pages 127 and 128, *Activity 1:* **A.** 1, 2, 3. **B.** 1. Yes; 2. No; 3. Yes; 4. No. **C.** 1. F; 2. F; 3. F; 4. T; 5. T. **D.** 1. T; 2. T; 3. F; 4. F. **E.** 1. T; 2. T; 3. F; 4. T; 5. F.
Activity 2: 1. No; 2. Yes; 3. No; 4. Yes; 5. Yes.
Activity 3: 1. Choice 2; 2. Choice 1; 3. Choice 2; 4. Choice 2; 5. Choice 1.

Page 129, *Activity 4:* 1. Yes; 2. Yes; 3. No; 4. Yes; 5. No; 6. Yes.
Activity 5: 4.

Page 130, *Activity 6:* 2, 5.
Activity 7: 1. F; 2. T; 3. T; 4. T; 5. T.

Page 140, *Activity 1:* **A.** 4. **B.** 2. **C.** 1. **D.** 1. Do not; 2. Do not; 3. Do; 4. Do not; 5. Do not; 6. Do not; 7. Do.

Page 141, *Activity 2:* 3, 4.
Activity 3: 1. T; 2. T; 3. T; 4. T.

Page 155, *Activity 1:* 1. No; 2. Yes; 3. Yes; 4. No; 5. No; 6. Yes; 7. Yes; 8. No.
Activity 2: 1. Yes; 2. No; 3. Yes; 4. No; 5. No; 6. Yes; 7. Yes; 8. Yes.

Page 156, *Activity 3:* **A.** 1. Choice 1; 2. Choice 1; 3. Choice 2. **B.** 1. 2; 2. 1; 3. 1; 4. 2; 5. 2. **C.** 3, 4.

Page 175, *Activity 1:* 1. Yes; 2. Yes; 3. Yes; 4. No; 5. No.
Activity 2: **A.** 1, 3, 4. **B.** 1. T; 2. T; 3. F; 4. F.

Page 176, *Activity 3:* 1. F; 2. T; 3. F; 4. T; 5. T; 6. F; 7. T; 8. T.
Activity 4: 1. F; 2. T; 3. T; 4. T; 5. F; 6. T; 7. F; 8. T.

Pages 191 and 192, *Activity 1:* **A.** 1, 3, 4. **B.** 1. Yes; 2. No; 3. No; 4. Yes; 5. Yes; 6. Yes.
Activity 2: **A.** 1, 2, 4, and 6. **B.** 1. Yes; 2. No; 3. Yes; 4. Yes. **C.** 1. B; 2. A; 3. A; 4. B; 5. B.
Activity 3: 1. Yes; 2. No; 3. No; 4. Yes.

Page 193, *Activity 4:* 1. No; 2. No; 3. No; 4. Yes; 5. Yes; 6. Yes; 7. Yes; 8. Yes.
Activity 5: 1. T; 2. F; 3. T; 4. T; 5. F; 6. F.

Quick Emergency Index

Abdominal:
    injury   79
Amputation   61
Animal bites   62
Ankle injuries   165
Asthma   184
Bandaging   195
Bee stings   111
Bites:
    animal   63
    insect   109
    snake   112
Bleeding   53
Blisters   86
Breathing problems   184
Broken bone   157
Bruises   55
Burns:
    chemical   74, 135
    electrical   136
    thermal   131
Butterfly bandage   58
Carbon monoxide   118
Cardiopulmonary resuscitation
    (CPR)   17
Charley horse   167
Chemical:
    burns   135
    in the eye   74
    ingested/swallowed   105
Chest injury   78
Choking   21
Cold injuries   143
Concussions   72
Convulsions   73
Cramps, muscle   167
Cravat bandages   196
Cuts   53
Dental emergencies   77
Diabetic emergencies   180

Dislocations   161
Dog bites   62
Drowning   215
Electrical burns   136
Epilepsy   182
Examination, victim   8
Exposure:
    cold   143
    heat   148
Eye injuries   73
Fainting   46
Finger injuries   84, 164
Fishhook   83
Foreign objects:
    abdomen   80
    cheek   83
    chest   83
    ear   82
    eye   81
    nose   82
Fractures   158
Frostbite   143
Hand injuries   84
Head injuries   71
Heart attack   177
Heat injuries:
    cramps   148
    exhaustion   148
    stroke   149
Heimlich Maneuver   21
Hypothermia   146
Infection   60
Insect bites and stings   109
Knee injuries   163
Mouth-to-mouth resuscitation   18
Muscle:
    contusions   167
    cramps   167
    strains   166

Neck injuries   160
Nose:
    bleeding   75
    foreign objects   82
Nosebleeds   75
Poison, ingested   105
    inhaled   118
    insect   109
    plants   117
    snakes   112
    spiders   114
Rescue:
    carries   209
    water   215
Respiratory and cardiac
    resuscitation   17
Scorpion stings   115
Seizures   182
Shock:
    anaphylactic   44
    due to injury   43
    fainting   44
Shortness of breath   184
Shoulder injuries   161
Snakebites   112
Spinal injuries   160
Splinting   202
Sprains   165
Stings, insects   109
Strains   166
Stroke   179
Tetanus   61
Tick removal   115
Tooth:
    broken   78
    loss   77
Triangular bandages   196
Victim assessment   7